Orthodontics: Current Principles and Techniques

Orthodontics: Current Principles and Techniques

Edited by Amy Reed

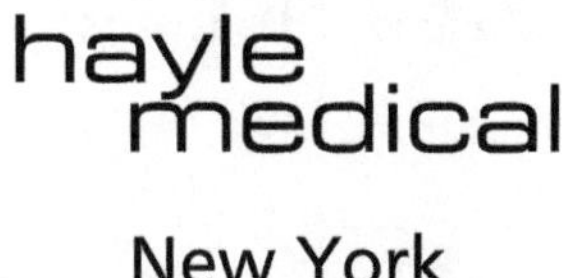

New York

Hayle Medical,
750 Third Avenue, 9th Floor,
New York, NY 10017, USA

Visit us on the World Wide Web at:
www.haylemedical.com

© Hayle Medical, 2019

This book contains information obtained from authentic and highly regarded sources. Copyright for all individual chapters remain with the respective authors as indicated. All chapters are published with permission under the Creative Commons Attribution License or equivalent. A wide variety of references are listed. Permission and sources are indicated; for detailed attributions, please refer to the permissions page and list of contributors. Reasonable efforts have been made to publish reliable data and information, but the authors, editors and publisher cannot assume any responsibility for the validity of all materials or the consequences of their use.

ISBN: 978-1-63241-572-1

Trademark Notice: Registered trademark of products or corporate names are used only for explanation and identification without intent to infringe.

Cataloging-in-Publication Data

Orthodontics : current principles and techniques / edited by Amy Reed.
p. cm.
Includes bibliographical references and index.
ISBN 978-1-63241-572-1
1. Orthodontics. 2. Orthodontics--Technique. 3. Dentistry.
4. Orthopedics. I. Reed, Amy.
RK521 .O78 2019
617.643--dc23

Table of Contents

Preface

In my initial years as a student, I used to run to the library at every possible instance to grab a book and learn something new. Books were my primary source of knowledge and I would not have come such a long way without all that I learnt from them. Thus, when I was approached to edit this book; I became understandably nostalgic. It was an absolute honor to be considered worthy of guiding the current generation as well as those to come. I put all my knowledge and hard work into making this book most beneficial for its readers.

Orthodontics, also known as orthodontia, is a specialty in the field of dentistry. It is concerned with the diagnosis of malpositioned teeth and jaws along with their correction and prevention. The abnormal deviation of teeth from the ideal occlusion is known as malocclusion. Orthodontic camouflage and growth modification are two common methods for treating malocclusions with underlying skeletal problems. A combination of orthodontic and orthognathic surgical treatment may also be used to correct jaw discrepancy. Orthodontic indices such as angle's classification, malignment index, occlusal feature index, Handicapping Labiolingual Deviation Index (HLDI), etc. are used to grade and assess malocclusions. This book is a valuable compilation of topics, ranging from the basic to the most complex advancements in the field of orthodontics. From theories to research to practical applications, case studies related to all contemporary topics of relevance to this field have been included herein. This book attempts to assist those with a goal of delving into the field of orthodontics.

I wish to thank my publisher for supporting me at every step. I would also like to thank all the authors who have contributed their researches in this book. I hope this book will be a valuable contribution to the progress of the field.

Editor

1

Impact of Malocclusions on Quality of Life from Childhood to Adulthood

Raquel Gonçalves Vieira-Andrade,
Saul Martins de Paiva and Leandro Silva Marques

1. Introduction

Malocclusions constitute a misalignment of the dental arches related to changes in the growth and development of the craniofacial system that affects both function and aesthetics and therefore exerts an influence on quality of life and social interactions [1-3]. High prevalence rates make malocclusions a worldwide public health problem [4].

Over the years, oral health-related quality of life (OHRQoL) measures have been used as a complement to the assessment of treatment needs as well as the prioritization of dental care and the evaluation of the outcomes of treatment strategies [5]. According to the World Health Organization [4], quality of life is the perception one has regarding one's position in life in the cultural context and the system of values in which one lives in relation to one's goals, expectations, standards and concerns. As oral health is an integral part of general health, OHRQoL is a multidimensional concept related to the impact of adverse oral conditions on psychosocial and functional well-being [6-8].

A number of assessment tools consider self-reported OHRQoL in different age groups. The use of such measures is of utmost importance, as the analysis of the results complements clinical indicators and allows the identification of the impact of oral problems, such as malocclusions, which can affect one's general well-being [9]. These assessment tools allow orthodontists to determine the consequences of malocclusion, which favors the prevention or early treatment of conditions that exert a negative impact on quality of life [10]. Indeed, orthodontic treatment is generally associated with gains in quality of life due to improvements in physical, social and psychosocial aspects [11]. As the assessment of quality of life has become an integral part of health programs, addressing this issue can contribute to the expansion of knowledge on the importance of preventive and/or interceptive orthodontics to reduce the negative impact of malocclusions on quality of life in different age groups.

1.1. Aim of the chapter

The aim of this chapter is to give a detailed description of the negative impact of malocclusions on the quality of life of individuals in different age groups (children, adolescents and adults) as well as the effect of orthodontic treatment on OHRQoL. Some of the main tools used to measure OHRQoL and the influence of the severity and type of malocclusion on quality of life are also discussed.

2. Problem statement

Like other adverse oral conditions, malocclusions are highly prevalent and can have consequences that affect physical and economic well-being, thereby exerting a negative impact on quality of life [12-14]. It is common for individuals with malocclusion to develop strategies, such as hiding their teeth and avoiding smiling, and develop social anxiety, emotional insecurity, fear and difficulty regarding personal relationships [15, 16]. These aspects increase the negative impact on quality of life. Indeed, recent studies report that malocclusions stand out among the main problems that affect OHRQoL due to the impact on function, appearance, interpersonal relationships, socialization, self-esteem, and psychological well-being [12, 13].

Individuals with attractive physical characteristics make a better impression on others and obtain more privileges due to their appearance [17]. In contrast, individuals who do not display the aesthetic standards imposed by society tend to provoke negative expectations and are often forced to support greater burdens of responsibility. Studies in the field of psychology demonstrate that individuals with a more attractive appearance are considered more capable, have more friends and attain greater professional success, all of which exerts a direct influence on quality of life [16, 17, 18].

The investigation into the physical, psychological, and social impacts of malocclusions on OHRQoL allows a better understanding of the desire for orthodontic treatment. Thus, OHRQoL may be considered the best subjective measure for orthodontic treatment needs [13], as the social and psychological effects of malocclusion are often the main reason for seeking treatment. Moreover, the results of subjective measures can contribute to the establishment of public health policies and the allocation of financial resources directed at the treatment of malocclusions [14].

3. Application area

Subjective measures for the assessment of OHRQoL should complement clinical indicators for the evaluation of treatment needs in oral health as well as the prioritization of care and the evaluation of the outcomes of treatment strategies [5]. Indeed, the sole use of normative clinical measures for the evaluation of treatment needs poses limits on the reliability of the findings by overlooking psychosocial and behavioral aspects [1-3, 5, 9-15]. The assessment of orthodontic treatment needs is traditionally performed using measures such as the Index of Orthodontic Treatment Need (IOTN) [14, 18]. However, orthodontists should consider the fact that malocclusion can be perceived differently by the affected person. Therefore, when evaluating the impact of malocclusion, it is important to consider the different aspects of life that can be affected and the individual's perception of the severity of the condition, as some individuals with severe malocclusion may be satisfied with or indifferent to their dental aesthetics, whereas others may be concerned about minor irregularities [14].

4. Method used

Retrospective and prospective longitudinal studies, randomized control trials, cross-sectional studies, systematic reviews, and meta-analyses that evaluated the impact of malocclusions and/or orthodontic treatment on the OHRQoL of children, adolescents, and adults were used in the drafting of this chapter. Studies were selected from electronic databases (MEDLINE, EMBASE, Cochrane, Web of Science and others) with no language restriction. Thus, the information presented is comprehensive.

5. Research course, status, and results

The criteria employed for the selection of articles led to the most important recently published studies. Most of the studies cited in this chapter have a cross-sectional design, which offers a low degree of scientific evidence and does not allow the precise prediction of the interaction between malocclusion/orthodontic treatment and OHRQoL. Part of this insufficient evidence may be explained by the different methodological criteria employed, such as different sample sizes, study populations, and OHRQoL assessment tools. The lack of longitudinal studies that determine the causal relationship between malocclusion/orthodontic treatment and OHRQoL is partially due to the recent development of assessment tools used to investigate the impact of adverse oral conditions on quality of life. Thus, over time, well-designed studies should contribute toward scientific evidence on this issue.

In the literature, most studies involving preschool children state that malocclusions are often not associated with a negative impact on OHRQoL [17-23]. In schoolchildren and adolescents, however, the position of one's teeth is reported to exert an impact on smiling, socializing and speaking [24]. Malocclusion in these age groups is also associated with functional limitations, psychological discomfort and psychological disability [25]. Moreover, severe malocclusion exerts a greater impact on social, emotional, and functional aspects [12, 26, 27]. Impaired aesthetics due to malocclusion has been reported to affect the quality of life in schoolchildren [28]. Moreover, the desire for orthodontic treatment among adolescents is associated with most types of malocclusion [29]. Malocclusions can also have a significant negative impact on OHRQoL among adults [30]. A recent study reports that the improvement in aesthetic satisfaction due to the treatment of severe malocclusion improves OHRQoL mainly by reducing levels of psychological discomfort and psychological disability [31].

5.1. Impact of malocclusions on the OHRQoL of preschool children

According to the literature, the prevalence of malocclusion ranges from 26.0% [32] to as high as 87.0% [33]. Anterior open bite (Figure 1), anterior crossbite (Figure 2), and posterior crossbite (Figure 3) are the most common types of malocclusion found in the primary dentition [34, 35]. Anterior open bite is defined as a lack of vertical overlap between the primary incisors not less than 3 mm [36]. Anterior crossbite is a vestibular-lingual alteration in the positioning of the upper and lower incisors, with an inversion of the occlusion in which the upper incisors occupies a lingual position in relation to the lower incisors [37]. Posterior crossbite is defined as a transverse discrepancy in the relationship between dental arches, in which the palatal cusps of one or more upper primary teeth do not occlude in the central fossa of the lower teeth [38].

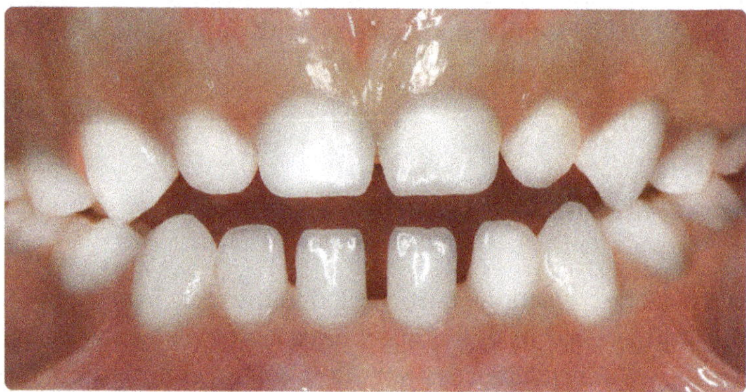

Figure 1. Anterior open bite in deciduous teeth

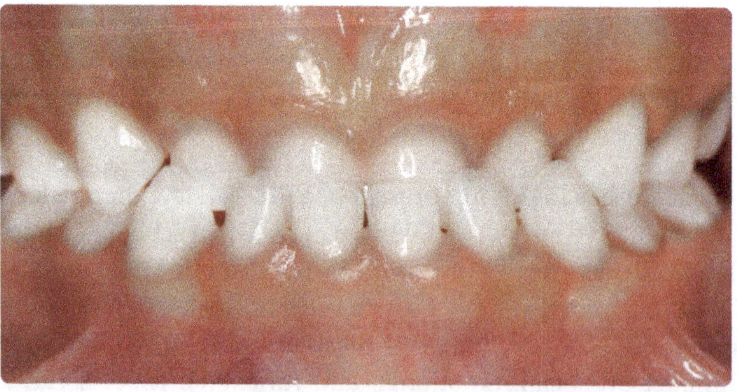

Figure 2. Anterior crossbite in deciduous teeth

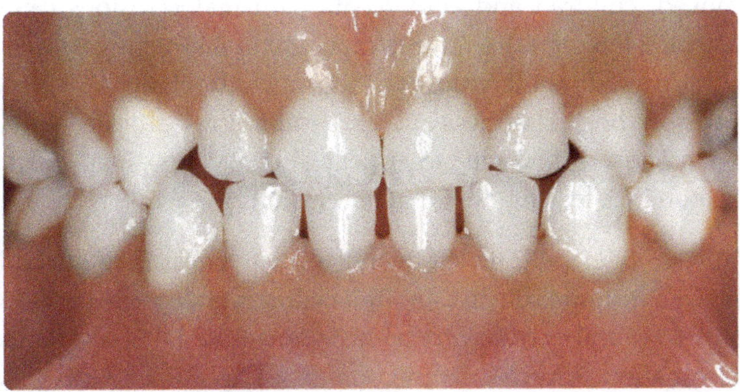

Figure 3. Posterior crossbite in deciduous teeth

The majority of studies that evaluate the impact of malocclusion on OHRQoL among preschool children employ the Early Childhood Oral Health Impact Scale (ECOHIS) [8]. This questionnaire has been translated, tested, and validated for use in different countries [39-47] and is administered to parents/caregivers in interview form. The ECOHIS is composed of 13 items distributed between the Child Impact Section, which has four subscales (symptoms, function, psychology, and social interaction/self-image), and Family Impact Section, which has two subscales (parental distress and family function). Each item is scored using a five-point scale, with responses ranging from "never" (0) to "very often" (4). The individual subscales scores are calculated through the sum of the response codes and the total score ranges from 0 to 52, with higher scores denoting a greater negative impact on quality of life. 'I don't know' responses (score 5) are excluded from the total ECOHIS score.

A number of studies report that parents/caregivers may have a limited view of the oral health status of their children [48-50]. Thus, parents/caregivers interviewed in studies involving the use of the ECOHIS may have had difficulty recognizing the contribution of malocclusion to a reduction in the quality of life of their children, since the items on this questionnaire seem to have greater sensitivity to the detection of the impact of early childhood caries, as demonstrated in previous studies [21, 22, 51-53]. Moreover, parents may not feel that malocclusions are as worrisome as other oral conditions and generally only perceive impact when an abnormality is obvious and has a psychological and/or social impact on the child.

5.2. Impact of malocclusion and orthodontic treatment on OHRQoL among children and adolescents

Most orthodontic patients are children and adolescents [54, 55], who are directly influenced by the school environment, and those with better interpersonal relationships achieve a higher level of learning and academic development [56]. Moreover, attractive individuals are regarded as friendlier, more interesting and more social [57, 58].

Irregularities in the position of the teeth and jaws exert a significant impact on the attractiveness of the smile and quality of life. In the school setting, such irregularities can affect social interactions, interpersonal relationships and mental well-being and may lead to a feeling of inferiority [59]. Indeed, children and adolescents with malocclusions can be the target of teasing and name calling [56]. Studies have demonstrated that young people with unsatisfactory dental aesthetics are sadder than those without such problems [58-62]. A disharmonious smile is the main reason for this sadness and can lead to low self-esteem, thereby impacting quality of life [58-62]. Thus, orthodontic treatment can have a positive effect on children and adolescents who experience teasing due to malocclusions [63, 64].

The face is a slightly stronger indicator of overall attractiveness than the body [65] and most parents seek specialized orthodontic care for their children to improve dental aesthetics as well as overall appearance. A number of studies have demonstrated that normative clinical criteria lead to an underestimation of problems in comparison to the subjective assessment of the affected individual [56, 57, 66]. It is therefore important for orthodontists to identify factors that directly motivate parents in order to design a treatment plan that meets the real needs of the patient and is not merely based on normative clinical indicators.

The main reasons children and adolescents seek orthodontic treatment are dissatisfaction with their dentofacial appearance, recommendations from a dentist, and the influence of schoolmates who wear braces [28, 58, 67, 68]. Gender, age, intellectual level, social class, malocclusion severity, and self-perceived facial aesthetics have also been found to be associated with the desire for orthodontic care [56, 69, 70]. Studies report that upper anterior crowding > 2 mm and parents' perceptions of their child's need for treatment are also factors associated with the desire for orthodontic treatment in adolescents [29]. In the study cited, the authors state that this type of malocclusion has an impact on quality of life of adolescents.

The first assessment tool designed to measure the impact of oral problems on the life of children was designed by Jokovic et al. (2002) and denominated the Child Oral Health Quality of Life Questionnaire (COHQoL). The COHQoL scales were designed to be generic assessment tools to be used as indicators in examinations, tests, and clinical practice and it is therefore necessary to investigate the performance of the COHQoL in different populations and clinical situations [7]. The Child Perceptions Questionnaire for children aged 8–10 years ($CPQ_{8\text{-}10}$) and adolescents aged 11–14 years ($CPQ_{11\text{-}14}$) make up part of the COHQoL [71, 72]. According to Locker et al. (2007) [73], the CPQ allows the discrimination of different clinical situations in groups of children and can be used with children in need of orthodontic treatment. The $CPQ_{8\text{-}10}$ has 29 items divided among 4 subscales (oral symptoms, functional limitations, emotional well-being, and social well-being) and addresses the influence of oral health status in the previous month.

A recent systematic review reports that there is strong scientific evidence that malocclusions have negative effects on the OHRQOL of children and adolescents, especially with regard to emotional and social well-being [74]. According to Martins-Júnior et al. (2012) [12], more severe malocclusions, such as upper anterior irregularity ≥ 2 mm, anterior open bite ≥ 2 mm and diastema ≥ 2 mm, have a greater impact with regard to social, emotional, and functional aspects among children aged 8–10 years. A recent study using the $CPQ_{8\text{-}10}$ found that anterior segment spacing and anterior mandibular overjet were significantly associated with a negative impact on OHRQoL in schoolchildren [27]. In another study, increased overjet and a spaced dentition were the malocclusions with the greatest impact on OHRQoL [75].

Orthodontic treatment is associated with gains in physical, social, and psychosocial aspects of quality of life [63, 64, 76]. According to Agou et al. (2008) [77], COHQoL assessment tools are adequate for the evaluation of changes in the OHRQoL of children following orthodontic treatment. However, poor oral hygiene, speech impairment, and tooth mobility have been associated with the use of fixed orthodontic appliances, demonstrating a negative influence on the quality of life of adolescents during treatment [78].

Besides the CPQ, other measures have been used to assess whether orthodontic treatment affects OHRQol among adolescents. A study involving the Oral Impacts on Daily Performance (OIDP) [79] and the shortened version of the Oral Health Impact Profile (OHIP-14) [80]) evaluated OHRQoL among adolescents using the Index of Orthodontic Treatment Need (IOTN) and found that adolescents who had completed orthodontic treatment had better OHRQoL than those under treatment and those who had not been submitted to treatment.

A recent study compared normative methods of orthodontic treatment needs with the sociodental approach in 12-year-old students and correlated normative measures of malocclusion with the impact of oral health on daily activities [81]. The authors determined normative orthodontic treatment needs using the IOTN and DAI. The sociodental approach combines normative measures, the impact of malocclusion on daily activities (OIDP), and a propensity-related orthodontic treatment assessment. Substantial reductions in normative need estimates for orthodontic treatment were observed using the sociodental approach. According to the authors, the sociodental approach for orthodontic treatment needs can optimize the use of resources at oral health services.

5.3. Impact of malocclusion and orthodontic treatment on OHRQoL among adults

The impact of oral health on quality of life among the adult population is of the utmost importance to health assessments. For young people, physical attractiveness is an important factor that affects social relationships, as abnormal facial aesthetic alterations can affect quality of life, leading to psychological discomfort [30, 82].

Malocclusions affect approximately 46% of young adults, the most common types of which are incisor crowding and misalignment of lower incisors [82]. Moreover, individuals with severe malocclusion are more likely to have a poor self-perception of their attractiveness in comparison to those with minor malocclusions [82]. The psychosocial impact of dental aesthetics is also related to malocclusion severity [83]. A recent study states that other dentofacial deformities, such as a class III occlusal relation, are associated with lower degrees of self-esteem and a greater impact on OHRQoL among adults [84].

The Oral Health Impact Profile (OHIP) and its short form, the OHIP-14, are among the most often employed OHRQoL assessment tools for adults. The OHIP-14 is the method of choice for measuring an individual's perceptions and feelings regarding his/her oral health status and expectations with respect to dental treatment. For such, each response option is attributed a score: never = 0; hardly ever = 1; occasionally = 2; fairly often = 3; very often = 4; and don't know (exclusion). This figure is multiplied by the weight of each item (Item 1: weight = 0.51; Item 2: weight = 0.49; Item 3: weight = 0.34; Item 4: weight = 0.66; Item 5: weight = 0.45; Item 6: weight = 0.55; Item 7: weight = 0.52; Item 8: weight = 0.48; Item 9: weight = 0.60; Item 10: weight = 0.40; Item 11: weight = 0.62; Item 12: weight = 0.38; Item 13: weight = 0.59; Item 14: weight = 0.41). The final score ranges from 0 to 28 points, with higher scores denoting a greater perception of impact [80, 85-88].

The dental literature involving the OHIP-14 provides evidence of the functional and psychosocial benefits of orthodontic treatment. A recent study concluded that young adults aged 18–30 years who received orthodontic treatment had significantly better OHRQoL scores in the retention phase (after the completion of treatment) than untreated individuals [88]. The most frequent impacts in the treated and untreated groups were "painful aching" and "been self-conscious," respectively. Another study investigated dental aesthetics and quality of life among adults aged 18–61 years before and after orthodontic treatment for severe malocclusion [31]. The authors concluded that improvements in aesthetic satisfaction due to the treatment of severe malocclusion lead to an improvement in OHRQoL, particularly by decreasing psychological discomfort and psychological disability. However, another study found that fixed orthodontic therapy had a negative impact on overall OHRQoL during the first 3 months of treatment, which then improved to pre-treatment scores [89]. Moreover, a significant increase in self-esteem is observed as a final result of the treatment.

A recent systematic review with a meta-analysis summarized evidence regarding the impact of malocclusion and its treatment on quality of life of adults in studies that employed the OHIP-14 [90]. The review included studies involving groups before and after treatment (pre-post design), studies involving groups with and without malocclusion (independent groups design), and studies comparing a group that had undergone orthodontic treatment to an independent group that required treatment (treated–untreated groups design). OHIP-14 scores were significantly lower among individuals after receiving treatment for malocclusion and individuals without malocclusion compared to those with malocclusion and treatment needs (independent groups).

Thus, the evidence strongly suggests that orthodontic treatment improves OHRQoL among adults. The sociodental approach, which combines normative and psychosocial perceptions of the dentition, is also recommended for the routine evaluation of treatment needs so that measures of patients' views complement clinical measures in adults.

6. Further research

The scientific evidence is strong regarding the negative impact of malocclusions on the OHRQoL of children, adolescents, and adults, with the greatest impact on emotional and social well-being. There is also strong evidence that orthodontic treatment leads to gains in quality of life, with improvements in physical, social, and psychosocial aspects. However, it is important to stress that the majority of studies presented in this chapter have a cross-sectional design, which does not allow the establishment of causality due to the fact that data are collected at a single moment in time. Thus, some of the findings should be interpreted with caution. The scarcity of longitudinal studies involving preschool children demonstrates a lack of scientific evidence on the actual impact of malocclusions on quality of life and the effectiveness of orthodontic treatment in this specific age group.

Further longitudinal studies should be carried out to determine the cause-and-effect relationship between malocclusion/orthodontic treatment and the impact on OHRQoL. It is also important to consider the diversity of assessment tools as well as the lack of uniformity and clarity in the administration of these tools. Studies are needed to compare the different measures used to evaluate OHRQoL, thereby allowing the improvement of such measures.

Since the assessment of quality of life has become an integral part of health programs, studies with a higher level of scientific evidence are fundamental to understanding how malocclusions and orthodontic treatment can affect the quality of life of children, adolescents, and adults. Such studies also contribute to strategies aimed at promoting health.

7. Conclusions

The analysis of studies found in the dental literature reveals that malocclusions exert a negative impact on the quality of life of children, adolescents, and adults. Among young people, psychological well-being, social interactions, and functional aspects are impacted the most. Moreover, the desire for orthodontic treatment among adolescents is associated with most types of malocclusion. Among adults, the impact on OHRQoL is often related to psychological discomfort and psychological disability. Thus, orthodontic treatment for severe malocclusion leads to an improvement in OHRQoL.

Orthodontists should be encouraged to employ OHRQoL assessment tools to measure the subjective perceptions of patients and their families as a complement to normative clinical indicators. The combination of objective and subjective evaluation methods can contribute to the establishment of a broader-scoped treatment plan as well as the determination of the best approach for each patient.

Acknowledgements

The authors are grateful to the Brazilian fostering agencies Coordination of Higher Education, Ministry of Education (CAPES), the Research Foundation of the State of Minas Gerais (FAPEMIG), and the National Council for Scientific and Technological Development (CNPQ).

Author details

Raquel Gonçalves Vieira-Andrade[1], Saul Martins de Paiva[2] and Leandro Silva Marques[3*]

*Address all correspondence to: lsmarques.prof@gmail.com

1 Department of Pediatric Dentistry and Orthodontics, Federal University of Minas Gerais, Belo Horizonte, Minas Gerais, Brazil

2 Department of Pediatric Dentistry and Orthodontics, Federal University of Minas Gerais, Belo Horizonte, Minas Gerais, Brazil

3 Department of Pediatric Dentistry and Orthodontics, Federal University of the Jequitinhonha and Mucuri Valleys, Diamantina, Minas Gerais, Brazil

References

[1] Cunningham SJ, Hunt NP. Quality of life and its importance in orthodontics. J Orthod. 2001;28:152-8.

[2] Marques LS, Barbosa CC, Ramos-Jorge ML, Pordeus IA, Paiva SM. Malocclusion prevalence and orthodontic treatment need in 10–14-year-old schoolchildren in Belo Horizonte, Minas Gerais: a psychosocial focus. Cad Saude Publica. 2005;21:1099-106.

[3] Liu Z, McGrath C, Ha°gg U. The impact of malocclusion/orthodontic treatment need on the quality of life: a systematic review. Angle Orthod. 2009;79:585-91.

[4] WHO: oral health surveys—basic methods. 4th edn. Geneva: World Health Organization, 1997:30.

[5] Sheiham A, Maizels JE, Cushing AM. The concept of need in dental care. Int Dent J. 1982;32:265-70.

[6] McGrath C, Broder H, Wilson-Genderson M. Assessing the impact of oral health on the life quality of children: implications for research and practice. Community Dent Oral Epidemiol. 2004;32:81-5.

[7] Locker D, Allen F. What do measures of 'oral health-related quality of life' measure? Community Dent Oral Epidemiol. 2007;35:401-11.

[8] Pahel BT, Rozier RG, Slade GD. Parental perceptions of children's oral health: The Early Childhood Oral Health Impact Scale (ECOHIS). Health Qual Life Outcomes. 2007;5:6.

[9] Jokovic A, Locker D, Guyatt G. Short forms of the Child Perceptions Questionnaire for 11–14-year-old children (CPQ11–14): development and initial evaluation. Health Qual Life Outcomes. 2006;19:4.

[10] Goursand D, Paiva SM, Zarzar PM, Ramos-Jorge ML, Cornacchia GM, Pordeus IA et al. Cross-cultural adaptation of the Child Perceptions Questionnaire 11–14 (CPQ11–14) for the Brazilian Portuguese language. Health Qual Life Outcomes. 2008;6:2.

[11] Zhang, McGrath, Hagg. Changes in oral health-related quality of life during fixed orthodontic appliance therapy. Am J Orthod Dentofacial Orthop. 2008;133:25-9.

[12] Martins-Junior PA, Marques LS, Ramos-Jorge ML. Malocclusion: Social, Functional and Emotional Influence on Children. J Clin Pediatr Dent. 2012;37:103-8.

[13] Masood M, Masood Y, Saub R, Newton JT. Need of minimal important difference for oral health-related quality of life measures. J Public Health Dent. 2014;74:13-20.

[14] Feu D, de Oliveira BH, de Oliveira Almeida MA, Kiyak HA, Miguel JA. Oral health related quality of life and orthodontic treatment seeking. Am J Orthod Dentofacial Orthop. 2010;138:152-9.

[15] O'Brien C, Benson PE, Marshman Z. Evaluation of a quality of life measure for children with malocclusion. J Orthod. 2007;34:185-93.

[16] Bellucci CC, Kapp-Simon KA. Psychological considerations in orthognathic surgery. Clin Plast Surg. 2007;34:11-6.

[17] Keruso H, Hausen H, Laine T, Shaw WC. The influence of incisal malocclusion on the social attractiveness of young adults in Finland. Eur J Orthod. 1995;17:505-12.

[18] Onyeaso CO. Orthodontic treatment complexity and need with associated oral health-related quality of life in Nigerian adolescents. Oral Health Prev Dent. 2009;7:235-41.

[19] Sousa RV, Clementino MA, Gomes MC, Martins CC, Granville-Garcia AF, Paiva SM. Malocclusion and quality of life in Brazilian preschoolers. Eur J Oral Sci. 2014;122:223-9.

[20] [20]Carvalho AC, Paiva SM, Viegas CM, Scarpelli AC, Ferreira FM, Pordeus IA. Impacto of malocclusion on oral health-related quality of life among Brazilian preschool children: a population-based study. Braz Dent J. 2013;24:655-61.

[21] Scarpelli AC, Paiva SM, Viegas CM, Carvalho AC, Ferreira FM, Pordeus IA. Oral health-related quality of life among Brazilian preschool children. Community Dent Oral Epidemiol. 2013;41:336-44.

[22] Abanto J, Carvalho TS, Mendes FM, Wanderley MT, Bönecker M, Raggio DP. Impact of oral diseases and disorders on oral health-related quality of life of preschool children. Community Dent Oral Epidemiol. 2011;39:105-14.

[23] Aldrigui JM, Abanto J, Carvalho TS, Mendes FM, Wanderley MT, Bönecker M, Raggio DP. Impact of traumatic dental injuries and malocclusions on quality of life of young children. Health Qual Life Outcomes. 2011;9:78.

[24] Naidoo S, Sheiham A, Tsakos G. The relation between oral impacts on daily performances and perceived clinical oral conditions in primary school children in the Ugu District, Kwazulu Natal, South Africa. SADJ. 2013;68:214-8.

[25] Oziegbe EO, Esan TA, Adesina BA. Impact of oral conditions on the quality of life of secondary schoolchildren in Nigeria. J Dent Child (Chic). 2012;79:159-64.

[26] Bernabé E, Sheiham A, de Oliveira CM. Impacts on daily performances attributed to malocclusions by British adolescents. J Oral Rehabil. 2009;36:26-31.

[27] Sardenberg F, Martins MT, Bendo CB, Pordeus IA, Paiva SM, Auad SM, Vale MP. Malocclusion and oral health-related quality of life in Brazilian school children. Angle Orthod. 2013;83:83-9.

[28] Marques LS, Ramos-Jorge ML, Paiva SM, Pordeus IA. Malocclusion: esthetic impact and quality of life among Brazilian schoolchildren. Am J Orthod Dentofacial Orthop. 2006;129:424-7.

[29] Marques LS, Pordeus IA, Ramos-Jorge ML, Filogônio CA, Filogônio CB, Pereira LJ, Paiva SM. Factors associated with the desire for orthodontic treatment among Brazilian adolescents and their parents. BMC Oral Health. 2009;9:34.

[30] Masood Y, Masood M, Zainul NN, Araby NB, Hussain SF, Newton T. Impact of malocclusion on oral health related quality of life in young people. Health Qual Life Outcomes. 2013;11:25.

[31] Silvola AS, Varimo M, Tolvanen M, Rusanen J, Lahti S, Pirttiniemi P. Dental esthetics and quality of life in adults with severe malocclusion before and after treatment. Angle Orthod. 2014;84:594-9.

[32] Dhar V, Van Jain A, Dyke TE, Kohli A. Prevalence of gingival diseases, malocclusion and fluorosis in school-going children of rural areas in Udaipur district. J Indian Soc Pedod Prev Dent. 2007;25:103-5.

[33] Leite-Cavalcanti A, Medeiros-Bezerra PK, Moura C. Breast-feeding, bottlefeeding, sucking habits and malocclusion in Brazilian preschool children. Rev Salud Publica. 2007;9:194-204.

[34] Hebling SRF, Cortellazzi KL, Tagliferro EPS, et al. Relationship between malocclusion and behavioral, demographic and socioeconomic variables: a cross-sectional study of 5-year-olds. J Clin Pediatr Dent. 2008;33:75-80.

[35] Carvalho AC, Paiva SM, Scarpelli AC, Viegas CM, Ferreira FM, Pordeus IA. Prevalence of malocclusion in primary dentition in a population-based sample of Brazilian preschool children. Eur J Paediatr Dent. 201;12:107-11.

[36] Katz CR, Rosenblatt A, Gondim PP. Nonnutritive sucking habits in Brazilian children: effects on deciduous dentition and relationship with facial morphology. Am J Orthod Dentofacial Orthop. 2004;126:53-7.

[37] Corrêa-Faria P, Ramos-Jorge ML, Martins-Júnior PA, Vieira-Andrade RG, Marques LS. Malocclusion in preschool children: prevalence and determinant factors. Eur Arch Paediatr Dent. 2014;15:89-96.

[38] Malandris M, Mahoney EK. Aetiology, diagnosis and treatment of posterior crossbites in the primary dentition. Int J Paediatr Dent. 2004;14:155-66.

[39] Tesch FC, Oliveira BH, Leão A. [Measuring the impact of oral health problems on children's quality of life: conceptual and methodological issues]. Cad Saude Publica. 2007;23:2555-64.

[40] Martins-Júnior PA, Ramos-Jorge J, Paiva SM, Marques LS, Ramos-Jorge ML. Validations of the Brazilian version of the Early Childhood Oral Health Impact Scale (ECOHIS). Cad Saude Publica. 2012;28:367-74.

[41] Scarpelli AC, Oliveira BH, Tesch FC, Leão AT, Pordeus IA, Paiva SM. Psychometric properties of the Brazilian version of the Early Childhood Oral Health Impact Scale (B-ECOHIS). BMC Oral Health. 2011;11:19.

[42] López Ramos RP, García Rupaya CR, Villena-Sarmiento R, Bordoni NE. Cross cultural adaptation and validation of the Early Childhood Health Impact Scale (ECOHIS) in Peruvian preschoolers. Acta Odontol Latinoam. 2013;26:60-7.

[43] Bordoni N, Ciaravino O, Zambrano O, Villena R, Beltran-Aguilar E, Squassi A. Early Childhood Oral Health Impact Scale (ECOHIS). Translation and validation in Spanish language. Acta Odontol Latinoam. 2012;25:270-8.

[44] Jankauskienė B, Narbutaitė J, Kubilius R, Gleiznys A. Adaptation and validation of the early childhood oral health impact scale in Lithuania. Stomatologija. 2012;14:108-13.

[45] Peker K, Uysal Ö, Bermek G. Cross-cultural adaptation and preliminary validation of the Turkish version of the early childhood oral health impact scale among 5-6-year-old children. Health Qual Life Outcomes. 2011;9:118.

[46] Wong HM, McGrath CP, King NM. Rasch validation of the early childhood oral health impact scale. Community Dent Oral Epidemiol. 2011;39:449-57.

[47] Lee GH, McGrath C, Yiu CK, King NM. Sensitivity and responsiveness of the Chinese ECOHIS to dental treatment under general anaesthesia. Community Dent Oral Epidemiol. 2011;39:372-7.

[48] Jokovic A, Locker D, Guyatt G. How well do parents know their children? Implications for proxy reporting of child health-related quality of life. Qual Life Res. 2004;13:1297-307.

[49] Wilson-Genderson M, Broder HL, Phillips C. Concordance between caregiver and child reports of children's oral health-related quality of life. Community Dent Oral Epidemiol. 2007;35:32-40.

[50] Barbosa TS, Gavião MB. Oral health-related quality of life in children: part III. Is there agreement between parents in rating their children's oral health-related quality of life? A systematic review. Int J Dent Hyg. 2008;6:108-13.

[51] Leal SC, Bronkhorst EM, Fan M, Frencken JE. Untreated cavitated dentine lesions: impact on children's quality of life. Caries Res. 2012;46:102-6.

[52] Vieira-Andrade RG, Martins-Júnior PA, Corrêa-Faria P, Marques LS, Paiva SM, Ramos-Jorge ML. Impact of oral mucosal conditions on oral health-related quality of life in preschool children: a hierarchical approach. Int J Paediatr Dent. 2014 Apr 15. [Epub ahead of print]

[53] Martins-Júnior PA, Vieira-Andrade RG, Corrêa-Faria P, Oliveira-Ferreira F, Marques LS, Ramos-Jorge ML. Impact of early childhood caries on the oral health-related quality of life of preschool children and their parents. Caries Res. 2013;47:211-8.

[54] Berk NW, Bush HD, Cavalier J, Kapur R, Studen-Pavlovich D, Sciote J, Weyant RJ. Perception of orthodontic treatment need: opinion comparisons of orthodontists, pediatric dentists, and general practitioners. J Orthod. 2002;29:287-91.

[55] Pratelli P, Gelbier S, Gibbons DE. Parental perceptions and attitudes on orthodontic care. Br J Orthod. 1998;25:41-6.

[56] Shaw WC, Meek SC, Jones DS. Nicknames, teasing harassment and the salience of dental features among school children. Br Dent J. 1980,7:75-80.

[57] Peres KG, Traebert ESA, Marcenes W. Diferenças entre autopercepção e critérios normativos na identificação das oclusopatias. Rev Saúde Pública. 2002;36:230-6.

[58] Oliveira CM, Sheiham A. Orthodontic treatment and its impact on oral health-related quality of life in Brazilian adolescents. J Orthod. 2004;31:20-7.

[59] Nanda RS, Ghosh J. Facial soft tissue harmony and growth in orthodontic treatment. Semin Orthod. 1995;1:67-81.

[60] Tung AW, Kiyak HA. Psychological influences on the timing of orthodontic treatment. Am J Orthod Dentofacial Orthop. 1998;113:29-39.

[61] DiBiase AT, Sandler PJ. Malocclusion, orthodontics and bullying. Dent Update. 2001;28:464-6.

[62] Seehra J, Newton JT, DiBiase AT. Bullying in schoolchildren - its relationship to dental appearance and psychosocial implications: an update for GDPs. Br Dent J. 2011;210:411-5.

[63] Seehra J, Newton JT, Dibiase AT. Interceptive orthodontic treatment in bullied adolescents and its impact on self-esteem and oral-health-related quality of life. Eur J Orthod. 2013;35:615-21.

[64] Seehra J, Fleming PS, Newton T, DiBiase AT. Bullying in orthodontic patients and its relationship to malocclusion, self-esteem and oral health-related quality of life. J Orthod. 2011;38:247-56.

[65] Ong E, Brown RA, Richmond S. Peer assessment of dental attractiveness. Am J Orthod Dentofacial Orthop. 2006;130:163-9.

[66] [66]. Mandall NA, McCord JF, Blinkhorn AS, Worthington HV, O'Brien KD. Perceived aesthetic impact of malocclusion and oral self-perceptions in 14-15- year-old Asian and Caucasian children in greater Manchester. Eur J Orthod. 1999;22:175-83.

[67] Bos A, Hoogstraten J, Prahl-Andersen B. Expectations of treatment and satisfaction with dentofacial appearance in orthodontic patients. Am J Orthod Dentofacial Orthop. 2003;123:127-32.

[68] Samsonyanová L, Broukal Z. A systematic review of individual motivational factors in orthodontic treatment: facial attractiveness as the main motivational factor in orthodontic treatment. Int J Dent. 2014;2014:938274.

[69] Kiyak HA. Comparison of esthetic values among Caucasians and Pacific-Asians. Community Dent Oral Epidemiol. 1981;9:219-23.

[70] Baldwin DC. Appearance and aesthetics in oral health. Community Dent Oral Epidemiol. 1980;8:244-56.

[71] Jokovic A, Locker D, Stephens M, Kenny D, Tompson B, Guyatt G. Validity and reliability of a questionnaire for measuring child oral-health-related quality of life. J Dent Res. 2002;81:459-63.

[72] [72]Foster Page LA, Boyd D, Thomson WM. Do we need more than one Child Perceptions Questionnaire for children and adolescents? BMC Oral Health. 2013;13:26.

[73] Locker D, Jokovic A, Tompson B, Prakash P. Is the Child Perceptions Questionnaire for 11-14- year olds sensitive to clinical and self-perceived variations in orthodontic status? Community Dent Oral Epidemiol. 2007;35:179-85.

[74] Dimberg L, Arnrup K, Bondemark L. The impact of malocclusion on the quality of life among children and adolescents: a systematic review of quantitative studies. Eur J Orthod. 2014 Sep 11. [Epub ahead of print]

[75] Johal A, Cheung MY, Marcene W. The impact of two different malocclusion traits on quality of life. Br Dent J. 2007;202:E2.

[76] Zhang M, McGrath C, Hägg U. Changes in oral health-related quality of life during fixed orthodontic appliance therapy. Am J Orthod Dentofacial Orthop. 2008;133:25-9.

[77] Agou S, Malhotra M, Tompson B, Prakash P, Locker D. Is the child oral health quality of life questionnaire sensitive to change in the context of orthodontic treatment? A brief communication. J Public Health Dent. 2008;68:246-8.

[78] Marques LS, Paiva SM, Vieira-Andrade RG, Pereira LJ, Ramos-Jorge ML. Discomfort associated with fixed orthodontic appliances: determinant factors and influence on quality of life. Dental Press J Orthod. 2014;19:102-7.

[79] Adulyanon S, Vourapukjaru J, Sheiham A. Oral impacts affecting daily performance in a low dental disease Thai population. Community Dent Oral Epidemiol. 1996;24:385-9.

[80] Slade GD. Derivation and validation of a short-form oral health impact profile. Community Dent Oral Epidemiol. 1997;25:284-90.

[81] Herkrath FJ, Rebelo MA, Herkrath AP, Vettore MV. Comparison of normative methods and the sociodental approach to assessing orthodontic treatment needs in 12-year-old schoolchildren. Oral Health Prev Dent. 2013;11:211-20.

[82] Claudino D, Traebert J. Malocclusion, dental aesthetic self-perception and quality of life in a 18 to 21 year-old population: a cross section study. BMC Oral Health. 2013;13:3.

[83] Kolawole KA, Agbaje HO, Otuyemi OD. Impact of malocclusion on oral health related quality of life of final year dental students. Odontostomatol Trop. 2014;37:64-74.

[84] Frejman MW, Vargas IA, Rösing CK, Closs LQ. Dentofacial deformities are associated with lower degrees of self-esteem and higher impact on oral health-related quality of life: results from an observational study involving adults. J Oral Maxillofac Surg. 2013;71:763-7.

[85] Allen PF, Locker D. Do item weights matter? An assessment using the oral health impact profile. Community Dent Health. 1997;14:133-8.

[86] Robinson PG, Gibson B, Khan FA, Birnbaum W. Validity of two oral health-related quality of life measures. Community Dent Oral Epidemiol. 2003;31:90-9.

[87] Oliveira BH, Nadanovsky P. Psychometric properties of the Brazilian version of the Oral Health Impact Profile-short form. Community Dent Oral Epidemiol. 2005;33:307-14.

[88] Palomares NB, Celeste RK, Oliveira BH, Miguel JA. How does orthodontic treatment affect young adults' oral health-related quality of life? Am J Orthod Dentofacial Orthop. 2012;141:751-8.

[89] Johal A, Alyaqoobi I, Patel R, Cox S. The impact of orthodontic treatment on quality of life and self-esteem in adult patients. Eur J Orthod. 2014 Sep 11. [Epub ahead of print]

[90] Andiappan M, Gao W, Bernabé E, Kandala NB, Donaldson AN. Malocclusion, orthodontic treatment, and the Oral Health Impact Profile (OHIP-14) Systematic review and meta-analysis. Angle Orthod. 2014 Aug 26. [Epub ahead of print]

2

Study of the Relationship of Smile Esthetics Between Torque and Dental Arch Width of Posterior Teeth in Orthodontics

Gaastra Carolin, Zamora Natalia, Paredes Vanessa,
Tarazona Beatriz and Jose Luis Gandía

1. Introduction

There are different factors affecting smile aesthetics, with posterior dental torque and dental arch width as two of the most important ones [1-3]. Sarver et al.[4] affirmed that the orthodontic expansion of a compressed arch improved the smile transversal dimension, and that a wider arch shape in the premolar area resulted in lower buccal corridors and buccolingual inclinations of posterior teeth (or posterior torque) [4, 5].

There is few scientific evidence about the most favourable torque from an aesthetic point of view [5, 6], although it has been showed that the most appropriate one should extend up to the latest visible teeth in the smile. Therefore, a posterior torque close to 0º contributes greatly to this smile aesthetics. On the other hand, a negative torque in posterior sectors gives a compression appearance to the arch, with a negative effect on its aesthetics [6].

Torque can be defined from a mechanical point of view or from a clinical standpoint. From a mechanical standpoint, it relates to a structure torque through its longitudinal axis, resulting in the twist angle. Clinically, refers to bucopalatal or buccolingual inclination of the crown or root of a tooth, and is adapted explanation used to describe the rotation along an axial axis [7]. When applied to an interaction between an archwire and a slot of a bracket, it describes the activation generated when twisting an archwire in the slot of a bracket [7].

Preadjusted bracket systems allow the clinician preset torque values obtained directly from the information contained therein. Today there is a wide availability of brackets, and each of them has an individual prescription, according to the orthodontic technique followed.

Sometimes these differences are minimal, sometimes the differences are greater. But it is known that all existing prescriptions currently available allow the brackets to get a negative coronal-palatine torque in posterior teeth [8], especially when the existing torque before treatment is remarkably negative [5].

According to authors such as Zachrisson [5, 6], to have a good occlusion there should not be a great difference between the molar and premolar lingual and buccal cusps. Hence, if posterior teeth present a high negative torque they would not allow a good posterior occlusion [5, 6]. As showed in Zachrisson [5, 6] research, a neutral posterior torque should be achieved, as it is a key factor for smile and face aesthetics. In accordance with the conclusions in the works of Zachrisson [5] and Badawi et al.[9], a negative torque in posterior sectors gives a compression appearance to the maxillary arch, as the crown inclination of this posterior superior area is a key factor for a bright and full smile [6].

2. Problem statement

Torque control is one of the weaknesses of the preadjusted bracket systems [6], and there is little data about what is the real capacity of the bracket systems to express the torque prescribed in brackets. Studies like Streva et al. [10] agree that the information that fails to express torque can exceed manufacturer estimated values by obtaining lower precision than expected. According Brauchli et al. [11] the time of treatment with high diameter archwires could influence the amount of torque expressed 6, but there are still no concrete data in the literature about this topic.

According Morina et al. [12] in self-ligating brackets torque is expressed in smaller amounts (up to seven times less) comparing with convencional brackets. However, these authors believe more importantly the use of a wire that completely fills the slot and have stiffness for proper expression torque [13]. Other authors have concluded in their studies that there are no clinical differences in the expression of torque between self-ligating brackets and convencional brackets [11].

Patient age and duration of treatment may be factors affecting the increase in the interdental widths and the final torque values, but there are few data in the literature to support this relationship.

On the other hand, some authors showed the added aesthetic value of wide smiles compared to narrow smiles [14, 15]. However, the ideal arch shape is not just one, as individual biologic diversity has an influence on it [16]. Some orthodontic techniques tend to increase dental arch width, which can cause instability (especially in intercanine and interpremolar areas), therefore it is recommended to individualize dental arches to their initial shape as possible [16].

Expansion due to orthodontic wires is dentoalveolar, and its effects are similar to those of the tipping described for quick expansion or disjunction [17]. This tipping movement implies that crowns in teeth of posterior sectors show a higher buccal inclination that at the beginning of the treatment. Authors such as Fleming et al. [18] observed that a higher increase in transversal expansion (0.91 mm more) occurred in cases with initial narrower arches [18]. This change in crown buccolingual inclinations of posterior teeth is a considering point when posterior neutral torques have to be achieved. However, few data referring to this concept can be found in the scientific literature.

Due to the lack of studies considering these aspects, the aims in our study where: firstly, to compare the tooth variation in torque depending on the type of bracket used among different bracket prescription techniques, and secondly, to compare the torque and arch width changes after orthodontic treatment, and to analyze the relationship between these changes with smile aesthetics.

3. Application area

A comparative, retrospective clinical study was carried out at the Orthodontics Teaching Unit of the University of Valencia, Spain from January to May 2012. This research was approved by the Ethics Committee on Human Research of the University of Valencia, Spain. Rights have been protected by an appropriate Institutional Review Board and written informed consent was granted from all subjects. The Helsinki declaration was considered and its guidelines were followed in our investigation. All patients agreed to participate in the study, even though the diagnosis material was gathered as part of their treatment protocol.

The present study is a cross-sectional observational human study and it has been conformed to the STROBE guidelines.

4. Material and methods

4.1. Sample

Two hundred and fifty patients attending the Orthodontics Department were randomly selected. Initial and final treatment plaster study models were available for all of them as part of their orthodontic records.

Inclusion criteria were as follows:

1. Permanent dentition from the first permanent molar, from one side to the other.
2. Absence of anomalies in number, size and dental shape.
3. Good quality of study models.
4. Patients previously treated with multibracket fixed appliances.

Exclusion criteria were:

1. Orthodontic treatment with extractions.
2. Use of two band expansive appliances through the treatment.

Subjects' age was not included as exclusion criteria, as it was initially supposed that it would not affect research results.

Of the initial 250 patients, a subsample of 76 was found to meet the described criteria.

The average age in the sample at the beginning of the treatment was 18.8 ± 8.8 years, ranging between 10.9 and 55.5 years. The average treatment length was 18.2 ± 7.0 months.

4.2. Material

Accordingly with the used orthodontic technique, the sample was divided in four groups (n=19): A, B, C and D:

Prescription A=brackets Victory® (3M Unitek©)

Prescription B=Tip-Edge® (TP Orthodontics©)

Prescription C=Smart Clip® (3M Unitek©)

Prescription D=Mini-Taurus® (Rocky Mountain©).

Bracket prescription for each of the techniques is showed in table 1. All brackets had a slot of 0.22 inches and the last used wire was a 0.021 x 0.025 inches stainless steel archwire. In all cases O-ring ligatures were used, except in technique C where the self-ligating system was applied.

TEETH	TECHNIQUE		
	A / C	B	D
Canines	0º	-4º	0º
First Premolar	-7º	-7º	0º
Second Premolar	-7º	-7º	0º
First Molar	-14º	-11º	0º

Table 1. Bracket prescription for each of the techniques of the study. Prescription A=brackets Victory® (3M Unitek©); Prescription B=Tip-Edge® (TP Orthodontics©); Prescription C=Smart Clip® (3M Unitek©); Prescription D=Mini-Taurus® (Rocky Mountain©).

The archwires in technique B are comparatively wider than the rest, particularly in the premolar area, and conversely, the technique D uses a narrower shape in the subsequent sectors. The archwires in A and C correspond to a form that could be considered intermediate between that of B and D.

4.3. Method

Occlusal and frontal photographs corresponding to the superior arch of all subjects were taken for the initial and final plaster study models (Figures 1 and 2). Initial and final plaster study models were cast through the same method, following the measures proposed by the Spanish Orthodontic Society (SEDO). Photographs were taken with a Canon EOS 400D camera, with a 100 mm Macro objective. A "ring" flash was used in order to avoid shadows in posterior sectors, and all the photographs were taken by the same operator.

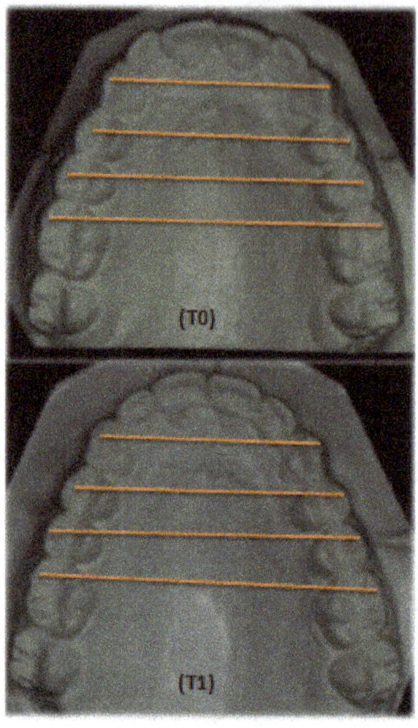

Figure 1. Dental arch widths (mm) in occlusal images of initial (T0) and final (T1) models.

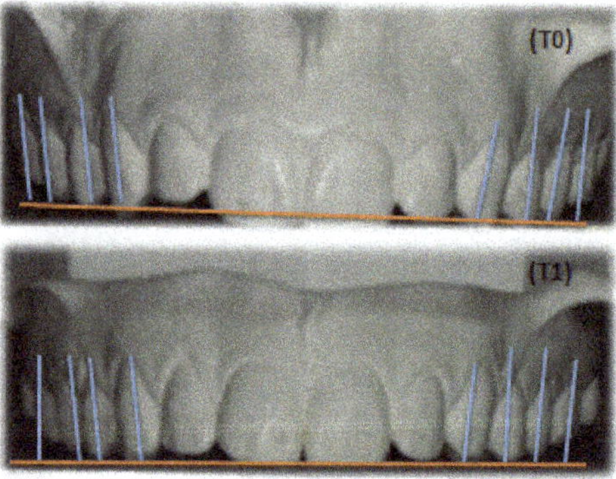

Figure 2. Initial (T0) and final (T1) torques (º) in both sides of canines, first premolars, second premolars and molars.

Occlusal images were used to measure intercanine, interpremolar and intermolar widths, whereas frontal photographs were used for the measuring of torques in bilateral posterior sectors. Images were taken perpendicularly to the ground, and a caliper was used for this purpose. A millimeter caliper was included in order to take scale measurements afterwards.

All measurements were carried out by the same operator (C.G). Interarch widths and torques for maxillary arches were measured before and after the treatment. T0 was assigned to values before treatment and T1 to values postreatment.

4.3.1. Occlusal photographs

Dental arch widths (mm) were measured in occlusal images of initial (T0) and final (T1) models (Figure 1):

- Intercanine width: distance between the cusp tips of bilateral canines.
- First interpremolar width: distance between the vestibular cusp tips of first bilateral premolars.
- Second interpremolar width: distance between the vestibular cusp tips of second bilateral premolars.
- Intermolar width: distance between mesiovestibular cusps of first bilateral molars.

4.3.2. Frontal photographs

- Initial (T0) and final (T1) torques (º) were measured by the same observer in both side of canines, first premolars, second premolars and molars (Figure 2).
- Parallel lines to the vestibular contour of the crown of canines, premolars and molars, going through the vestibular cusp and the highest point in the gingival margin visible from the frontal projection, were drawn in order to measure torques. Imaginary lines were designed to have a reference for the measurement of the different angles. The first line went through the mesiovestibular cusps of both first superior molars (right and left), and the second line, perpendicular to the first one, went through the centre of the papilla located between the two superior central incisors. The resulting angles in the intersection between the line going through the middle line and the crown axis previously described were measured with a Leone goniometer. Torque was measured with a positive, negative or 0º angle. Positive or negative values were assigned based on the clockwise or counterclockwise divergence of the lines. Whereas a 0 value was given when they were coincident or parallel. Angles were measured for both sides, right and left.

In order to estimate the measurement error and determine intraexaminer correlation, 5 cases of each bracket prescription system were randomly selected (a total subsample of 20 cases) and the main examiner repeated the measurements with an interval of two weeks after the first measurement. To estimate interexaminer correlation, 5 cases in each bracket system were randomly selected (a total subsample of 20 cases) and the same parameters described previously were measured with the same method by a second examiner (P.P). Both examiners performed the measurements blinded, without the knowledge of the examiners of each patient prescription.

4.3.3. Statistical analysis

The response variables in the research were: torques of the mentioned teeth (13, 23, 14, 24, 15, 25, 16, 26) and widths between pairs of teeth of the same kind (canines, first premolars, second premolars and first molars), measured before and after the treatment (T0 and T1).

Model application hypotheses were verified: variance homogeneity (Levene and M-Box) and residuals normality (Kolmogorov test). Bonferroni test was used for multiple comparisons (post-hoc).

A general linear model (GLM) of repeated measures was developed to assess changes produced by the different techniques. A GLM of repeated measures was estimated for the variable chosen response. It was a mixed design (split-plot), including time as intrasubject factor, or of repeated measures (with 2 levels, T0 basal and T1 final), and technique as inter-subject factor (with 4 levels).

For this MLG model, and considering a size of 0.25 (medium) in the effect to detect, the reached power was of 0.99 in intrasubject contrast and of 0.51 in intersubject contrast, with a confidence level of 95%. The linear correlation between torque variation and width was assessed through Pearson coefficient, whereas the assessment within each technique was performed through Spearman coefficient, due to sample reduction. Reference significance level was of 5% in all the analysis.

Through Kolmogorov-Smirnov test, all measurements, including T1-T0 differences, were shown to follow a normal distribution.

5. Results

5.1. Analysis intra and intersubjects

Intraexaminer and interexaminer errors are shown in Table 2 and 3.

Intraexaminer measurement error (d Dahlberg) ranged from 0.5 mm to 1.5 mm approximately in width measurements, increasing to ranges of 1.5º-3.0º for torques. Variability in measurement differences was higher in torques than in widths.

In interexaminer analysis, the measurement error (d Dahlberg) ranged from 0.8 mm to 2.0 mm approximately in width measurements, increasing to ranges of 2.0º-4.0º for torques. Variability in measurement differences was higher in torques than in widths.

	Intraexaminer			**Interexaminer**		
	Difference 1ª – 2ª measurement		**d Dahlberg**	**Difference measurements**		**d Dahlberg**
	Mean	**SD**		**Mean**	**SD**	
Torque 13 T0	-2,00º	2,53º	2,25º	-0,45º	3,43º	2,38º
Torque 13 T1	-0,35º	2,46º	1,71º	0,30º	3,37º	2,33º
Torque 23 T0	-0,70º	2,20º	1,60º	0,43º	2,74º	1,91º
Torque 23 T1	-1,20º	2,07º	1,66º	1,23º	2,90º	2,18º
Torque 14 T0	-0,45º	3,32º	2,31º	-1,85º	4,06º	3,09º

	Intraexaminer			Interexaminer		
	Difference 1ª – 2ª measurement		d Dahlberg	Difference measurements		d Dahlberg
	Mean	SD		Mean	SD	
Torque 14 T1	-0,10º	3,04º	2,10º	-2,20º	3,90º	3,11º
Torque 24 T0	-1,25º	3,13º	2,33º	-1,35º	5,36º	3,82º
Torque 24 T1	-1,25º	2,24º	1,78º	1,28º	2,78º	2,12º
Torque 15 T0	-1,30º	3,56º	2,62º	-1,53º	3,63º	2,73º
Torque 15 T1	-0,30º	2,32º	1,61º	-2,43º	4,49º	3,54º
Torque 25 T0	-1,55º	2,86º	2,25º	-1,45º	5,33º	3,81º
Torque 25 T1	-1,05º	2,44º	1,84º	0,35º	3,94º	2,72º
Torque 16 T0	-1,15º	4,00º	2,88º	-1,63º	3,57º	2,72º
Torque 16 T1	-0,85º	2,81º	2,03º	-0,95º	4,59º	3,24º
Torque 26 T0	-1,30º	4,13º	2,99º	-0,70º	5,66º	3,93º
Torque 26 T1	-1,55º	3,27º	2,50º	0,45º	3,53º	2,45º

Table 2. Intra and inter-examiner differences between torque measurements and D Dahlberg's method error in T0 and T1. All values are expressed in degrees.

	Intraexaminer			Interexaminer		
	Difference 1ª – 2ª measurement		d Dahlberg	Difference measurements		d Dahlberg
	Mean	SD		Mean	SD	
Canine width T0	-0,68mm	2,08mm	1,51mm	0,20mm	1,49mm	1,03mm
Canine width T1	-0,30mm	0,54mm	0,43mm	0,04mm	1,17mm	0,81mm
1st premolar width T0	-0,58mm	1,46mm	1,09mm	0,22mm	1,46mm	1,02mm
1st premolar width T1	-0,09mm	1,70mm	1,17mm	0,33mm	1,23mm	0,88mm
2nd premolar width T0	-0,38mm	2,08mm	1,46mm	0,60mm	1,00mm	0,81mm
2nd premolar width T1	0,42mm	1,49mm	1,07mm	0,79mm	1,30mm	1,06mm
1st molar width T0	-0,20mm	2,48mm	1,71mm	2,39mm	0,96mm	1,82mm
1st molar width T1	-0,33mm	0,76mm	0,57mm	1,65mm	2,26mm	1,95mm

Table 3. Intra and inter-examiner differences between width measurements and D Dahlberg's method error in T0 and T1. All values are expressed in mm.

5.2. Torque changes from T0 to T1 depending on the technique

The average difference between T0/T1 was estimated as main result in patient torque variation through the treatment. Success in treatment was defined as achieving a close value to 0º torque or achieving a 0º torque value. Maintaining a stable torque from T0 to T1, invariable, was also considered for measuring the success rate.

Depending on the initial torque values at T0, the classification of the improvement in torque variation would be achieved as follows:

- Achieving a negative torque value close to 0, when higher negative values were measured at T0 (e.g. from-5º (T0) to-2º (T1)).
- Achieving a positive torque value close to 0, when higher positive values were measured at T0 (e.g. from 5º (T0) to 2º (T1)).
- Depending on the initial torque values at T0, the classification of the worsening in torque variation would be achieved as follows:
- Achieving a negative torque value away to 0, when lower negative values, closer to 0, were measured at T0 (e.g. from-2º (T0) to-5º (T1)).
- Achieving a positive torque value away to 0, when lower positive values, closer to 0, were measured at T0 (e.g. from 5º (T0) to 2º (T1)).

Results can be observed in Figure 3.

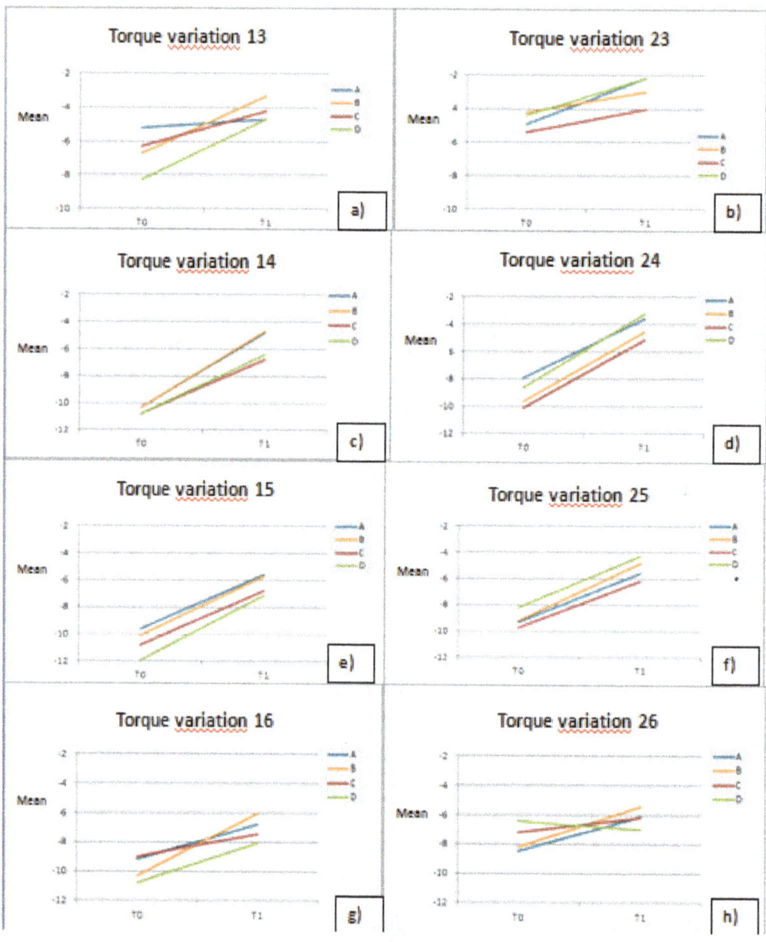

Figure 3. Maxillary torque changes between T0 and T1 depending on the technique. a) and b) left and right canine torque variation; c) and d) left and right 1st premolar torque variation; e) an f) left and right 2nd premolar torque variation; g) and h) lenf and right 1st molar torque variation.

5.3. Dentoalveolar maxillary width changes between T0 and T1 depending on the technique

Figure 4 shows the variation in width changes of the different posterior tooth analyzed (canines, 1st premolars, 2nd premolars, 1st molars) according to the technique used.

In the region of canines with techniques C and D there were no changes from T0 to T1 ($p > 0.05$); we found, though, changes in techniques A and B.

The increase in width at first premolars was significant from T0 to T1 ($p < 0.001$), but not of the same magnitude in all techniques ($p < 0.001$). In technique D the change was of low magnitude. In the region of second premolars, there was an increase in the width ($p < 0.05$) with all techniques. Finally, with respect to the width of the first molars, differences between T0 and T1 ($p < 0.0019$) in all techniques except technique D ($p = 0.149$, Bonferroni) were observed.

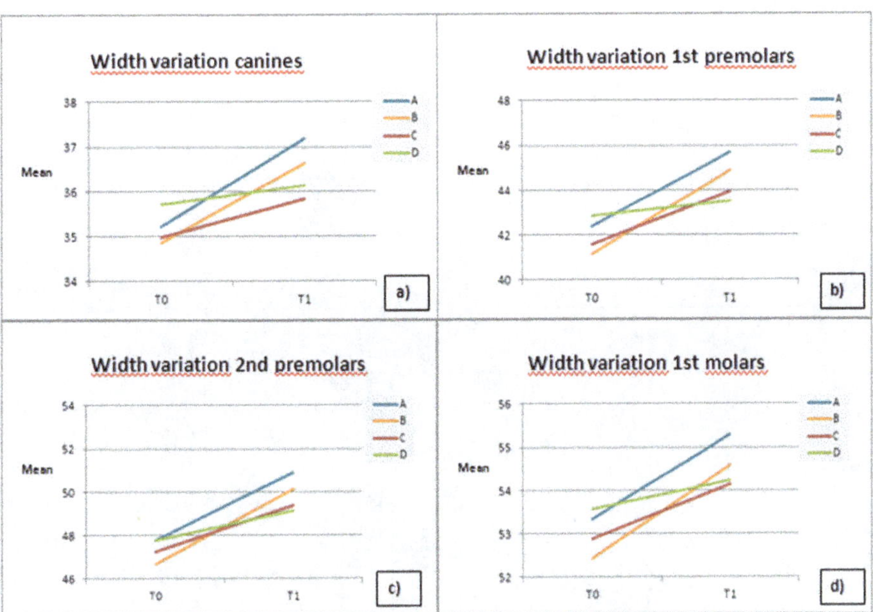

Figure 4. Dentoalveolar maxillary width changes between T0 and T1 depending on the technique. a) Canine width variation; b) 1st premolar width variation; c) 2nd premolar width variation; d) 1st molar width variation.

5.4. Relationship between torque and width variations between T0 and T1 depending on the technique

Table 4 shows the relationship between torque variation and the different interdental widths.

Correlation between torque changes and widths can also be observed in Figure 5 (a,b,c,d).

It also was determined whether these correlations are maintained within each of the techniques. When calculating correlations in small samples ($n=19$) is preferable to use the nonlinear coefficient of Spearman (table 5)

	Width variation 1st premolars	Width variation 2nd premolars	Width variation 1st molars	Width variation canines
Torque variation canines	n.s.	n.s.		<0,001 (r=0,436)
Torque variation 1st premolars	<0,001 (r=0,392)	0,002 (r=0,352)	0,001 (r=0,363)	0,049 (r=0,226)
Torque variation 2nd premolars	0,023 (r=0,261)	<0,001 (r=0,399)	0,004 (r=0,330)	0,350 (r=0,109)
Torque variation 1st molars	0,008 (r=0,304)	0,048 (r=0,227)	0,011 (r=0,290)	n.s.

n.s. non significant

Table 4. Lineal correlation between torque and width variation (r Pearson's coefficient)

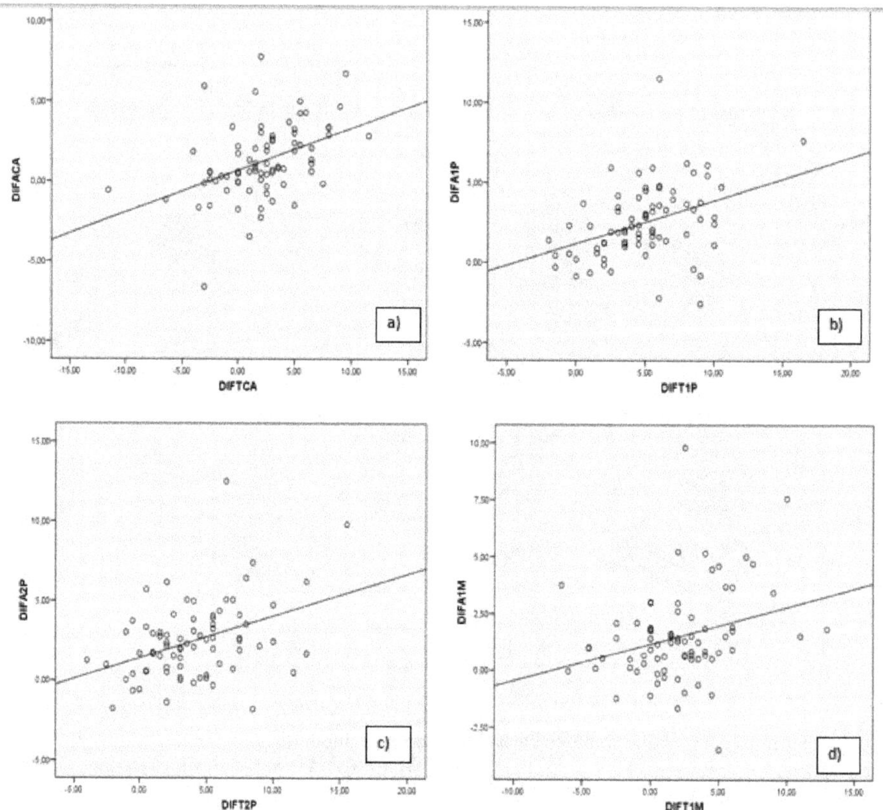

Figure 5. Relationships between changes in a) intercanine widths (DIFWCA) and torques in canines (DIFTCA), b) 1st inter-premolar widths (DIFW1P) and torques in 1st premolars (DIFT1P), c) 2nd interpremolar widths (DIFW2P) and torques in 2nd premolars (DIFT2P) and d) 1st intermolar widths (DIFW1M) and torques in 1st molars (DIFT1M), respectively.

Correlations between torque and witdh variation were found to be frequent for A and B techniques, lower for C and almost insignificant for D technique. The strongest correlation between torque variation and width was found in the canine area, with the C prescription technique. Correlations were also detected at first premolar and canine areas for subjects treated with B technique.

TECHNIQUE		Width variation 1st premolars	Width variation 2nd premolars	Width variation 1st molars	Width variation canines
A	Torque variation 1st premolars	0,043 (r=0,468)	n.s.	0,036 (r=0,484)	0,006 (r=0,605)
	Torque variation 2nd premolars	n.s.	n.s.	0,015 (r=0,551)	n.s.
	Torque variation 1st molars	0,043 (r=0,469)	n.s.	0,019 (r=0,531)	n.s.
	Torque variation canines	n.s.	n.s.	n.s.	n.s.
B	Torque variation 1st premolars	**0,001 (r=0,676)**	**0,002 (r=0,673)**	n.s.	n.s.
	Torque variation 2nd premolars	0,035 (r=0,485)	0,005 (r=0,614)	n.s.	n.s.
	Torque variation 1st molars	n.s.	n.s.	n.s.	n.s.
	Torque variation canines	**0,003 (r=0,643)**	0,049 (r=0,456)	n.s.	0,034 (r=0,488)
C	Torque variation 1st premolars	n.s.	0,039 (r=0,478)	0,005 (r=0,613)	n.s.
	Torque variation 2nd premolars	n.s.	n.s.	n.s.	n.s.
	Torque variation 1st molars	n.s.	n.s.	n.s.	n.s.
	Torque variation canines	n.s.	n.s.	n.s.	**<0,001 (r=0,792)**
D	Torque variation 1st premolars	n.s.	n.s.	n.s.	n.s.
	Torque variation 2nd premolars	n.s.	n.s.	n.s.	n.s.
	Torque variation 1st molars	n.s.	n.s.	n.s.	n.s.
	Torque variation canines	0,043 (r=0,469)	n.s.	n.s.	n.s.

n.s. non significant

Table 5. No lineal correlation between torque and width variation. (Spearman´s Rho Coefficient)

6. Further research

It has been shown that proper torque should be extended to the last visible tooth when smiling [5, 6], reason why in this research the torque from the canine to the first molar has been studied.

In this work, no cases previously treated with extractions in the maxillary arch were included, due to the controversy of the impact of dental extractions and their possible effect on the final aesthetic result [6, 19-22]. Therefore, a possible bias was eliminated.

The initial torque before and after treatment in different orthodontic techniques was measured. We chose to use pictures because it was intended to measure the coronal torque or 'apparent' torque that is seen when the patient smiles and not the 'real' torque, which corresponds to the angle between the long axis of root with a horizontal reference axis. Coronary torques were measured with the aim of observing whether these tend to approach a neutral value (close to 0 degrees) or, conversely, if the torques were kept still negative values after treatment in any of the techniques.

All measurements were taken from photographs of plaster models carried out before and after the orthodontic treatment. All the images were taken with the same camera, parallel to the same horizontal plane, with the same light conditions, and with the plaster models correctly positioned. However, intra and interexaminer errors have been detected, especially in torque measurements. This could be due to the lack, in frontal photographs, of clear reference points marking the line of the dental crown buccolingual axis.

Intraexaminer analysis determined that values were higher in the second round of measurements, both in torque and width. Variability in measurement differences was higher in torques than in widths.

In interexaminer analysis, no observer measured systematically more than the other. The measurement error (d Dahlberg) ranged from 0.8 mm to 2.0 mm approximately in width measurements, increasing to ranges of 2.0º-4.0º for torques. Again, variability in measurement differences was higher in torques than in widths.

6.1. Analysis of T0 to T1 changes in torque according to the technique

The differences between T0 and T1 as a result of variation of torque of the subjects during treatment were calculated. Treatment success was defined as the approximation of zero torque values without being positive.

Changes in torque were assessed as favorable when they went from a negative value to a less negative value or ideally zero. Not sought to find positive values, but close to zero or neutral. For example, the difference in degrees of a tooth torque when going from-5º to-1 º is 4º, the same as a tooth that go from-2° to+2º, or from 0º to+4º. However, not all situations are reflecting the same degree of success.

Three possible scenarios regarding the evolution of torque were defined: Favorable, unfavorable or stable. The favorable situation was the one in which the torque went to values close to zero, either from a situation with negative torque or (less often) positive torque. The stable situation was the one in which the torque did not varied, and the unfavorable was that in which the torque went away from zero, either from negative values or from positive values.

In the results, rarely the torques of the posterior teeth were 0º absolute value, but a remarkable tendency to obtain torque of 0 ° was observed in all teeth, especially the premolars (78-85% for premolars, 60-70% for canines and between 63 and 73% for molars), which according to Zachrisson [5] is favorable for obtaining an aesthetic and functional smile [5,6]. Despite this overall improvement, there was significant variation in the final torque values when analyzed between techniques and within each of them, which is consistent with that observed by authors like Streva et al. [10] or Brauchli et al. [11].

Watching the torque of canines, most experienced a favorable outcome, they tended to evolve after treatment at values closer to 0 ° Specifically, techniques C and D showed a higher percentage of improvement, and techniques A and B the least. However, the technique B obtained the average torque values closest to 0 degrees. For cases that evolved unfavorably, the technique that showed fewer incidences was the technique B. With technique A no improvement in torque in this tooth was detected. After assessing the evolution of the torques of the canines in the four techniques, we can add that there is no statistically significant difference between the four techniques. However, we can see that there is no symmetry between the two sides in the case of canines.

At first premolars, in more than 80% of cases the torque from both sides improved. In these teeth a more homogeneous relationship between sides was observed, and all techniques improved significantly their torque. However, these differences were not statistically significant, although that it could impact clinically. The technique B obtained average values closer to 0 ° torque at end of treatment, and it was obtained more positive values of torque. Observing the evolution of the torque in the four techniques, techniques A and B showed higher percentages of improvement. Statistically, it was observed that all the techniques worked well with the torque of the premolars. The homogeneity in the results was significantly higher than for canines.

In the case of the second premolars, in about 80% of cases the techniques favorably modify the torque getting very obvious way. Again, not statistically significant differences between techniques regarding the improvement of the torque were found, and the situation is similar to that shown above. Although not statistically significant, a difference in the average torque at end of treatment was proven, and technique C presented the more negative torques.

In the case of the first molars, around 63% and 73% of patients showed improvement of torque in these teeth in the left and right side, respectively. As with the other teeth, the torque variation was significant during treatment. In general, we observed that the four techniques managed to improve the torque of the first molars but no statistically significant differences between techniques were found. However, in this case, differences which could have clinical significance were also observed. The technique B was the one that showed less negative torques at the end of treatment in these teeth, despite having very negative torques prior to treatment. Technique D presented the lowest percentage of improvement (50-57%).

It was also studied if the variation value of torque experienced by a particular tooth was similar to that of the contralateral. It was observed that the buccolingual inclination of the crowns were not symmetrical in most cases, however, the statistical results obtained allowed to conclude that the average change in torque on either side could be considered similar. The largest discrepancy occurred in the molars, but without being statistically significant. Despite not showing statistical significance, these differences between the two sides could itself have clinical significance, because they may affect the final aesthetic smile of the subjects. As suggested by Zachrisson et al. [5, 6] for optimal smile aesthetics, a normal canine of the maxillary arch should have a slight symmetrical lingual inclination and the first and second premolars should be straight and show also symmetrical torques [5,6]. Authors like Hulsey et al. [23] showed that attention must be paid to asymmetric variables, since alterations in symmetry negatively affect the aesthetics of the smile [23]. As has been explained above, the torque values of both sides were not uniform in many cases, indicating that preadjusted brackets systems do not meet the purpose of symmetry in many cases, although the same information on both sides is contained.

This diversity of results in torques could be explained by the presence of multiple factors that have influenced this research and are difficult to control in a clinical context. It should be remembered that this is a retrospective study, so there are treatment variables that could not be controlled. As Zachrisson [6] said, torque control is one of the weaknesses of the preadjusted bracket systems [6]. And, as many authors have suggested, the expression of torque is the result of interaction of many factors [9, 11, 24]. In this research, variables, such as individual biological variation, the deformation of the slot of the bracket during treatment, the amount of resin between the bracket base and the tooth, possible defects in wires and brackets or the starting torque of the posterior teeth, could not be controlled.

It is known that expression of the torque is achieved by filling the slot of the bracket and progressively increasing the size of the wires during treatment (wires sequence) [9]. In this study, all cases were applied a progressive increase in the sequence of archwires used during treatment. Initially, Nickel-Titanium wires of small-caliber were used, followed by intermediate wires of medium caliber and finishing with stainless-steel wires that filled completely the slot of the bracket. However, in this study the amount of time these arches remained in the mouth of the patient was variable and indefinite. According to authors like Brauchli et al,[11] the amount of time of treatment with high diameter arches as well as the materials used could influence the amount of expressed torque in teeth [11]. In all cases of the present study, the material of the bracket and the wires were the same.

Although the brackets in technique C contain the same torque information that in technique A, different results were obtained with both techniques. The observed differences could be due to the bracket ligation. While technique A uses is a conventional bracket ligation method (Victory®) technique C uses a passive self-ligating bracket (Smart Clip®). This confirms what suggested Morina et al. [12] or other authors as Huang et al. [25] about the different expression of torque depending on the way of the bracket ligation method.

Some authors like Badawi et al [9] observed that passive self-ligating brackets (such as technique C) got a lower expression of torque than their counterparts: active self-ligating brackets [9]. Other authors have demonstrated the absence of such relationship, stating that the basic system of self-ligation did not influence clinically the expression of torque [11]. Therefore, one might assume that if active self-ligating brackets were been used, the final torque would have been similar to that obtained with brackets of technique A (conventional ligatures). However, we do not have enough data to support this claim.

Observing the results, and coinciding with authors like Archambault et al. [7], one could assume that it is difficult to predict the final torque to be obtained at the end of treatment only from a certain system of brackets.

6.2. Analysis of T0 to T1 changes in twidth according to the technique

At this point, the differences obtained in the width between the two times T0 and T1 and the dependence of the technique used were analyzed. Techniques A and B showed significant changes from T0 to T1 in the interdental width of posterior teeth analyzed, B being the most, while technique D showed no significant changes in intermolar or interpremolar widths. This coincides with the different archforms used. In technique B, the archwire was the widest of the four techniques. Instead, in technique D the archwire was the one that least width presented.

6.3. Correlation between torque changes and widths

A general correlation between torque variations and widths was found. These relationships were direct, with a higher torque variation meaning a higher width variation.

Correlations were found to be frequent, especially for techniques A and B, lower for technique C and almost disappeared for technique D. Therefore, in this last technique (D), torque variation was completely independent from width variation, whereas with techniques A and B, torque variation could be considered dependent on width variation. With technique B, the achieved width in premolars and canines allowed a good prediction of torque variation in these teeth.

At the end of the treatment, a general direct relationship between width change and torque change was detected. This implies that higher expected width changes will mean a higher change in posterior torques into close to neutral values. No literature supporting this observation has been found, but it could open new research lines.

A direct relationship between the level of performed dentoalveolar expansion and the achieved negative torque reduction has been shown. This was specially visible at premolar level where, according to Zachrisson[5,6], the torque must be closer to 0º. It could be inferred from these results that a way of changing the initial negative torque would be by incrementing the interpremolar width dentoalveolarly. However, there is not scientific literature to date relating maxillary width variation with final torque value.

The tipping movement described for quick expansion or disjunction [17,11] implies that dental crowns in posterior sectors present a higher buccal inclination at the end of treatment than at the beginning of the treatment. This could be one of the causes explaining the previously described relationship. Therefore, it can be concluded that the use of wires to achieve a dentoalveolar expansion in posterior sectors would help in getting a neutral torque in these sectors. Specifically, with technique B, at the end of treatment, the relationship between width gain and torque change close to 0º was higher than with the other techniques, especially in the premolar area, where a higher trend to neutral torque and a higher expansion could be observed. In accordance with authors such as Fleming et al.[18,12] and the findings in this study, in cases with a higher dentoalveolar compression, the gain of close to 0º torque could also be higher.

As described by Sarver et al.[4], treatment with ovoid or expanded arches should increase maxillary width and promote neutral torques in posterior sectors, and thus cause an aesthetic improvement. However, it has to be noted, that works of authors such as Mutinelli et al.[25,17] showed that the original width should be kept in order to achieve a long term stability of the orthodontic treatment. Accordingly to these authors, an arch shapes assessment prior to the orthodontics treatment is essential to choose the most appropriate arch shapes[25,17].

In our study, in cases treated with technique D, torque changes were found to be completely independent of width changes. Through the results, it can be observed that with this technique the change in final width was low, especially in the molar area. From these results, it can be inferred that the torque achieved at the treatment end was mainly related with the torsion forces applied individually to the wire in each posterior tooth, and not with the expansion. In such cases torque could be individualized by bending the wires, and an appropriate torque was achieved for each individual.

Thus, it can be concluded that the highest torque change is not only caused by the fact of filling the slot completely, as stated by Brauchli et al.[11,18], but also by the use of a strong and rigid wire that can generate a greatest dentoalveolar expansion. Therefore, with a tipping movement a negative torque becomes closer to 0º simply by changing the dentoalveolar width.

Considering the great variety in torque level of expression in posterior maxillary sectors found in literature and in the present study, it could be inferred that torque present in the different bracket system is irrelevant, and that the individualization of cases in order to achieve an appropriate torque close to 0º in posterior sectors would be more recommendable. Securing an ideal arch shape applying the appropriate torsion in each case would help in the achievement of neutral torques at the end of treatment.

7. Conclusions

Conclusions derived from our study are:

1. The four orthodontic techniques (A, B, C and D) showed a reduction on posterior dental torque with the orthodontic treatment, although this reduction is not related to the prescription used.

2. Between 70 and 90% of the subjects achieved an improvement in the value of torque in first and second premolars. These ratios decrease for canines and first molars.

3. The results in reducing the torque are not significantly different according to the technique used. The type of treatment hardly influenced the quality of the correction.

4. Increases occurred in the widths of the maxillary arches after treatment were related to improvements to neutral torques (to values closer to 0º), especially in subjects treated with the A and B techniques. In technique D no such relationship was observed.

Author details

Gaastra Carolin, Zamora Natalia*, Paredes Vanessa, Tarazona Beatriz and Jose Luis Gandía

*Address all correspondence to: natalia.zamora@uv.es

Department of Orthodontics, Faculty of Medicine and Dentistry, University of Valencia, Valencia, Spain

References

[1] Yang IIH, Nahm DS, Baek SH. Wich hard and soft tissue factors relate with the amount of buccal corridor space during smiling?. Angle Orthod. 2008; 78(1):5-11.

[2] Janson G, Castello Branco N, Freire Fernandes TM, Sathler R, Garib D, Pereira Lauris JR. Influence of othodontic treatment, midline position, buccal corridor and smile arc on smile attractiveness. Angle Orthod. 2011; 81(1):153-161.

[3] Mackley RJ. An evaluation of smiles before and after treatment. Angle Orthod. 1993;63 (3):183-189.

[4] Sarver DM, Ackerman MB. Dynamic visualization and quantification: Part 2. Smile analysis and treatment strategies. Am J Orthod Dentofacial Orthop. 2003; 124(2): 116-127.

[5] Zachrisson BU. Buccal uprighting of canines and premolars for improved esthetics and stability. World J Orthod. 2006; 7(4):406-12.

[6] Zachrisson BU. Premolar extraction and smile esthetics. Am J Orthod Dentofacial Orthop. 2003; 124(6):11A-12A.

[7] Archambault A, Lacoursière R, Badawi H, Major PW, Carey J, Flores-Mir C. Torque expression in Stainless Steel Orthodontic Brackets. Angle Orthod. 2010;80(1):201-210.

[8] Ügur T, Yukay F. Normal faciolingual inclinations of Toth Clowns compared with treatment groups of standard and pretorqued brackets. Am J Orthod Dentofacial Orthop. 1997; 112(1):50-57.

[9] Badawi HM, Toogood RW, Carey JPR, Heo G, Major PW. Torque expression in self-ligating brackets. Am J Orthod Dentofacial Orthop. 2008;133(5):721-728.

[10] Streva AM, Cotrim-Ferreira FA, Garib DG, Carvalho PEG. Are torque values of preadjusted brackets precise? J Appl Oral Sci. 2010; 9(4):313-7.

[11] Brauchli LM, Steineck M, Wichelhaus A. Active and passive self-ligation: a myth? Part 1: torque control. Angle Orthod. 2011;81:1-7.

[12] Morina E, Eliades T, Pandis N, Jäger A, Bourauel C. Torque expression of self-ligation brackets compared with convencional metallic, ceramic, and plastic brackets. Eur J Orthod. 2008; 30:233-238.

[13] Moore T, Southard KA, Casko JS, Qian F, Southard TE. Buccal corridors and smile esthetics. Am J Orthod Dentofacial Orthop. 2005; 127(2):208-213.

[14] Gioka C, Eliades T. Materials-induced variation in the torque expresión of preadjusted appliances. Am J Orthod Dentofacial Orthop. 2004; 125(3):323-328.

[15] Roden-Johnson D, Gallerano R, English J. The effects of buccal corridor spaces and arch form on smile esthetics. Am J Orthod Dentofacial Orthop. 2005; 127(3):343-350.

[16] Erum G, Fida M. Changes in smile parameters as perceived by orthodontists, dentists, artists, and laypeople. World J Orthod. 2008; 9(2):132-140.

[17] Graber LW, Lucker GW. Dental esthetic self-evaluation and satisfaction. Am J Orthod Dentofacial Orthop. 1980; 77(2):163-173.

[18] Fleming PS, Dibiase AT, Sarri G, Lee RT. Comparison of mandibular arch changes during alignment and leveling with 2 preadjusted edgewise appliances. Am J Orthod Dentofacial Orthop. 2009; 136(3):340-347.

[19] Be Gole EA, Fox DL, Sadowsky C. Analysis of change in arch form with premolar extraction. Am J Orthod Dentofacial Orthop. 1998;113(3):307-315.

[20] Isiksal E, Hazar S, Akyalcin S. Smile esthetics: Perception and comparison of treated and untreated smiles. Am J Orthod Dentofacial Orthop. 2006; 129(1):8-16.

[21] Kim E, Gianelly A. Extraction vs nonextraction: Arch widths and smile esthetics. Angle Orthod. 2003; 73(4):354-358.

[22] Ritter DE, Gonzaga L, Dos Santos A, Locks A. Esthetic influence of negative space in the buccal corridor during smiling. Angle Orthod. 2006; 76(2):198-203.

[23] Hulsey CM. An esthetic evaluation of lip-teeth relationships present in the smile. Am J Orthod Dentofacial Orthop. 1970; 57(2):132-144.

[24] Archambault A, Major TW, Graber JP, Heo G, Badawi H, Major PW. A comparison of torque expresión between stainless steel, titanium molybdenum alloy, and cooper nickel titanium wires in metalic self-ligating brackets. Angle Orthod. 2010;80(5): 884-889.

[25] Huang Y, Keilig L, Rahimi A, Reimann S, Eliades T, Jäger A, Bourauel C. Numeric modeling of torque capabilities of self-ligating and convencional brackets. Am J Orthod Dentofacial Orthop. 2009; 136(5):638-643.

[26] Mutinelli S, Manfredi M, Cozzani M. A mathematic-geometric model to calculate variation in mandibular arch form. Eur J Orthod. 2000; 22:113-125.

3

Prevention, Diagnosis and Treatment of Caries and Non-Carious Lesions in Orthodontic Patients

Andréa Cristina Barbosa da Silva,
Diego Romário da Silva, Ana Marly Araújo Maia,
Pierre Andrade Pereira de Oliveira,
Daniela Correia Cavalcante Souza and
Fábio Correia Sampaio

1. Introduction

1.1. Caries risks and orthodontic treatment

Although orthodontic treatment has many recognized benefits, including improvement in dental health, function, appearance, and self-esteem; nevertheless, orthodontic appliances can cause unwanted complications if adequate care is not taken during the treatment.

It is important that patients are aware of these potential risks so that they can know their responsibilities and expectations on them during the treatment. This ensures in achieving successful results without any adverse effects after the completion of orthodontic treatment [1].

Some of potential intraoral risks that orthodontic treatment carries with it are enamel demineralization/caries, adverse effects to the periodontal tissues, tissues damage, enamel fractures, enamel wear (abrasion/erosion), root resorption, pulp reactions, and allergic reactions to nickel and latex.

These potential complications are easily avoidable by undertaking certain precautions and timely interventions by both the orthodontist and the patient [1]. However, the lack of patient's cooperation and consequent poor oral hygiene is one of the main challenges in orthodontic practice [2].

The irregular surfaces of brackets, bands, wires and other attachments also limit naturally occurring self-cleansing mechanisms, such as the movement of the oral musculature and saliva [3, 4, 5]. The insertion of fixed orthodontic appliances creates stagnation areas for plaque and makes tooth cleaning more difficult [6, 7]. These promote retention niches that pose an increased risk of caries [5, 8].

Enamel demineralization around the brackets and bands is one adverse side effect of major clinical relevance [4, 7, 9, 10, 11]. White spot lesions develop as a result of prolonged plaque accumulation on the affected surface, commonly due to inadequate oral hygiene [6].

All these changes in the local environment appear to favor colonization of aciduric bacteria such as *Streptococcus mutans* and *lactobacilli* [3].

Clinically, formation of white spots around orthodontic attachments can occur as early as 4 weeks into treatment [6, 12] and their prevalence among orthodontic patients ranges from 2% to 96% [4, 5, 8, 12, 13].

Several studies have reported significant increase in the prevalence and severity of demineralization in patients after orthodontic treatment [12, 14, 15, 16].

Whilst the demineralized surface remains intact, there is a possibility of remineralization and lesion reversal [17]. It is generally believed that, when the appliances are removed and oral hygiene is restored, these lesions regress [9].

Some white spot lesions may remineralize and return to normal conditions or at least to a visually acceptable appearance. However, white spot lesions may also persist, resulting in aesthetically unacceptable result, as opaque and/or hypoplastic areas [18, 19]. In severe cases, restorative treatment may be required [20].

Besides incipient carious lesions, common damage that also needs attention from the orthodontist includes enamel wear by abrasion and erosion. Wear of enamel against both metal and ceramic brackets may occur. Stainless steel brackets tend to induce less enamel abrasion than ceramic brackets [21]. In patients with deep bite, use of bite planes is advocated to minimize interference and the subsequent risk of enamel abrasion [22]. Any enamel erosion must be recorded prior to treatment commencing and appropriate dietary advice should be given to minimize further tooth substance loss. Carbonated drinks and acid pure juices are the commonest causes of erosion and should be avoided in patients with fixed appliances [17].

Treatment can only be justified and success can only be ensured thanks to thorough understanding and controlled management of the potential associated risks, including those of carious and non-carious lesions. Preventive measures are available and have been scientifically validated and therefore, they should be implemented before and during orthodontic treatment [20].

Among the most common and effective preventive measures are special oral hygiene instructions, including a recommendation for using high-fluoride toothpaste, fluoride mouth rinse, and products with high-fluoride content [23].

Just importantly as preventing, intercepting and correcting problems related to tooth alignment and bone growth, is to provide patients undergoing orthodontic treatment, the maintenance of their oral health as a whole [18].

The provision of oral hygiene instruction, monitoring and motivation of all patients under orthodontic treatment is the responsibility of the orthodontist, the General practitioner and his/her entire team.

In this context, professionals in the field of orthodontics should be prepared to prevent and recognize the risks and diseases that may arise due to the use of orthodontic apparatus for their patients, as well as properly dealing with possible complications with appropriate measures.

2. Etiology and diagnosis of carious and non-carious lesions

Despite the still high prevalence of dental caries in the world population [24], increase in the prevalence of non-carious lesions has also been observed in recent years [25]. Especially, the carious white spot lesions may present increased risk of developing in teeth during orthodontic treatment due to the installation of devices in orthodontic patients [26].

The carious and non-carious lesions differ in their etiology, basically due to the former being associated with bacteria, while the latter have no relationship with microorganisms. Thus, the term dental caries is used to describe the results of a chemical dissolution of tooth structure caused by the metabolic events that occur in the biofilm, which covers the affected areas [27]. In non-carious lesions, loss of tooth structure is caused by multiple factors and of complex diagnosis due to difficulty in identifying the primary cause; however, it is not associated with the presence of microorganisms [28, 29].

In other words, the dental caries result from a change in the ecology and metabolic activity of the biofilm, in which a balance between tooth mineral and biofilm is established. Importantly, the biofilm formed that grows ubiquitously in solid surfaces does not necessarily result in the development of clinically visible caries. However, the biofilm is a prerequisite for the occurrence of these injuries. In general, the dental caries are result of physiological imbalance between the tooth mineral and biofilm fluid [27].

Initially, carious lesions can develop into any dental site of the oral cavity, where a biofilm can develop and remain for a period. It is erroneous talk on surfaces more or less susceptible to decay, since it can generate the belief that certain tooth parts are "tougher" or "less prone" to developing dental caries in function of variations in the chemical and structural composition [30, 31].

However, it is worth noting that the risk factor to the onset of tooth decay is higher in orthodontic patients, due to mechanical propensity of greater accumulation of waste associated with the presence of brackets and bands in the development of lesions. These "protected" sites are relatively protected areas of the mechanical influence of the tongue, cheeks, abrasive foods and brushing. Thus, these are the most likely sites to develop the lesion, because biofilms can stagnate for a long time [27]. Thus, some tests for risk assessment of caries can be useful in these patients, as the computerized program Cariograma® [32], as well as others developed especially for these patients, as an immediate chair-side test, displaying the intraoral lactic acid production of cariogenic bacteria. Recently, this test was considered useful to evaluate the risk for dental caries in patients with orthodontic treatment. Furthermore, specific clinical approaches for this group of patients are required [33].

In this context, it becomes important for the patient, prior to installation of the appliance, to have a dental and periodontal examination adequate for a correct diagnosis of dental and/or periodontal injuries [34], with referral for some specialists in periodontics and/or dentistry, if necessary.

Overall, the tactile–visual examination of the teeth is currently considered sufficient for a proper diagnosis of caries. Thus, it should be conducted systematically after each quadrant of the mouth has been isolated with cotton rolls and with a suction device for preventing the teeth wetting by saliva. This type of examination requires good lighting and clean and dry teeth. The teeth can be examined with the help of a mirror and a probe with a blunt tip, whose purpose is to remove biofilm and verify the lesion surface texture [35].

Moreover, the increased knowledge of the dynamic chemical processes of caries has stimulated the development of a new method for visual–tactile diagnosis of caries based on verification of the lesion activity. This method evaluates the surface features of the lesion: the activity, reflected by the surface texture, and surface integrity, expressed by the presence and absence of a cavity or microcavity on the surface [36]. The pathobiological principle of the method is based on the observation that enamel surface characteristics change in response to changes in the biofilm activity covering the tooth surface [37].

It is noteworthy that one should not force the tooth tissue with the probe, as there is a risk of causing irreversible damage to the surface area of incipient lesion [38] damage. Additional resources in tactile–visual diagnosis of caries include fiber optic transillumination, tooth separation and teeth expansion, especially for professionals in the labor market for longer [35].

Regarding the use of radiography in the diagnosis of carious lesions, the most commonly used is the *bitewing*. Although routine use of bitewing radiography could help identify teeth with hidden caries to allow early and conservative treatment, it is inaccurate in diagnosing occlusal enamel caries [39]. However, small mineral loss cannot be detected in the radiographs, and the additional diagnostic yield in bitewing radiography is confined to lesions diagnosed at the level of cavity\dentin. In addition, the radiographic examination fails to determine the lesion activity and cavity formation, and suffers from a high number of false-positive diagnoses [35].

Among the unknown carious lesions, the most important and can be associated to orthodontic treatment is tooth erosion that is caused by dissolution and removal of an ultrathin layer of enamel whenever exposed to the acidic challenge. In early enamel caries with the tipical subsurface lesion, mineral loss and changes predominantly occur in the body of the lesion below the pseudo-intact surface layer [40].

Only the surfaces directly exposed to acid are affected. The teeth are eroded and where foods and fresh and acidic beverages reach the enamel surfaces prior to being neutralized and diluted by saliva [40]. In addition, tooth erosion can also be caused by acid stomach content that can return to the mouth due to an eating disorder or gastroesophageal reflux [41, 42]. Vomit may be a feature of an eating disorder, which can cause erosion and bulimia [43].

Early identification of patients with erosion is important, and thus the dentist may assist the patient in establishing the cause. Sometimes, the patient's complaint about tooth sensitivity directs attention to the problem because the dentin is exposed. However, the dentist may have diagnosed even early lesions. In particular, lingual surfaces of the maxillary incisors should be examined because they are the most eroded. Thus, a careful anamnesis is essential to try to determine the probable cause, and counseling is mandatory [40]. Even if the cause is not identified in the anamnesis, for being difficult to determine [44], counseling is provided to the patient [40].

Enamel erosion (decalcification) around orthodontic brackets bonded to the teeth has been a concern for orthodontists, since this decalcification is the first step to more greater damage to the enamel. These erosive lesions can also lead to infiltration of resin restorations and shear of orthodontic brackets [45].

Finally, it is interesting to note that despite the self-ligated brackets being considered more hygienic than those with elastic, no differences in terms of white spot lesion formation were found between conventional and self-ligating wire brackets straight; no differences in terms of white spot lesion formation were found between conventional straight wire and self-ligating brackets; and white spot lesion formation does depend largely on patients' oral hygiene status, the type of bracket or ligation used [46].

3. Control of dental biofilm associated with orthodontic treatment

It is known that the goal of orthodontic treatment is to make corrections to the occlusion and also provide improvements in dental aesthetics. However, this treatment can provide increased chances of developing dental caries and/or periodontal disease, which can harm the patient and the progress of treatment. The development of these diseases may be mainly associated with a deficient biofilm removal due to the impediment of a proper hygiene, caused by intraoral devices [47]. Wires, brackets and orthodontic bands serve as a biofilm reserve and source of infections since it provides increased biofilm retainer niches due to its configuration and surface. Factors such as the type of material of the bracket, the type of ligature used, taping or gluing of orthodontic accessories, diet and biofilm control can influence the capacity of proliferation of microorganisms and subsequent development of caries [48, 49, 50].

Wires, brackets and bands can become centers of tooth decay if the patient fails to maintain oral hygiene. Studies have shown increased prevalence of great severity of enamel demineralization after orthodontic treatment when compared to individuals not subjected to this treatment. However, once active orthodontic treatment has been completed, the demineralization process is normally expected to decelerate due to a change in local environmental factors [9].

Diet can be defined as the usual intake of food and drinks daily taken by any person, and may have a local effect in the mouth by its reaction with the tooth enamel surface, serving as a substrate for cariogenic microorganisms, particularly if it is rich in sucrose [51]. The frequency of intake, the sugar content and consistency of meals are decisive for caries formation [52]. On this basis, it is easy to observe that a poor diet associated with poor hygiene and the use of orthodontic appliance may be potential factors that influence the development of caries and inflammatory processes. It is the responsibility of the orthodontist to instruct the patient regarding these factors, especially at the point that relates to oral hygiene and plaque control. In addition, the orthodontist must have diagnostic accuracy to know when to refer the patient to the periodontist, when necessary.

Regarding the biofilm control, it is known that this procedure may be performed by mechanical and chemical means. The mechanical control consists of the biofilm removal using a proper brushing technique associated with the use of toothpaste and auxiliary materials, such as dental floss or tape [53]. Brushing, although extremely important, it is a relatively simple technique. There is no ideal brushing; however, there are features that facilitate oral hygiene procedures, such as the presence of multi-tufts, small head, rounded soft bristles, according to [54]. Brushing is extremely effective in controlling biofilm and reducing the risk of caries; however, to obtain maximum effectiveness in hygiene is necessary to consider factors such as the frequency and technique of brushing, hand skills and motivation of patients [55]. It is for the orthodontist to motivate the patient, who is considered to have a potential for developing caries and inflammation, to have a proper hygiene for oral health during and after treatment. The plaque disclosure can be a valuable alternative to help this motivation.

Chemical control is only an adjunct to mechanical control. Thus, it should not be used as a substitute for mechanical control. Chemical control can be performed in the prophylactic or therapeutic sense, depending on the patient's oral health status [56]. Generally, mouthwashes containing sodium fluoride [57], chlorhexidine [58], cetylpyridinium chloride [59] and essential oils [60] are used. Studies have shown that the use of commercial mouthwashes along with mechanical oral hygiene, guidance and motivation is the most appropriate management for maintenance of oral health in orthodontic patients [61]. Furthermore, the use of fluorides, in its various forms of presentation, is extremely important for dental remineralization and prevention of demineralization that might cause carious lesions [62]. It is important that the orthodontist can make use of these resources, adapting to the reality of each patient to provide orthodontic treatment free of complications.

4. Treatment of carious and non-carious lesions in orthodontics patients

Regarding all factors previously discussed, it is also important to the orthodontist to be aware of techniques and products that can prevent and treat, as a nonoperative procedure, the development of carious and non-carious lesions during orthodontics treatment. Management of white spot lesions begins with a good oral hygiene regime and needs to be associated with use of fluoride agents, as fluoridated toothpaste, fluoride-containing mouth rinse, gel, varnish, bonding materials, elastic ligature, CPP-ACP, antiseptics, LASER, tooth whitening, resin infiltration and micro-abrasion [63]. As demonstrated, the patient's behavior before the increased risk is very important, although the professional should supervise and also choose the better technique for each patient.

One of the first important points, which only depends on the orthodontist technique, is to choose the best adhesive composite type to bracket bonding, and also control and reduce the adhesive composite excess around the brackets. Incorporating preventive agents in orthodontic bonding composite seems to be a potential method to reduce white spot lesions during orthodontic treatment [64]. Bioavailable minerals from cement-containing amorphous calcium phosphate (ACP), as the Aegis–Ortho with 28% ACP fillers (Bosworth, Skokie Companies) [65], have been described to facilitate remineralization and also inhibit lesion development. There are also other cements-containing fluorides, as Pro-seal and Quick Cure (Reliance Orthodontic Products), and Light cure composite without fluoride or ACP, as Transbond XT (3M Unitek) has been also used followed by application of Varnish fluoride [66].

Researches are fundamental to compare and establish better options for each patient, [64], comparing different cements under similar in-vitro conditions to prevent incipient caries lesions next to brackets on teeth, observed that ACP into orthodontics adhesive material provided reduction in bacterial adhesion and lesion depth formation, with similar results to the Quick Cure adhesive with fluoride. Although Behnan et al., (2010) [66] having demonstrated that both light-cured filled resin (Pro-seal) and fluoride varnish (Varnish) might prevent enamel demineralization, even positive effects of Aegis-Ortho and MI Paste were not significant. The development of cements with preventive agents that can be effectively delivered in the long term encourages further investigation and also *in vivo* performance to evaluate these materials in clinical application, and also their importance to be applied in the orthodontic patient who lacks compliance with oral hygiene.

Attention is fundamental to position braces accurately, but it is also fundamental to remove composite excess between brackets and teeth with a scalar or another instrument, avoiding adding more area to plaque retention. One other option to this objective, commonly used when braces are placed on the lingual surface, is the indirect transfer system. This technique was evaluated in vivo during 4 months, if it could help reducing plaque accumulation around the brackets and consequently, the surrounding enamel demineralization. Concerning the differences between direct and indirect bonding, there was a significantly greater presence of white spots at the end of the treatment and a greater plaque accumulation around the braces where the direct bonding was used [67]. It was concluded by authors that, in a clinical point of view, the indirect bonding technique could help to reduce the enamel demineralization.

The bracket model has been also changed through the years, and the use of elastic ligatures has been also discussed about the association with white spot lesions development. The self-ligation bracket that does not require elastic ligatures was firstly introduced also as a hygienic option to minimize dental plaque retention and microbial flora. Although a clinical trial that evaluated 20 boys about plaque index, bleeding on probing and others, before bonding, after

1 week and 3 months after bonding, found that all clinical parameters showed statistically significant increases from before bonding, although self-ligation brackets and conventional brackets ligated with stainless steel ligatures did not differ with regard to dental plaque retention [68]. These results are similar to [46], that also revealed no statistically significant differences on white spot lesion development between conventional straight wire and self-ligating brackets, and also highlighted that WSL formation does depend largely on patients' oral hygiene status, not the type of bracket or ligation used.

In the light of the difficulties involved in clinically detecting, monitoring and managing dental demineralization, researchers are actively searching for new agents for prevention as preventive programs should be implemented to avoid the potentially detrimental [69]. The basic home care oral hygiene with manual toothbrush and fluoride toothpaste (1100ppm of fluoride), dental floss use, and patient's compliance seem to be an efficient preventive procedure, although it is also necessary to individualize and consider high risk of patients that even before and after some months do not have a satisfactory oral hygiene. For these patients, it is necessary to add some other alternatives such as the association of antimicrobial therapies.

The application of antimicrobial therapies with common commercially produced antibacterial agents such as varnishes, mouthwashes, or dentifrice gel formulations, particularly with chlorhexidine (CHX), have been found as beneficial preventive strategy for reducing undesirable outcomes of fixed orthodontic appliances [70, 71]. Some studies investigated the effects of various concentrations of chlorhexidine on oral microflora [72], and also fluoride varnish [73]. The combination of chlorhexidine–fluoride-containing dentifrice and fluoride varnish has also been investigated, and shown to be successful and promising alternative for improving oral hygiene features of patients lacking sufficient oral hygiene characteristics during orthodontic treatment. It was also observed that a one-visit chlorhexidine varnish treatment combined with a home-based chlorhexidine–fluoride gel formulation may be implemented as a caries-prevention strategy for patients undergoing fixed appliance treatment and particularly under high risk of caries [74].

The application of clinical procedures of each material is also fundamental to effectiveness. The Cervitec®Plus (1% chlorhexidine diacetate and 1% thymol, Ivoclar Vivadent) application procedures recommends that tooth surfaces should be cleaned thoroughly dry with air syringe and isolated with cotton rolls. Three drops of Cervitec®Plus poured into a dapper dish and a thin coat of varnish applied to all of the surfaces of the bonded teeth (buccal, lingual, occlusal and proximal areas). The varnish should be dispersed with air and allowed to dry, and the cotton rolls were removed after 30 seconds. After application, patients should be instructed not to rinse, eat/drink or brush for one hour. The Cervitec Plus can also be associated with Cervitec®Gel (Ivoclar Vivadent), 0.2% chlorhexidine digluconate and 0.2% sodium fluoride (900 ppm fluoride) to brush their teeth with as a dentifrice for four weeks at home, three times a day for 2 min.

The Fluor Protector (Ivoclar Vivadent) contents 5 wt% difluorosilane corresponding to 0.7 wt % F-; application procedure also consists of tooth surface cleaned thoroughly and dried with air syringe and isolated with cotton rolls. A thin layer of Fluor Protector should be applied to all tooth surfaces (buccal, lingual, occlusal and proximal areas) using applicator, dispersed with air and allowed to dry, and cotton rolls but just removed after 60 seconds. After the application of varnish, patients should be told not to eat/drink or brush for 45 minutes.

Many studies have investigated the protective effect of fluoride on erosion using fluoride compounds that are widely used in caries prevention such as NaF, AmF, SnF_2, or acidulated phosphate fluoride [75]. Fluorides has also been associated to ACP (amorphous calcium phosphate), commercially as MI Paste Plus(GC Corporation, Tokyo, Japan), that use the nano-complex of the milk protein casein phosphor-peptide (CPP); this product has demonstrated preventive and remineralization properties in the caries process [76] and suggested as a mechanism to prevent or reduce enamel demineralization also in orthodontics patients [77], that following for 3 months, demonstrated that the use of MI Paste Plus for a minimum of 3 to 5 minutes each day at night after brushing helped prevent the development of new white spot lesions during orthodontics treatment and decreased the number of white spot lesions already present.

Another technique to prevent enamel demineralization for the full duration of orthodontics treatment with fixed appliances is the tooth sealant polish, as Biscover LV (Bisco), and a clinically small but statistically significant ability to prevent white spot lesion was demonstrated [66]. To apply BisCover LV, the cleaned tooth surface should be etched for 15 seconds, rinsed copiously, air-dry thoroughly. After, one thin coat of BisCover LV should be applied, evaporated for 15 seconds without air, and then light-cured for 30 seconds with a LED.

The high risk of permanent damage to the enamel structure makes the orthodontic bracket debonding and subsequent clean-up extremely important to maintain the integrity of the enamel surface [78]. Many instruments have been proposed for bracket debonding and subsequent enamel clean-up, such as Arkansas points, diamond points, multiblade burs, pliers and others. However, once none of these instruments can achieve complete clean-up without affecting the enamel surface, several protocols have been proposed [79]. Instruments and protocols must be developed and tested in order to avoid possible iatrogenic damage to the enamel structure, leaving it as close as possible to its pretreatment condition. [80].

Associated to the risk, the presence of white spot or non-carious lesion appearance around brackets increased the risk of damage and also became a disappointment to the patient after debonding. Even with all homemade care, sometimes preventive procedures are not sufficient at all. Thus, the first option after debonding brackets that should be applied as soon as possible is remineralization agent procedures. There are also several techniques that have been evaluated by in vitro and in vivo experiments that each orthodontist should be aware, although no systematic review specifically addressing remineralization of WSLs after orthodontic treatment has been published [81]. Even not being possible to review all options, this chapter presents a small review about this topic and aims at discussing the strengths and limitations of the techniques and certainly helping clinicians weigh the effectiveness of various remineralization agents.

One of the most used preventive agents is the sodium fluoride, common used in toothpaste and also in varnish. To remineralize effects, the fluoride varnish Duraphat (5 % sodium fluoride) has been applied and analyzed through a clinical trial of 110 participants followed by 3 and 6 months, and it has been demonstrated that its effective in reversing WSLs after debonding every month during the first 6 months after debonding [16]. Authors also commented on the topical fluoride varnish that should be advocated as a routine caries prevention during orthodontic treatment.

The fluoride Varnish Duraphat application consists of this sequence, as preconized by [16]. Firstly, the subject's teeth should be clean with a toothbrush, especially the surfaces with WSLs. Secondly, excessive saliva in one or two quadrants of the mouth should be removed by cotton rolls or by using air syringe. It was not necessary to keep the tooth surface extremely dry because Duraphat could set in the presence of saliva. Thirdly, fluoride varnish should be applied onto the tooth surfaces with WSLs using a miniature cotton swab or brush, with the applicator dabbed repeatedly onto the tooth surface without contacting soft tissues. After a few minutes, a thin and clear layer is formed. Then, the next quadrants were treated in the same manner. After application, the patient should be advised not brushing their teeth or chewing food for at least 4 h after treatment; during this time, soft food and liquid might be consumed.

The casein phosphopeptide-amorphous calcium phosphate previously discussed, associated in cements and as a preventive treatment, has been also recommended to post–orthodontic population [82]. The product applied twice daily after fluoride toothpaste use for 12 weeks showed significantly regressed post–orthodontic white spot lesions [82]. The application preconized in this clinical test is very simple; after normal oral hygiene procedures using fluoridated dentifrice and a soft texture toothbrush, the patient uses a finger to apply 1g of the cream to the buccal/labial surfaces of teeth in the morning and night for 12 consecutive weeks.

However, the recently conducted research of [81] comparing the effectiveness of MI Paste Plus and PreviDent fluoride varnish (22,600 ppm of fluoride) with a standard oral hygiene regimen using toothpaste (1100 ppm of fluoride; Colgate Oral Pharmaceuticals) in terms of improving the appearance of WSLs after orthodontic treatment, found no difference of MI Paste Plus or PreviDent fluoride varnish compared to a standard oral hygiene and toothpaste regimen for ameliorating WSLs during an 8-week period. For more details, see [83].

Another new approach in treating incipient caries lesions and also non-carious lesion is the resin infiltration technique that became a treatment option for non-cavitated lesions not expected to arrest or remineralize it [45]. Infiltrate caries with low viscosity penetrate the porous body and are optimized for rapid capillary penetration [84]. The resin completely fills the pores within the tooth, replacing lost tooth structure and stopping caries and erosion progression by blocking further introduction of any nutrients into the pore system [85]. The resin infiltration is recommended for teeth that present obvious area of WSL found around the fixed orthodontic brackets but non-cavitated enamel surface. The applications procedures of the resin infiltrate (Icon caries infiltrant-Smooth Surfaces), according to the manufacturer's instructions and described by Hammad and Enan (2013) [45], recommend that firstly, a rubber dam as well as the OptraGate Lip and Cheek Retractor should be placed to protect the gingiva and to provide a dry working field to ensure the best treatment result as possible. Mylar strips should be placed securely with wedges distal to protect the neighboring teeth. Next, the pseudo-intact enamel surface layer is eroded using a 15% HCl gel (Icon-Etch), which is applied with a specially developed smooth surface applicator tip (mini-brush head), attached to the syringe containing the etching gel. By twisting the syringe top, an ample amount of the acid (Icon- Etch) is dispensed through an opening in the center of the applicator. The flocked tip is used to spread the gel evenly on the enamel surface by moving it in a circular motion, resulting in a homogenous etching pattern, extending 2 mm beyond the edges of the lesion. After 2 minutes of contact time, the etchant was rinsed off with water spray for at least 30 seconds, and dried with oil- and water-free air, resulting in a chalky white appearance of the etched area. To free the enamel microporosities of any remaining water, a 99% ethanol (Icon-Drya) should be applied, using roughly half the syringe content, onto the lesion site surface and left for 30 seconds, after which it is air dried. The resin infiltrate should be applied in two steps: a clean Smooth Surface Tip was attached onto the Icon-Infiltrate syringe, and an ample amount of the Icon-Infiltrate should be applied onto the etched lesion surface and left for 3 minutes to infiltrate and spread into the microporosities and then light-cured (output of 450 nm and a light intensity of 800 mW/cm2 for 40 seconds). A second layer of Icon-Infiltrate should be applied, for an additional minute, and then excess material removed and light-cured again for 40 seconds. Finally, after removing the rubber dam, polishing cups were used to finish the surface to a smooth luster. For further information see [86].

Another prevention method involves improving the effect of different fluoride compounds by applying high-intensity (~100–200 J/cm^2) laser radiation. [87]. According to [88], laser irradiation can significantly alter the permeability, crystallinity and acid solubility of enamel, and lead to increased resistance to demineralization. Furthermore, the absorption of fluoride is improved by laser irradiation [89].

As it was discussed, conservative treatment options for WSLs aim at bypassing the superficial layer and remineralizing the subsurface zone of the lesion. This is accomplished in two distinct ways: with the application of low levels of fluoride and calcium ions, which can penetrate deep into the WSL [90], or by reactivating the superficial enamel substrate via mechanical and chemical abrasion [91].

Considered as a minimally invasive treatment, microabrasion consists of the application of acidic and abrasive compound to the enamel surface and white spot lesion [92]. The microabrasion process abrades the surface enamel while also polishing it, causing it to reflect light differently than natural enamel. The application of a microabrasion technique results in significant regression of WSLs. [93].

One option of microabrasion procedure, preconized experimentally by [93], suggested applying 2-minute 35% phosphoric acid etch applied with Gel-Etch Semi Gel (Temrex Corp, Freeport, NY) and rinse, followed by a 20-second pumice with Topex Prep & Polish Paste (Sultan Dental Products Inc, Englewood, NJ) with a rubber cup, attached to a slow-speed handpiece, in a clockwise direction followed by a rinse. The same microabrasion application can be followed by twice-daily application of 1:1 diluted MI Paste and deionized water for 20 seconds.

The procedures preconized by Akin and Basciftci (2012) [94], recommends the application of 18% of hydrochloric acid mixed with fine pumice powder to obtain a slurry form to be applied on the affected teeth, by using a rubber cup in a contra angle handpiece. A rubber dam should be used to isolate these teeth from the rest so as to eliminate the chemical effects of microabrasion. The slurry should be agitated into the tooth surface for 30 seconds and then washed off with an air-water spray. The cycle of microabrasion procedure and washing can be repeated three to four times on each affected tooth. The patients underwent four or five sessions of the microabrasion therapy at 2-week interval when necessary.

The association between microabrasion and subsequently, the application of CPP-ACP cream has also been described, and suggested microabrasion to remove the hypermineralized superficial layer of enamel, followed by daily home application of CPP-ACP, could eliminate WSLs without involving invasive restorative procedures [91]. Akin and Basciftci (2012) [94], also concluded that CPP-ACP and fluoride agents support increased remineralization of the demineralized enamel, but the microabrasion is the best method for the cosmetic treatment of these post–orthodontic demineralized white spot lesions.

5. Final remarks

The demineralization occurring in teeth during orthodontic treatment is a significant clinical problem. Thus, in view of the etiological factors related to the development of carious and non-carious lesions, the best preventive strategy seems to be assessing the risk factors prior to banding, coupled with fluoride rinses, regular reinforcement of oral hygiene and dietary advice throughout the course of treatment.

Author details

Andréa Cristina Barbosa da Silva[1*], Diego Romário da Silva[1], Ana Marly Araújo Maia[1], Pierre Andrade Pereira de Oliveira[1], Daniela Correia Cavalcante Souza[2] and Fábio Correia Sampaio[2]

*Address all correspondence to: andreacbsilva@gmail.com

1 Center of Sciences, Technology and Health, State University of Paraiba, UEPB, Paraíba, Brazil

2 Center of Health Sciences, Federal University of Paraiba, Paraíba, Brazil

References

[1] Meeran NA. Iatrogenic possibilities of orthodontic treatment and modalities of prevention. J Orthod Sci 2013;2(3) 73-86.

[2] White LW. Oral hygiene for orthodontic patients. J Clin Orthod 1996;30 340-341.

[3] Rosenbloom RG, Tinanoff N. Salivary *Streptococcus mutans* levels in patients before, during, and after orthodontic treatment. Am J Orthod Dentofacial Orthop 1991;100(1) 35-37.

[4] Gorelick L, Geiger AM, Gwinnett AJ. Incidence of white spot formation after bonding and banding. Am J Orthod Dentofacial Orthop 1982;81(2) 93–98.

[5] Mizrahi, E. Enamel demineralization following orthodontic treatment. Am J Orthod 1982;82(1) 62-67.

[6] O'Reilly MM, Featherstone JD. Demineralization and remineralization around orthodontic appliances: an in vivo study. Am J Orthod Dentofacial Orthop 1987;92(1) 33-40.

[7] Gontijo L, Cruz RA, Brandão PRG. Dental enamel around fixed orthodontic appliances after fluoride varnish application. Braz Dent J 2007;18(1) 49-53.

[8] Lovrov S, Hertrich, K, Hirschfelder U. Enamel demineralization during fixed orthodontic treatment – incidence and correlation to various oral-hygiene parameters. J Orofac Orthop 2007;68(5) 353-356.

[9] Sudjalim TR, Woods MG, Manton DJ. Prevention of white spot lesion in orthodontics practice: a contemporary review. Aust Dent J 2006;51(4) 284-289.

[10] Olympio KPK, Bardal PAP, Henriques JFC, Bastos JRM. Prevenção de cáries dentária e doença periodontal em ortodontia: uma necessidade imprescindível. Revista Dental Press Ortop Facial 2006;11(2) 110-119.

[11] Chapman JA, Roberts WE, Eckert GJ, Kula KS, González-Cabezas C. Risk factors for incidence and severity of white spot lesions during treatment with fixed orthodontic appliances. Am J Orthod Dentofacial Orthop 2010;138(2) 188-194.

[12] Ogaard B, Rølla G, Arends J. Orthodontic appliances and enamel demineralization. Part 1. Lesion development. Am J Orthod Dentofacial Orthop 1988;94(1) 68-73.

[13] Enaia M, Bock N, Ruf S. White spot lesions during multibracket appliance treatment: A challenge for clinical excellence. Am J Orthod Dentofacial Orthop 2011;140(1) 17-24.

[14] Øgaard B. Prevalence of white spot lesions in 19-year-old: a study on untreated and orthodontically treated persons 5 years after treatment. Am J Orthod Dentofacial Orthop 1989;96(5) 423-427.

[15] Øgaard B, Larsson E, Henriksson T et al. Effects of combined application of antimicrobial and fluoride varnishes in orthodontic patients. Am J Orthod Dentofacial Orthop 2001;120(1) 28-35.

[16] Du M, Cheng N, Tai B, Jiang H, Li J, Bian Z. Randomized-controlled trial on fluoride varnish application for treatment of white spot lesion after fixed orthodontic treatment. Clin Oral Investig. 2012;16(2) 463-68. doi: 10.1007/s00784-011-0520-4.

[17] Travess H, Roberts-Harry D, Sandy J. Orthodontics. Part 6: Risks in orthodontic treatment. Br Dent J 2004;196(2) 71-77.

[18] Consolaro A, Consolaro MFM-O. Lesões cariosas incipientes e formação de cavidades durante o tratamento ortodôntico. É papel do ortodontista diagnosticar, prevenir e até tratar manchas brancas cariosas e não cariosas no esmalte? Rev Clín Ortodon Dental Press 2006;5(4) 104-111.

[19] Willmot D. White spot lesions after orthodontic treatment. Semin Orthod 2008;14(3) 209-219.

[20] Vital SO, Haignere-Rubinstein C, Lasfargues JJ, Chaussain C. Caries risk and orthodontic treatment. Int Orthod 2010;8(1) 28-45.

[21] Viazis AD, DeLong R, Bevis RR, Rudney JD, Pintado MR. Enamel abrasion from ceramin orthodontic brackets under an artificial oral environment. Am J Orthod 1990;98(2) 103-109.

[22] Chen YJ, Yao CC, Chang HF. Nonsurgical correction of skeletal deep overbite and class II division 2 malocclusion in an adult patient. Am J Orthod Dentofacial Orthop 2004;126(3) 371–378.

[23] Alexande SA, Ripa LW. Effects of self-applied topical fluoride preparations in orthodontic patients. Angle Orthod 2000;70(6) 424-430.

[24] Bagramian RA, Garcia-godoy F, Volpe AR. The global increase in dental caries. A pending public health crisis. Am J Dent 2009;21(1) 1-6.

[25] Caldeira EM, Fidalgo TKS, Passalini P, Marquezan M, Maia LC, Nojima MCG. Effect of fluoride on tooth erosion around orthodontic brackets. Braz Dent J 2012;23(5) 581-585.

[26] Julien KC, Buschang PH, Campbell PM. Prevalence of white spot lesion formation during orthodontic treatment. Angle Orthod 2013;83(4) 641-647.

[27] Fejerskov O, Kidd, E. Cárie dentária: a doença e seu tratamento clínico. 2 ed. São Paulo: Santos, 2011.

[28] Davies SJ, Gray RJ, Qualtrough AJ. Management of tooth surface loss. Br Dent J 2002;192(1) 11-16, 19-23.

[29] Hobkirk JA. Tooth surface loss: causes and effects. Int J Prosthodont 2007;20(4) 340-341.

[30] Black GV. Operative dentistry, Vol. 1 Pathology of the hard tissues of the teeth. London: Claudius Ash, Sons & Co., 1914.

[31] Weatherell JA, Robinson C, Hallsworth AS. The concept of enamel resistance: a critical review. In: Guggenheim B (ed) Cariology today. Basel: Karger, 1984, pp. 223–230.

[32] Bratthall D, Hänsel Petersson G. Cariogram: a multifactorial risk assessment model for a multifactorial disease. Community Dent Oral Epidemiol 2005;33(4) 256-264.

[33] Chaussain C, Opsahl VS, Viallon V, Vermelin L, Haignere C, Sixou M, Lasfargues JJ. Interest in a new test for caries risk in adolescents undergoing orthodontic treatment. Clin Oral Investig 2010;14(2) 177-185.

[34] Meade MJ, Millett DT. An audit of the caries status of patients about to start orthodontic treatment. J Ir Dent Assoc 2011;57(3) 156-160.

[35] Nyvad B, Machiulskiene V, Baelun V. Construct and predictive validity of clinical caries diagnostic criteria assessing lesion activity. J Dent Res 2003;82(2) 117-122.

[36] Nyvad B, Machiulskiene V, Baelum V. Reliability of a new caries diagnostic system differentiating between active and inactive caries lesions. Caries Res 1999;33(4) 252-260.

[37] Thylstrup A, Bruun C, Holmen L. In vivo caries models: mechanisms for caries initiation and arrestment. Adv Dent Res 1994;8(2) 144-157.

[38] Ekstrand KR, Qvist V, Thylstrup A. Light microscope study of the effect of probing in occlusal surfaces. Caries Res 1994;21(4) 368-374.

[39] Mejàre I, Kidd EAM. Radiography for caries diagnosis. In: Fejerskov O, Kidd EAM (Eds) Dental caries: the disease and its clinical management. Oxford: Blackwell Munksgaard, 2008, pp. 69-89.

[40] Fejerskov O, Nyvad B, Kidd EAM. Clinical and histological manifestations of dental caries. In: Fejerskov O, Kidd EAM (eds): Dental caries. The disease and its clinical management. Oxford: Blackwell Munksgaard, 2003, pp. 71–98.

[41] Holst JJ, Lange F. Perimylolysis. A contribution towards the genesis of tooth wasting from non-mechanical causes. Acta Odontol Scand 1939;1(1) 36–47.

[42] Scheutzel, P. Etiology of dental erosion – intrinsic factors. Eur J Oral Sci 1996;104 178-190.

[43] Corega C, Vaida L, Festila DG, Rigoni G, Albanese M, D'Agostino A, Pardo A, Rossetto A, Nocini PF, Bertossi D. Dental white spots associated with bulimia nervosa in orthodontic patients. Minerva Stomatol 2014; Jan 14. [Epub ahead of print].

[44] Kidd EAM et al. Occlusal caries diagnosis: a changing challenge for clinicians and epidemiologists. J Dent 1993;21(6) 323-337.

[45] Hammad SM, Enan ET. In vivo effects of two acidic soft drinks on shear bond strength of metal orthodontic brackets with and without resin infiltration treatment. Angle Orthod 2013;83(4) 648-652.

[46] Polat Ö, Gökçelik A, Arman A, Arhun N. A comparison of white spot lesion formation between a self-ligating bracket and a conventional preadjusted straight wire bracket. World J Orthod 2008;9(2) e46-e50.

[47] Bourzgui F, Sebbar M, Hamza M. Orthodontics and caries. In: Naretto S (Ed) Principles in contemporary orthodontics. InTech, 2011. ISBN: 978-953-307-687-4. Available from: http://www.intechopen.com/books/principles-in-contemporary-orthodontics/orthodontics-and-caries.

[48] Brusca M, Chara O, Sterin-Borda L, Rosa AC. Influence of different orthodontic brackets on adherence of microorganisms in vitro. Angle Orthod 2007;77(2) 331-336.

[49] Souza RA, Magnani MBBA, Nouer DF, Silva CO, Klein MI, Sallum EA et al. Periodontal and microbiologic evaluation of 2 methods of archwire ligation: ligature wires and elastomeric rings. Am J Orthod Dentofacial Orthop 2008;134(4) 506-512.

[50] Lidel ID, Elter C, Heuer W, Heidenblut T, Stiesch M, Schwestka- Polly R et al. Comparative analysis of long-term biofilm formation on metal and ceramic brackets. Angle Orthod 2011;81(5) 907-914.

[51] Newbrun E. Açúcar, substitutos do açúcar e agentes adoçantes não calóricos. In: Newbrun E (Ed) Cariologia. São Paulo: Santos, 1988.

[52] Dresti DVW, Waes HV. Prevenção coletiva, semicoletiva e individual em crianças e adolescentes. In: Waes HJMV, Stockli PW (Ed) Odontopediatria. Porto Alegre: Artmed, 2002. cap. 7, pp. 133-150.

[53] Owens J, Addy M, Faulkner J, Lockwood C, Adair R. A short-term clinical study design to investigate the chemical plaque inhibitory properties of mouthrinses when used as adjuncts to toothpastes: applied to chlorhexidine. J Clin Periodontol 1997;24(10) 732–737.

[54] Panzeri H, Lara EHG, Zaniquelli O, Schiavetto F. Avaliação de algumas características das escovas dentais do mercado nacional. Rev ABO Nac 1993;1(1) 23-29.

[55] Halla DA. Propósito das escovas dentárias. Rev Paul Odontol 1982;4(2) 42-47.

[56] Marsh PD. Microbiological aspects of the chemical control of plaque and gingivitis. J Dent Res 1992;71(7) 1431-1438.

[57] Bijella MFTB, Zanella NLM, Tarzia O, Bijella VT. Avaliação do efeito inibidor de bochechos diários com fluoreto de sódio neutro e acidulado a 0, 05 por cento sobre o metabolismo da placa dentária humana (fermentação e síntese de polissacarídeos extracelulares). Cecade News 1994;2(2) 1-19.

[58] Rodrigues LG, Zawadski PT, Calvete E. O efeito do plax na formação da placa bacteriana. Rev Periodontia1999;8(1) 39-44.

[59] Monfrin R, Ribeiro MC. Avaliação in vitro de anti-sépticos bucais sobre a microbiota da saliva. Rev Assoc Paul Cir Dent 2000;54(5) 400-407.

[60] Fine DH et al. Reducing bacteria in dental aerosols: pre-procedural use of an antiseptic mouth rinse. J Am Dent Assoc 1993;124(5) 56–58.

[61] Alves KM, Goursand D, Zenobio EG, Cruz RA. Effectiveness of procedures for the chemical-mechanical control of dental biofilm in orthodontic patients. J Contemp Dent Pract 2010;11(2) 41-48.

[62] Adriaens ML, Dermaut LR, Verbeeck RM. The use of 'Fluor Protector', a fluoride varnish, as a caries prevention method under orthodontic molar bands. Eur J Orthod 1990;12(3) 316-319.

[63] Morrier JJ. White spot lesions and orthodontic treatment. Prevention and treatment. Orthod Fr 2014;85(3) 235-244.

[64] Chow CKW, Wu CD, Evans CA. In vitro properties of orthodontic adhesives with fluoride or amorphous calcium phosphate. Int J Dent 2011; 2011 1-8.

[65] Rao A, Malhotra N. The role of remineralizing agents in dentistry: a review. Compend Contin Educ Dent 2011;32(6) 26-33.

[66] Behnan SM, Arruda AO, González-Cabezas C, Sohn W, Peters MC. In-vitro evaluation of various treatments to prevent demineralization next to orthodontic brackets. Am J Orthod Dentofacial Orthop 2010;138(6) 712.e1-712.e7; discussion 712-3. doi: 0.1016/j.ajodo.2010.05.014.

[67] Dalessandri D, Dalessandri M, Bonettic S, Viscontid L, Paganellie C. Effectiveness of an indirect bonding technique in reducing plaque accumulation around braces, Angle Orthod 2012;82(2) 313–318.

[68] Baka ZM, Basciftci FA, Arslan U. Effects of 2 bracket and ligation types on plaque retention: a quantitative microbiologic analysis with real-time polymerase chain reaction. Am J Orthod Dentofacial Orthop 2013;144(2) 260-267.

[69] Oltramari-Navarro PV, Titarelli JM, Marsicano JA, Henriques JF, Janson G, Lauris JR et al. Effectiveness of 0.50% and 0.75% chlorhexidine dentifrices in orthodontic patients: a double-blind and randomized controlled. Am J Orthod Dentofacial Orthop 2009;136(5) 651-656.

[70] Øgaard B, Alm AA, Larsson E, Adolfsson U. A prospective, randomized clinical study on the effects of an amine fluoride/stannous fluoride toothpaste/mouthrinse on plaque, gingivitis and initial caries lesion development in orthodontic patients. Eur J Orthod 2006;28(1) 8-12.

[71] Jenatschke F, Elsenberger E, Welte HD, Schlagenhauf U. Influence of repeated chlorhexidine varnish applications on mutans streptococci counts and caries increment in patients treated with fixed orthodontic appliances. J Orofac Orthop 2001;62(1) 36-45.

[72] Sari E, Birinci I. Microbiological evaluation of 0.2% chlorhexidine gluconate mouth rinse in orthodontic patients. Angle Orthod 2007;77(5) 881-884.

[73] Gatti A, Camargo LB, Imparato JC, Mendes FM, Raggio DP. Combination effect of fluoride dentifrices and varnish on deciduous enamel demineralization. Braz Oral Res 2011;25(5) 433-438.

[74] Baygin O, Tuzuner T, Ozel MB, Bostanoglu O. Comparison of combined application treatment with one-visit varnish treatments in an orthodontic population. Med Oral Patol Oral Cir Bucal 2013;18(2) 362-370.

[75] Schlueter N, Duran A, Klimek J, Ganss C. Investigation of the effect of various fluoride compounds and preparations thereof on erosive tissue loss in enamel in vitro. Caries Res 2009;43(1) 10-16.

[76] Reynolds EC. Calcium phosphate-based remineralization systems: scientific evidence? Aust Dent J 2008;53(3) 268-278.

[77] Robertson MA, Kau CH, English JD, Lee RP, Powers J, Nguyen JT. MI Paste Plus to prevent demineralization in orthodontic patients: a prospective randomized controlled trial. Am J Orthod Dentofacial Orthop 2011;140(5) 660-668.

[78] Eliades T, Gioka C, Eliades G, Makou M. Enamel surface roughness following debonding using two resin grinding methods. Euro J Orthod 2004;26(3) 333-338.

[79] Bonetti GA, Zanarini M, Incerti Parenti S, Lattuca M, Marchionni S, Gatto MR. Evaluation of enamel surfaces after bracket debonding: an in-vivo study with scanning electron microscopy. Am J Orthod Dentofacial Orthop 2011;140(5) 696-702.

[80] Karan S, Kircelli BH, Tasdelen B. Enamel surface roughness after debonding. Angle Orthod 2010;80(6) 1081-1088.

[81] Huang GJ, Roloff-Chiang B, Mills BE, Shalchi S, Spiekerman C, Korpak AM, Starrett JL, Greenlee GM, Drangsholt RJ, Matunas JC. Effectiveness of MI Paste Plus and PreviDent fluoride varnish for treatment of white spot lesions: a randomized controlled trial. Am J Orthod Dentofacial Orthop 2013;143(1) 31–41.

[82] Bailey DL, Adams GG, Tsao CE, Hyslop A, Escobar K, Manton DJ, Reynolds EC, Morgan MV. Regression of post-orthodontic lesions by a remineralizing cream. J Dent Res 2009;88(12) 1148-1153.

[83] Llena-Puy C. MI Paste Plus and PreviDent fluoride varnish appear no more effective than normal home care for improving the appearance of white spot lesions. J Evid Based Dent Pract 2013;13(3) 114-116.

[84] Kielbassa AM, Muller J, Gernhardt CR. Closing the gap between oral hygiene and minimally invasive dentistry: a review on the resin infiltration technique of incipient (proximal) enamel lesions. Quintessence Int 2009;40(8) 663-681.

[85] Attin R, Stawarczyk B, Kecik D, Knosel M, Wiechmann D, Attin T. Shear bond strength of brackets to demineralize enamel after different pretreatment methods. Angle Orthod 2012;82(1) 56-61.

[86] Shivanna V, Shivakumar B. Novel treatment of white spot lesions: a report of two cases Conserv Dent 2011;14(4) 423-426.

[87] Rios D, Magalhães AC, Machado MAAM, Silva SMB, Lizarelli RFZ, Bagnato VS, Buzalaf MAR. In vitro evaluation of enamel erosion after Nd:YAG laser irradiation and fluoride application. Photomed Laser Surg 2009;27(5) 743-747.

[88] Zezell DM, Boari HGD, Ana PA, Eduardo CP, Powell GL. Nd:YAG laser in caries prevention: a clinical trial. Lasers Surg Med 2009;41(1) 31–35.

[89] Tagomori S, Morioka T. Combined effects of laser and fluoride on acid resistance of human dental enamel. Caries Res 1989;23(4) 225–231.

[90] Bishara S, Ostby A. White spot lesions: formation, prevention, and treatment. Semin Orthod 2008;14(3) 174-182.

[91] Ardu S, Castioni NV, Benbachir N, Krejci I. Minimally invasive treatment of white spot enamel lesions. Quintessence Int 2007;38(8) 633-636.

[92] Murphy TC, Willmot DR, Rodd HD. Management of postorthodontic demineralized white lesions with microabrasion: a quantitative assessment. Am J Orthod Dentofacial Orthop 2007;131(1) 27-33.

[93] Pliska BT, Warner GA, Tantbirojn D, Larson BE. Treatment of white spot lesions with ACP paste and microabrasion. Angle Orthod 2012;82(5).

[94] Akin A, Basciftci FA. Can white spot lesions be treated effectively? Angle Orthod 2012;82(5) 770-775.

4

Effect of Allergy on Root Resorption Induced by Orthodontic Tooth Movement

Hideki Ioi, Mizuho A. Kido, Naohisa Murata,
Masato Nishioka, Mikari Asakawa,
Ryusuke Muroya and Ichiro Takahashi

1. Introduction

Orthodontic teeth movement results from the application of orthodontic forces to teeth through orthodontic appliances which transmit the forces to the surrounding tissues. However, an undesirable and unexpected result of orthodontic treatment is the orthodontically induced tooth resorption (Fig. 1). The development of excessive root resorption during orthodontic treatment is considered an adverse side effect of the orthodontic tooth movement. Many factors have been investigated to explain the orthodontically induced root resorption observed among orthodontic patients. However, there are still controversies over this issue.

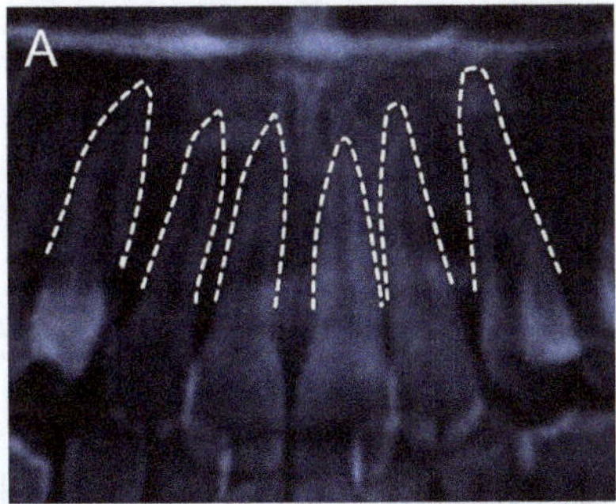

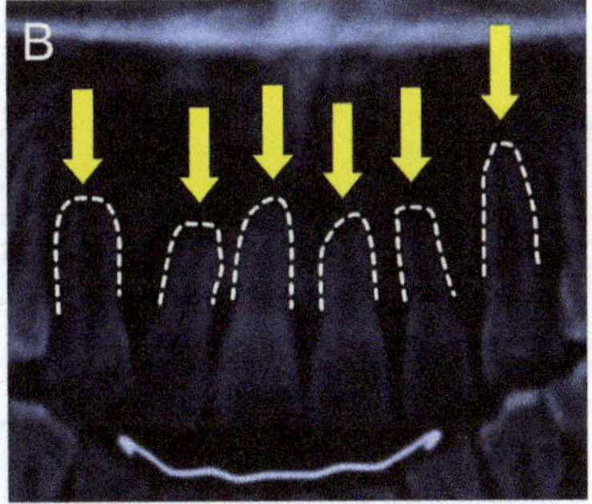

Figure 1. An undesirable and unexpected result of orthodontic treatment (A) Before treatment, (B) After treatment.

Davidovitch et al. [1] hypothesized that individuals who have a history of immune diseases including allergy, asthma, and systemic diseases may be at a high level of risk for developing excessive root resorption during the course of orthodontic treatment. To confirm the association between allergy and the orthodontically induced root resorption, we designed the epidemiological clinical study. Moreover, to extrapolate the direct effect of allergy on the orthodontically induced root resorption, which is difficult to prove in the clinical study design, we conducted experimental animal study using rats.

In this chapter, we refer at the beginning to the current knowledge of root resorption and then focus on the risk factors inherent in individuals to the external root resorption (ERR), especially allergic diseases as a possible risk factor of ERR.

2. Basic information

2.1. Prevalence

The presence of root resorption is common after orthodontic treatment [2]. Prevalence of root resorption following orthodontic treatment has been reported from 0% to 100% [3-5]. Thus, the prevalence varies widely due to differing methods of reporting root resorption, differing radiographic technique and interpretation, and individual susceptibility [2]. Close radiographic examination revealed that some loss of root length occurred in nearly every orthodontic patient. Moderate to severe apical root resorption (>2 mm, <1/3 of the root length) has been found in 10-17% of orthodontically treated patients [6,7] and excessive root resorption (>1/3 of the root length) in 1-5% [8,9]. Phillips [10] stated apical root resorption exceeding one-fourth of the original root length was shown in 1.5 % of maxillary central incisors and in 2.2 % of lateral incisors.

2.2. Site of root resorption

Regardless of patient-related or treatment-related factors, the maxillary incisors likely indicated more root resorption than the other teeth, followed by the mandibular incisors and first molars [11]. However, every tooth is capable of root resorption during orthodontic treatment.

2.3. Risk factors

2.3.1. *Orthodontic treatment-related risk factors*

Magnitude of force

Many studies have shown a distinct positive correlation between the applied orthodontic force and the amount of root resorption in both animal studies and clinical studies [12-16]. Owman-Mall et al. [17,18] reported that there were large individual variations in the amount of root resorption even when the same degree of orthodontic force was applied. They speculated that root resorption would not be very force-sensitive.

Duration of force

Several investigations revealed that the duration of force was one of the risk factors of orthodontically induced root resorption [19,20]. Some claimed that the duration of force application was an even more critical factor than the degree of orthodontic force [21,22]. Interaction between magnitude and duration of force would play an important role for orthodontic treatment-related risk factors. Large individual variations still existed even in well-controlled research design [17,18].

2.3.2. Patient-related risk factors (individual susceptibility)

Besides orthodontic treatment-related factors, patient-related risk factors have also been discussed previously. This includes systemic diseases [23], nutrition [24,25], age [26], trauma [10,27], previous root resorption [28,29], gender [20,28], nail biting habits [30], root morphology [31], endodontically treated teeth [32], gingivitis [9], allergy [33-35], and medications [36]. Al-Qawasmi et al. [37] identified an interleukin (IL)-1β polymorphism in orthodontically treated individuals as having a role in the genetic influence on external apical root resorption.

3. The role of allergy related to orthodontically induced root resorption

Teeth are relocated under the dynamic balance of bone metabolism. The role of bone cells, including osteocytes, osteoblasts, and osteoclasts, are to resorb alveolar bone in sites of mechanically compressed tissues, thus enabling dental roots in these locations to move in the direction of the applied orthodontic force [38]. In these sites of tissue compression, one finds infiltrations of inflammatory cells followed by multinucleated osteocalsts and odontoclasts engaged in resorbing the dental roots [39,40]. Osteoclasts and their mononucleated progenitors are derived from the monocyte/macrophage lineage [41]. Osteoclasts and odontoclasts have a similar histochemical appearance; we defined here the multinucleated cells faced to tooth root as odontoclasts.

Patients with asthma and rhinitis share common physiology including heightened bronchial hyperresponsiveness and heightened reactivity to a variety of stimuli. Immunopathology of allergic rhinitis is also similar with a predominance of T-helper type 2 inflammation and tissue eosinophilia [42]. Allergy and asthma trigger the various associated biological, cellular, and molecular events with inflammation, such as increased vascular permeability, vasodilatation, cellular migration, increased mucus secretion, bronchoconstriction, structural changes of airway architecture, decline in pulmonary functions, release of intracellular mediators, increased formation of reactive oxygen species, cartilage degradation, and loss of function [43].

During orthodontic tooth movement, inflammation appears to be the main mechanism whereby immune cells and blood plasma reach the periodontal ligament of mechanically loaded teeth [44]. Apparently, strained sensory nerve endings in close proximity to periodontal ligament small blood vessels and capillaries release signal molecules such as substance P, vasoactive intestinal peptide, and calcitonin gene-related peptide [45]. Substance P stimulates endothelial cells to adhere to circulating leukocytes and promote their migration to the extravascular space, where they secrete a variety of cytokines, such as interleukins and tumor necrosis factors (TNFs).

TNF-α and IL-1β play an important role in bone pathophysiology [46,47] and have been suggested to be involved in orthodontic tooth movement [48]. These inflammatory cytokines induce local expression of receptor activator of nuclear factor-κB ligand (RANKL), which is critical for the terminal differentiation of osteoclast precursor cells [49].

Furthermore, leukotrienes, which are metabolites of arachidonic acid, are potent lipid mediators that play an important role in a variety of allergic and inflammatory reactions and comprise several products of the 5-lipoxygenase (5-LOX) pathway [50–52]. Leukotrienes are produced by activated leukocytes in inflammatory diseases such as bronchial asthma and rheumatoid arthritis [53,54]. LTB_4 is known to play an important role in the allergic reactions induced by ovalbumin (OVA) in rodents [55] and has been suggested to modulate bone metabolism by increasing osteoclastic bone resorption [56].

In light of these facts, we hypothesize that patients with allergic diseases such as food allergy, allergic asthma, allergic rhinitis, and allergic conjunctivitis are susceptible to orthodontic root resorption. We show the scheme to explain the hypothesis of orthodontically induced root resorption due to the risk factor of allergy (Fig. 2).

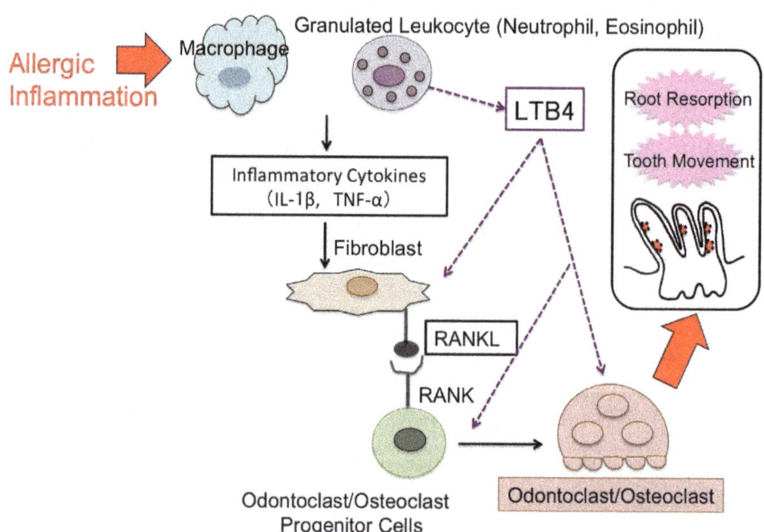

Figure 2. Scheme of possible explanation of the orthodontically induced root resorption due to the risk factor of allergy.

At first, we report the possible association between excessive root resorption during the orthodontic tooth movement and allergy using clinical study design. Next, we extrapolate the effect of allergy on orthodontically induced root resorption using animal models.

3.1. Epidemiological study

3.1.1. Sample

The records of 3500 patients were obtained from the Section of Orthodontics, Kyushu University Hospital, Fukuoka, Japan. All these patients have completed their course of orthodontic treatment. In this sample, 100 individuals were found to have developed excessive resorption of dental roots. In the root resorption group, 29 subjects were males and 71 were females (Table 1). A control group was selected from the remaining patients of this sample who did not display any significant radiographic evidence for dental root resorption in the light of root morphology at the end of their orthodontic treatment. Each individual in the control group was pair-matched with one in the root resorption group based on age, gender, treatment period, and the type of malocclusion (Table 1).

	Number	Age (y)	Treatment Period (y)
Root resorption group			
Male	29	18.9 ± 5.4	2.9 ± 0.8
Female	71	17.3 ± 6.5	3.1 ± 1.1
Total	100	17.8 ± 6.2	3.1 ± 1.1
Control group			
Male	29	17.9 ± 6.1	2.8 ± 0.8
Female	71	18.2 ± 4.8	2.9 ± 0.8
Total	100	18.1 ± 5.2	2.9 ± 0.8

Table 1. Comparison of Means and Standard Deviations of Age and Treatment Period in the Root Resorption and Control Groups

3.1.2. Methods

Determination of root resorption

Determination of the root resorption status of each patient was established by comparing the dental panoramic radiographs that had been taken before and after treatment. All teeth were measured along the tooth's longitudinal axis for root length (defined as cement-enamel junction to apex of root). This method was similar to that used by Linge & Linge [7]. Individuals were assigned to the root resorption group when it was disclosed that one or more of their dental roots had been shortened by more than 25% of the original root length in the time that had elapsed between the two radiographs. The root shape was recorded subjectively as normal or abnormal (shortened, blunt, eroded, pointed, bent, bottle shaped) (Fig. 3) by examining dental panoramic radiographs that had been taken before the onset of treatment.

Questionnaire

The questionnaire sought information on the following subjects: personal details, medical history, dental history, and oral habits. Information on medical history included local or systemic diseases, details on medication uptake, hospitalizations, allergies, health during

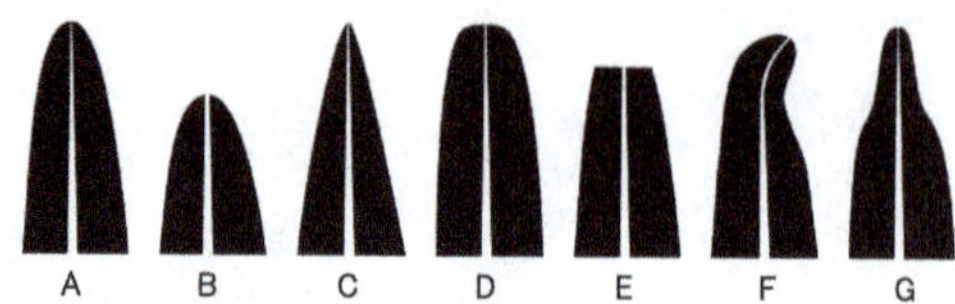

Figure 3. Morphology classification of the root (A) Normal, (B) Shortened, (C) Pointed, (D) Blunt, (E) Eroded, (F) Bent, (G) Bottle shaped.

gestation and first year of life, childhood diseases, other conditions, and developmental events in infancy and childhood. Dental history questions referred to details on previous dental treatment and information about past oral injuries. Habits listed in the questionnaire were nail biting, tongue thrusting, and mouth breathing.

Statistical analysis

The validity of our hypothesis was tested by the logistic regression analysis using the Stat View 5.0 pro- gram (SAS Institute Inc, Cary, NC). Logistic regression produces odds ratios associated with each predictor variables (root anomaly, extraction, trauma, gingivitis, allergy, asthma, systemic disease, medication use, thumb sucking, nail biting, tongue thrusting, mouth breathing).

3.1.3. Results

The prevalence of excessive root resorption was 7.8%. The distribution of each risk factor in the root resorption and the control groups is shown in Figure 4. The logistic regression analysis is shown in Table 2. The incidence of allergy and asthma was significantly higher in the root resorption group (P = 0.005), with a mean odds ratio of 2.54 and 95% confidence interval of 1.34–4.92. The incidence of root anomaly was significantly higher in the root resorption group (P = 0.001), with a mean odds ratio of 2.95 and 95% confidence interval of 1.53–5.83.

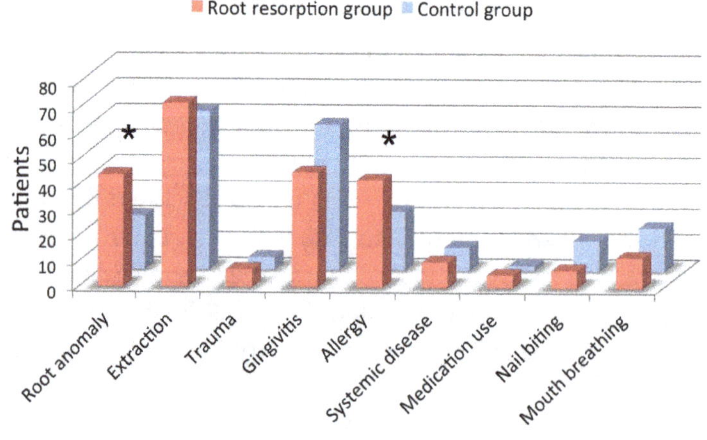

*: $P < 0.05$.

Figure 4. Prevalence of each risk factor in the root resorption and control groups.

Risk Factors	*P Value*	Odds Ratio	95% Confidence Interval
Root anomaly	0.001	2.95	1.53-5.83
Extraction	0.168	1.56	0.83-2.98
Trauma	0.473	1.59	0.45-5.97
Gingivitis	0.120	0.62	0.34-1.13
Allergy	0.005	2.54	1.34-4.92
Systemic disease	0.900	0.93	0.32-2.70
Medication use	0.344	2.31	0.45-17.2
Nail biting	0.311	1.57	0.66-3.84
Mouth breathing	0.539	0.76	0.31-1.81

Table 2. Logistic Regression Analysis of Each Risk Factor

3.1.4. Discussion

This clinical study showed that allergy might be an aetiological factor in increased root resorption. The same association was found in earlier studies [1,57]. However, those studies were primarily performed on Caucasian subjects. Our finding, derived from an examination of the clinical records of Japanese subjects, supports the hypothesis that allergy is a high risk factor for the development of excessive root resorption during orthodontic treatment.

Our results also indicate that abnormal root shape is probably associated with excessive root resorption (p=0.056). This finding is in agreement with the results of the previous study [23,58-60]. If the same orthodontic force is applied to the dental crown, the root apex is exposed to increasing stress as the root becomes shorter. Additionally, when the same orthodontic force is applied to the root apex, the distribution of the stress is different according to the types of root anatomy, and the dental root with pointed or bent shape may be exposed to larger stress than roots with normal morphological features. These increased stresses may traumatize the apical periodontal ligament, followed by an inflammatory/repair process, which includes resorption of the root apex.

Patients with periodontal disease have circulating primed monocytes, and sera of patients with periodontal disease contain high levels of proinflammatory cytokines [8]. In this study, however, gingivitis did not have a significant association to orthodontic root resorption. This is most likely due to the sample selection of young patients; mean age of 17.8 ± 6.2 years, and the method used to detect the status of periodontal health; examination of intra-oral photographs.

In cases requiring tooth extraction, the remaining teeth are usually moved relatively great distance, particularly when maxillary incisors are retracted in order to reduce large overjet [58,59,61]. Additionally, biologically, tooth extraction and the ensuing wound healing attract vast numbers of immune cells to the extraction site. These inflammatory cells may directly spread from the wound site to tissues surrounding adjacent teeth or, indirectly, produce large amounts of cytokines that enter the circulation and exit into the extravascular space in the periodontal ligament of neighboring mechanically stressed teeth, which regulate remodeling activities not only at extraction site but also in tissues surrounding adjacent teeth. However, in this study, we have not found a significant association between extraction of permanent teeth and orthodontic root resorption. Therefore, we conclude that healing of extraction sites is primarily a local event which does not promote the resorption of adjacent teeth.

One limitation of this study was using the panoramic radiographs in order to evaluate the amount of root resorption. Although this method of examination makes it possible to view the whole dentition, its main drawback is distortion of the tooth image, predominantly in the incisor region. Periapical radiographs would be preferable to determine the size and shape of dental roots, but these radiographs were not available to us this time.

3.2. Animal model study

In the experimental animal study, we used Brown–Norway (BN) rats, which are known to produce high levels of IgE after sensitization with OVA. BN rats have been used extensively as animal models of allergic asthma [62–64], atopic dermatitis [65], and food allergies [66,67].

This study aimed to determine whether systemic allergic inflammation had adverse effects on orthodontic tooth movement and bone and root resorption and, if so, to investigate the possible mechanisms of the acceleration. Furthermore, we examined the ability of aspirin, which has been reported to improve bone mineral density (BMD) in human epidemiological studies [68,69], to reverse tooth root resorption.

3.2.1. Allergen sensitization for rats and OF

Six-week-old male BN rats (weighing 110–140 g) were sensitized by a subcutaneous injection of saline (1 mL) containing 1 mg of OVA (grade V; Sigma-Aldrich, St. Louis, MO, USA) and 200 mg of aluminum hydroxide. A *Bordetella pertussis* vaccine containing 1×10^{10} heat-killed bacilli (Wako, Osaka, Japan) was given intraperitoneally as an adjuvant. After 7 days, OVA was injected for a booster effect. The serum IgE levels were measured using an IgE ELISA Kit (Shibayagi, Gunma, Japan). At 7 days after the second sensitization, an orthodontic appliance consisting of an Ni-Ti closed-coil spring (Sentalloy®, Ultra Light; Tomy International Inc., Tokyo, Japan) was inserted between the upper right first molar (M1) and the incisors. The orthodontic force (OF) level of the spring was set at approximately 0.1N (Fig. 5).

The animals were divided into four groups: OVA with OF group, OVA alone group (no OF), OF alone group (no OVA), and control group (no OVA or OF).

After 7 or 14 days of OF (at days 7 and 14, respectively), the animals were perfused transcardially. The two halves of the maxilla were decalcified in 10% ethylenediamine-tetraacetic acid and cut into 8-μm-thick parasagittal sections. The sections were stained for tartrate-resistant acid phosphatase (TRAP) (Sigma-Aldrich) and counterstained with toluidine blue.

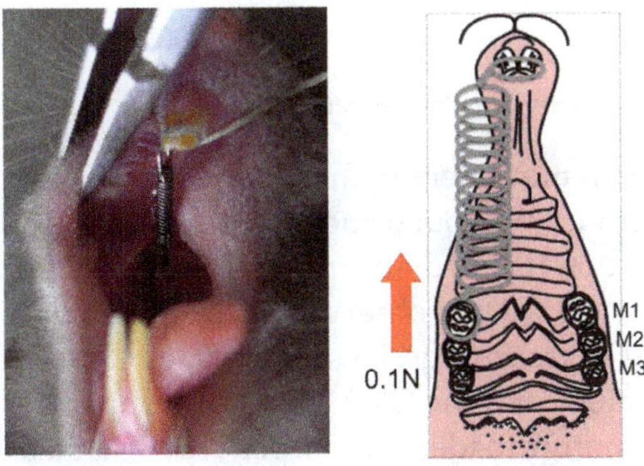

Figure 5. Maxillary first molar (M1) was moved medially with Ni-Ti Coil spring (0.1N) (Murata et al., 2013).

3.2.2. *Measurements and analyses*

We measured the area of ERR as well as the number of odontoclasts and osteoclasts within a defined area according to the method of Mavragani et al. [70]. TRAP-positive cells in resorption lacunae that faced the tooth roots were counted as odontoclasts, and other TRAP-positive cells (containing more than two nuclei) were counted as osteoclasts.

Proinflammatory cytokines were measured in the periodontal tissues, including the bone surrounding M1, after 24 hours of OF. The levels of TNF-α, IL-1β, and IL-6 were evaluated using a TNF-αELISA Kit (Shibayagi), IL-1β ELISA Kit, and IL-6 ELISA Kit (Biosource, Camarillo, CA, USA), respectively, according to the manufacturers' protocols.

The lipid components were extracted in 100% methanol at –30°C overnight.

The periodontal tissues around M1 after 24 hours of OF were rapidly frozen in liquid nitrogen and homogenized. After mRNA isolation, quantitative real-time PCR or conventional RT-PCR was performed with gene-specific primer sets as described previously [71].

Micro-CT images were acquired at a resolution of 9 μm using a SkyScan 1076 (SkyScan, Antwerp, Belgium) to assess the degree of OF. At day 14 (10 weeks of age), the hemi-maxilla samples were excised. The hemi-maxilla samples were directed parallel to the occlusal plane and scanned for 2.70 mm. The distance from the distal surface of M1 to the mesial surface of the second molar (M2) was measured using DataViewer software (ver. 1.4.3; SkyScan).

Aspirin dissolved in feed water (250 μg/kg/day) was administered orally to OVA-sensitized rats with orthodontic force application. For histologic experiments, aspirin was administered from the initiation of OF. For ELISA and RT-PCR analyses, aspirin was administered from 24 hours before OF.

3.2.3. *Statistical analysis*

The total serum IgE was compared using Student's *t*-test. The means of multiple groups were compared by one-way ANOVA. Other values were compared by ANOVA followed by Tukey's multiple comparison test. Values of $P < 0.05$ were considered to indicate statistical significance.

3.2.4. Results

OVA sensitization, OF, and root and bone resorption

At day 14, the degree of tooth movement in the OVA with OF group was significantly larger than that in the OF alone group. Without orthodontic force application, no osteoclasts and/or odontoclasts were observed on the medial surface of the alveolar bone in any of the groups (Fig. 6A, 6B). On day 7, marked ERR was observed on the pressured side in the OF alone group, especially in the OVA with OF group (Figs. 7A, 7B). On day 14, these tendencies became further significant in both the OF alone and the OVA with OF groups (Figs. 8A, 8B). The OVA with OF group exhibited significantly broader and deeper TRAP-stained areas compared to the OF alone group on days 7 as well as 14 (Fig. 9A). The number of odontoclasts and osteoclasts was significantly greater in the OVA with OF group than in the OF alone group on day 7 (Figs. 9B, 9C). The number of osteoclasts peaked on day 7 in the OVA with OF group and then decreased by day 14. While the area of ERR increased from day 7 to day 14, the number of odontoclasts was maintained through days 7 to 14 (Figs. 9A, 9C). The alveolar bone resorption and osteoclast number were significantly greater in the OVA with OF group than in the OF alone group on days 7 and 14 (Figs. 9D, 9E).

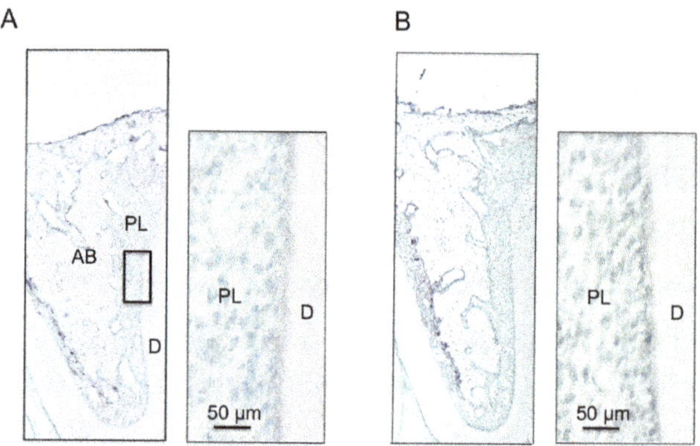

Figure 6. Histologic sections of periodontal tissues around the distopalatal root of the first molar stained for TRAP. (A) Control group (no treatment), (B) OVA-alone group (Murata et al., 2013).

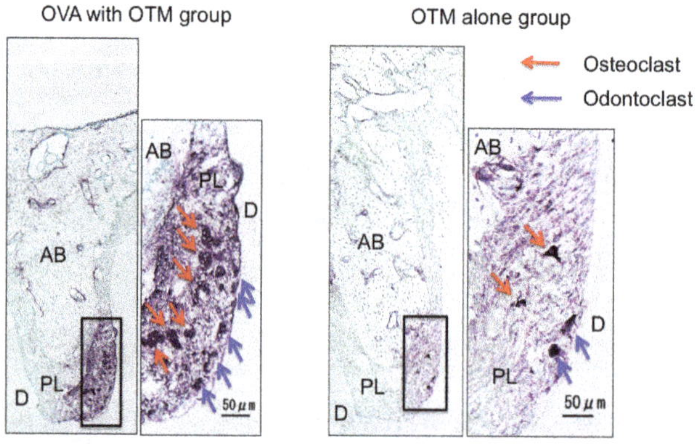

Figure 7. Histologic sections of periodontal tissues around the distopalatal root of the first molar stained for TRAP on day 7. (A) OVA with OTM group, (B) OTM-alone group (Murata et al., 2013).

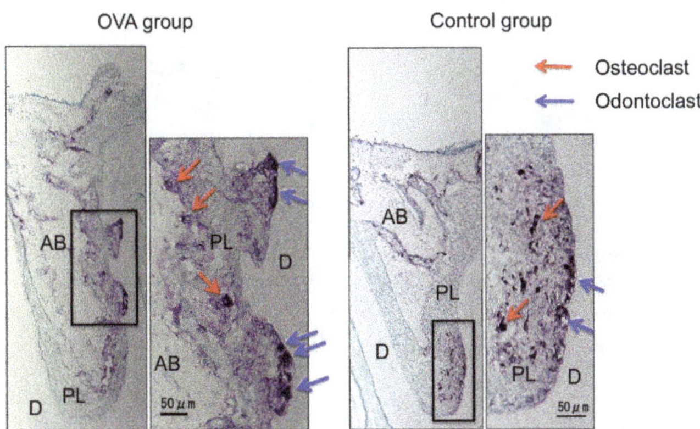

Figure 8. Histologic sections of periodontal tissues around the distopalatal root of the first molar stained for TRAP on day 14. (A) OVA with OTM group, (B) OTM-alone group (Murata et al., 2013).

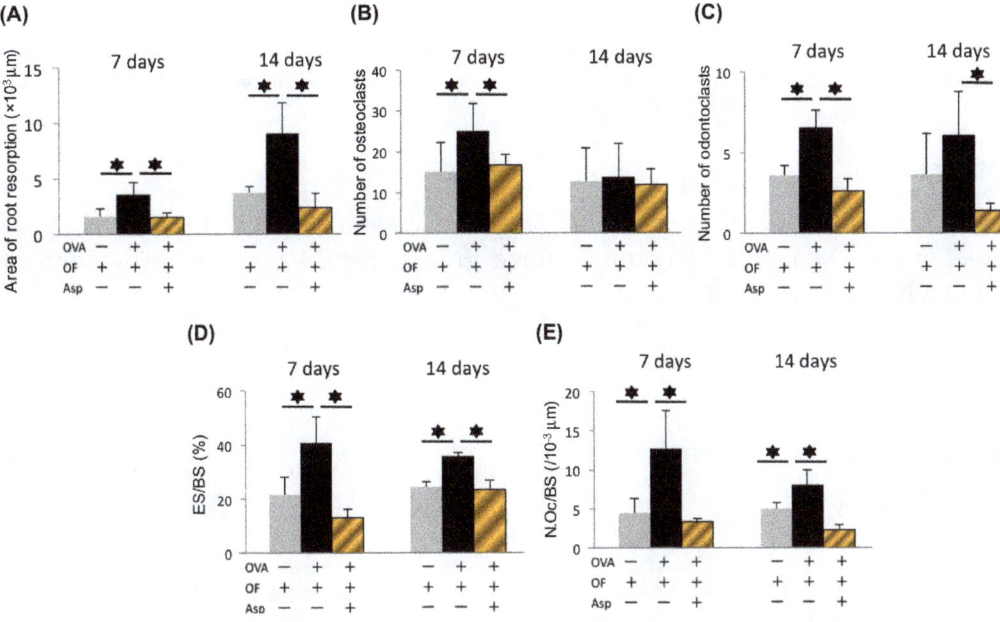

Figure 9. The numbers of osteoclasts/odontoclasts and amounts of root/bone resorption on the pressured side after tooth movement. (A) Area of root resorption (×103 μm2), (B) Number of osteoclasts, (C) Number of odontoclasts, (D) Eroded surface per alveolar bone surface (ES/ BS), (E) Number of osteoclasts per alveolar bone surface (N.Oc/BS). *: $P <$ 0.05. (Murata et al., 2013).

Pro-inflammatory cytokines

The expression levels of RANKL, TNF-α, and IL-1β were significantly higher in the OVA with OF group than in the other groups after 24 hours of OF (Figs. 10A–10C), while the difference in IL-6 was not significant (Fig. 10D). Although no significant differences were observed, the OF alone group showed tendencies toward higher levels of TNF-α and IL-1β (Figs. 10B, 10C).

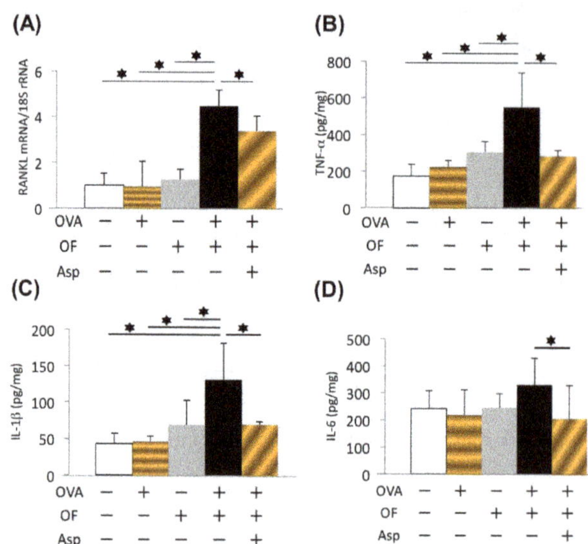

Figure 10. Concentrations of RANKL and inflammatory cytokines in rat periodontal tissues with or without OVA sensitization, after 24 h of orthodontic force application, and after aspirin administration. (A) RANKL, (B) TNF-α, (C) IL-1β, (D) IL-6. *: $P < 0.05$. (Murata et al., 2013).

Leukotrienes

The LTB_4 level and mRNA levels of the leukotriene synthases LTA4h were significantly increased in the OVA with orthodontic force group after 24 hours of orthodontic force compared with the other groups (Figs. 11A, 11B).

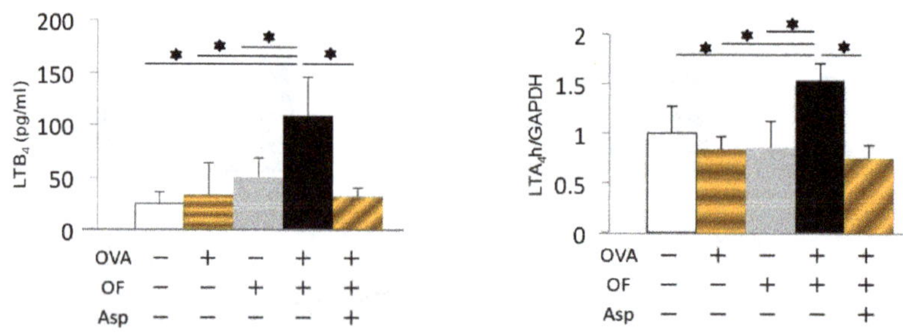

Figure 11. Effects of OVA sensitization, OF application for 24 h, and aspirin administration on the leukotriene synthases. (A) LTB_4, (B) LTA_4h. *: $P < 0.05$. (Murata et al., 2013).

Aspirin effects

Aspirin administration reversed the degree of tooth movement in the OVA with OF group to a similar level of the OF alone group on day 14. Histologic examinations revealed that the area of ERR and the numbers of odontoclasts and osteoclasts were decreased to the levels observed in the OF alone group (Figs. 9A–9E). The expression levels of RANKL mRNA and TNF-α,

IL-1β, and IL-6 proteins were also suppressed in the levels detected in the OF alone group (Figs. 10A–10D). Furthermore, the expression levels of LTB_4 and LTA_4h were suppressed by aspirin treatment (Fig. 11).

3.2.5. Discussion

We demonstrated that allergies affect ERR during orthodontic treatment using an animal model. It is notable that the degree of OF in the present study was greater in the OVA-sensitized animals, suggesting that allergies can affect OF. In the histological observations, we found that the OVA-sensitized rats showed increased numbers of odontoclasts and osteoclasts on the pressured side during OF. The present findings suggested that allergies enhanced both odontoclastogenesis and osteoclastogenesis under the condition of orthodontic force.

TNF-α, IL-1β, and IL-6, which are well-known proinflammatory cytokines, were detected at high levels in the periodontal tissues from the OVA with OF group. Recently, Polzer et al. [72] suggested that IL-1β contributes to TNF-mediated inflammatory osteopenia, reporting that TNF-α transgenic IL-1β-deleted mice were protected against bone loss. The elevated expression levels of TNF-α and IL-1β, together with RANKL as an essential cytokine for osteoclastogenesis, suggested boosts in the rates and magnitudes of ERR as well as orthodontic tooth movement due to the differentiation of osteoclasts and odontoclasts.

Lipid mediators derived from arachidonic acid through the lipoxygenase and cyclooxygenase pathways are known to act as important modulators of inflammation. Increased levels of leukotrienes are found in inflammatory diseases such as asthma, arthritis, and periodontal disease [73-75]. LTB4 has been reported to stimulate osteoclast formation and bone resorption in the mouse calvaria [55] and to inhibit osteogenesis [76]. In our model, the expression levels of the leukotriene synthases LTB_4 and LTA4h were increased in the periodontal tissues in OVA-sensitized rats with OF. The fact that mechanical loading with OVA sensitization elevated the expression of leukotriene synthases reveals a potential role for leukotrienes in bone and root resorption. Interestingly, these effects of mechanical OF suggest the involvement of the lipoxygenase pathway in response to mechanical loading. We assume that the present findings are compatible with our previous epidemiologic observations [33,34].

We further found that oral administration of aspirin was able to reverse the increases in ERR and degree of OF in the allergic model. The dose of aspirin in the present study, 250 μg/kg/day, was much lower than that for general use as a painkiller. A recent study showed that low-dose aspirin inhibited ovariectomy-induced osteoporosis by inhibiting T cell activation [77]. Our findings raise the possibility that low-dose aspirin administration inhibits osteoclastogenesis under inflammatory conditions.

Through the epidemiological and animal model studies, we have demonstrated that allergies would be possible risk factors of ERR in the course of orthodontic treatments. In the clinical study, the evidence would be strengthened using a prospective study involving a much larger sample, such as the randomized controlled test. Moreover, we need to investigate the unsolved mechanism of ERR, and the elucidation of the pharmacological targets for ERR during orthodontic tooth movement would be warranted.

4. Conclusions

In the clinical study, we found that allergy and root morphology abnormalities may be considered high-risk factors for the development of excessive root resorption during the course of orthodontic treatment.

We have proposed a model for studying the effects of allergen-induced inflammation and/or mechanical stress on ERR during OTM. This process was affected by pro-inflammatory cytokines, together with lipid mediators. Furthermore, our findings suggest that pro-inflammatory cytokines and leukotrienes, together with low-dose aspirin, may represent pharmacological targets for ERR during orthodontic treatment with allergic conditions.

Acknowledgements

This work was supported by grants-in-aid for Scientific Research (C) (no. 18592238 to H.I), Scientific Research (C) (no. 21592600 to H.I), and Scientific Research (C) (no. 24593095 to H.I) from the Ministry of Education, Culture, Sports, Science and Technology of Japan. We would like to express our sincere gratitude to Professor Ze'ev Davidovitch and Professor Amy L. Counts for continuing support to our research.

Author details

Hideki Ioi[1*], Mizuho A. Kido[2], Naohisa Murata[1], Masato Nishioka[3], Mikari Asakawa[4], Ryusuke Muroya[4] and Ichiro Takahashi[1]

*Address all correspondence to: ioi@dent.kyushu-u.ac.jp

1 Section of Orthodontics, Graduate School of Dental Science, Kyushu University, Fukuoka, Japan

2 Department of Molecular Cell Biology and Oral Anatomy, Graduate School of Dental Science, Kyushu University, Fukuoka, Japan

3 Nishioka Orthodontic Clinic, Fukuoka, Japan

4 Faculty of Dentistry, Kyushu University, Fukuoka, Japan

References

[1] Davidovitch Z, Lee YJ, Counts AL, Park YG and Bursac Z. The immune system possibly modulates orthodontic root resorption. In: Davidovitch Z. (ed.) Biological Mechanisms of Tooth Movement and Craniofacial Adaptation. Oklahoma City: University of Oklahoma; 2000. p207-217.

[2] Thilander B, Rygh P, Reitan K. Tissue reactions in orthodontics. In: Graber TM, Vanarsdall RL. (eds.) Orthodontics: Current Principles and Techniques. 3rd ed. St Louis: Mosby; 2000. p117-191.

[3] Henry J, Weinmann J. The pattern of resorption and repair of human cementum. Journal of the American Dental Association 1951;42(3) 270-290.

[4] Massler M, Perreault J. Root resorption in the permanent teeth of young adults. Journal of Dentistry for Children 1954;21 158-164.

[5] Copeland S, Green L. Root resorption in maxillary central incisors following active orthodontic treatment. American Journal of Orthodontics and Dentofacial Orthopedics 1986;89(1) 51-55.

[6] Hollender L, Rönnerman A, Thilander B. Root resorption, marginal bone support and clinical crown length in orthodontically treated patients. European Journal of Orthodontics 1980;2(4) 197-205.

[7] Linge L, Linge BL. Patients characteristics and treatment variables associated with apical root resorption during orthodontic treatment. American Journal of Orthodontics and Dentofacial Orthopedics 1991;99(1) 35-43.

[8] Levander E, Malmgren O. Evaluation of the risk of root resorption during orthodontic treatment: a study of upper incisors. European Journal of Orthodontics 1988;10(1) 30-38.

[9] Davidovitch Z. Etiologic factors in force-induced root resorption. In: Davidovitch Z, Norton LA. (eds.) Biological Mechanisms of Tooth Movement and Craniofacial Adaptation. Boston: Harvard Society for the Advancement of Orthodontics; 1996. p349-355.

[10] Phillips J. Apical Root Resorption under Orthodontic Therapy: University of Washington. Seattle; 1955.

[11] Weltman B, Vig KWL, Fields HW, Shanker S, Kaizar EE. Root resorption associated with orthodontic tooth movement. American Journal of Orthodontics and Dentofacial Orthopedics 2010;137(4) 462-476.

[12] Reitan K. Effects of force magnitude and direction of tooth movement on different alveolar bone types Angle Orthod. 1964;34(4) 244-255.

[13] Dellinger EL. A histologic and cephalometric investigation of premolar intrusion in the Macaca speciosa monkey. American Journal of Orthodontics. 1967;53(5) 325-355.

[14] Kvam E. Scanning electron microscopy of tissue changes on the pressure surface of human premolars following tooth movement Scandinavian. Journal of Dental Research 1972;80(5) 357-368.

[15] King GJ, Fischlschweiger W. The effect of force magnitude on extractable bone resorption activity and cemental cratering in orthodontic tooth movement. Journal of Dental Research 1982;61(6) 775-779.

[16] Pilon JJGM, Kuijpers-Jagtman AM, Maltha JC. Magnitude of orthodontic forces and rate of bodily tooth movement, an experimental study in beagle dogs. American Journal of Orthodontics and Dentofacial Orthopedics 1996;110(1) 16-23.

[17] Owman-Moll P, Kurol J, Lundgren D. Effects of doubled orthodontic force magnitude on tooth movement and root resorption. An interindividual study in adolescents. European Journal of Orthodontics 1996;18(2) 141-150.

[18] Owman-Moll P, Kurol J, Lundgren D. The effects of a four-fold increased force magnitude on tooth movement and root resorptions. An intraindividual study in adolescents. European Journal of Orthodontics 1996;18(3) 287-295.

[19] DeShields RW. A study of root resorption in treated Class II, division I malocclusions. Angle Orthodontist 1969;39(4) 231- 245.

[20] McFadden WM, Engstrom C, Engstrom H, Anholm JM. A study of the relationship between incisor intrusion and root shortening. American Journal of Orthodontics and Dentofacial Orthopedics 1989;96(5) 390-396.

[21] Stenvik A, Mjör IA. Pulp and dentine reactions to experimental tooth intrusion. A histological study of the initial changes. American Journal of Orthodontics 1970;57(4) 370-385.

[22] Harry MR, Sims MR. Root resorption in bicuspid intrusion. A scanning electron microscopy study. Angle Orthodontist 1982;52(3) 235-258.

[23] Newman WG. Possible etiological factors in external root resorption. American Journal of Orthodontics 1975;67(5) 522-539.

[24] Becks H. Root resorption and their relation to pathologic bone formation. Part 1. International Journal of Orthodontia and Oral Surgery 1936;22 445-482.

[25] Becks H. Orthodontic prognosis: evaluation of routine dentomedical examinations to determine "good and poor risks." American Journal of Orthodontics and Oral Surgery 1936;25(7) 610-624.

[26] Malmgren O, Goldson L, Hill C, Orwin A, Petrini L, Lundberg M. Root resorption after orthodontic treatment of traumatized teeth. American Journal of Orthodontics 1982;82(6) 487-491.

[27] Linge B, Linge L. Apical root resorption in upper anterior teeth. European Journal of Orthodontics 1983;5(3) 173-183.

[28] Massler M, Malone AJ. Root resorption in human permanent teeth: A roentgenographic study. American Journal of Orthodontics 1954;40(8) 619-633.

[29] Kalley J, Phillips C. Factors related to root resorption in edgewise practice. Angle Orthodontist 1991;61(2) 125-132.

[30] Odenrick L, Brattström V. The effect of nailbiting on root resorption during orthodontic treatment. European Journal of Orthodontics 1983;5(3) 185-188.

[31] Levander E, Malmgren O, Eliasson S. Evaluation of root resorption in relation to two orthodontic treatment regimes. A clinical experimental study. European Journal of Orthodontics 1994;16(3) 223-228.

[32] Mirabella AD, Årtun J. Prevalence and severity of apical root resorption of maxillary anterior teeth in adult orthodontic patients. European Journal of Orthodontics 1995;17(2) 93-99.

[33] Nishioka M, Ioi H, Nakata S, Nakasima A, Counts AL. Association between orthodontic root resorption and factors of the immune system in Japanese. In: Davidovitch Z, Norton LA. (eds.) Biological Mechanisms of Tooth Movement and Craniofacial Adaptation. Boston: Harvard Society for the Advancement of Orthodontics; 2004. P131-136.

[34] Nishioka M, Ioi H, Nakata S, Nakasima A, Counts AL. Root resorption and immune system factors in the Japanese. Angle Orthod 2006;76(1) 103-108.

[35] Murata N, Ioi H, Ouchi M, Takao T, Oida H, Aijima R, Yamaza T, Kido MA. Effects of allergen sensitization on external root resorption. Journal of Dental Research 2013;92(7) 641-647.

[36] Kameyama Y, Nakane S, Maeda H, Fujita M, Takesue M, Sato E. Inhibitory effect of aspirin on root resorption induced by mechanical injury of the soft periodontal tissue in rats. Journal of Periodontal Research 1994;29(2) 113-117.

[37] Al-Qawasmi RA, Hartsfield JK Jr, Everett ET, Flury L, Liu L, Foroud TM, Macri JV, Roberts WE. Genetic predisposition to external apical root resorption. American Journal of Orthodontics and Dentofacial Orthopedics 2003;123(3) 242-252.

[38] Reitan K. Tissue behavior during orthodontic tooth movement. American Journal of Orthodontics 1960;46(12) 881-890.

[39] Reitan K. Initial tissue behavior during apical root resorption. Angle Orthodontist 1974;44(1) 68-82.

[40] Brudvik P, Rygh P. The initial phase of orthodontic root resorption incident to local compression of the periodontal ligament. European Journal of Orthodontics 1993;15(4) 249-263.

[41] Rossi M, Whitcomb S, Lindemann R. Interleukin-1β and tumor necrosis factor-α production by human monocytes cultured with L-thyroxine and thyrocalcitonin: Relation to severe root resorption. American Journal of Orthodontics 1996;110(4) 399-404.

[42] Khan DA. Allergic rhinitis and asthma: Epidemiology and common pathophysiology. Allergy and Asthma Proceedings 2014;35(5) 357-361.

[43] Naik SR, Wala SM. Inflammation, Allergy and Asthma, Complex Immune Origin Diseases: Mechanisms and Therapeutic Agents. Recent Patents on Inflammation & Allergy Drug Discovery 2013;7(1) 62-95.

[44] Storey E. The nature of tooth movement. Am J Orthod 1970;63(3) 292-314.

[45] Davidovitch Z. Tooth movement. Crit Rev Oral Biol Med 1991;2(4) 411-35.

[46] Redlich K, Hayer S, Ricci R, David JP, Tohidast-Akrad M, Kollias G, Steiner G, Smolen JS, Wagner EF, Schett G. Osteoclasts are essential for TNF-alpha-mediated joint destruction. Journal of Clinical Investiment 2002;110(10) 1419-1427.

[47] Buchs N, Giovine FS di, Silvestri T, Vannier E, Duff GW, Miossec P. IL-1B and IL-1Ra gene polymorphisms and disease severity in rheumatoid arthritis: interaction with their plasma levels. Genes and Immunity 2001;2(4) 222-228.

[48] Tian YL, Xie JC, Zhao ZJ, Zhang Y. Changes of interleukin-1beta and tumor necrosis factor-alpha levels in gingival crevicular fluid during orthodontic tooth movement. Hua Xi Kou Qiang Yi Xue Za Zhi 2006;24(3) 243-245.

[49] Azuma Y, Kaji K, Katogi R, Takeshita S, Kudo A, Tumor necrosis factor-alpha induces differentiation of and bone resorption by osteoclasts, J. Biol. Chem 2000;275(7) 4858-4864.

[50] Samuelsson B. Leukotrienes: mediators of immediate hypersensitivity reactions and inflammation. Science 1983;220(4597) 568-575.

[51] Henderson WR Jr. The role of leukotrienes in inflammation, Annals of Internal Medicine 1994;121(9) 684-697.

[52] Murphy RC, Gijon MA. Biosynthesis and metabolism of leukotrienes. Biochemical Journal 2007;405(3) 379-395.

[53] Sala A, Folco G. Neutrophils, endothelial cells, and cysteinyl leukotrienes: a new approach to neutrophil-dependent inflammation? Biochemical Biophysical Research Communication 2001;283(5) 1003-1006.

[54] Yu W, Xu L, Martin JG, Powell WS. Cellular infiltration and eicosanoid synthesis in brown Norway rat lungs after allergen challenge. American Journal of Respiratory Cell and Molecular Biology 1995;13(4) 477-486.

[55] Garcia C, Boyce BF, Gilles J, Dallas M, Qiao M, Mundy GR, Bonewald LF. Leukotriene B4 stimulates osteoclastic bone resorption both in vitro and in vivo. Journal of Bone and Mineral Research 1996;11(11) 1619-1627.

[56] Hikiji H, Ishii S, Yokomizo T, Takato T, Shimizu T. A distinctive role of the leukotriene B4 receptor BLT1 in osteoclastic activity during bone loss, Proceedings of National Academy of Sciences of the United States of America 2009;106(50) 21294-21299.

[57] Owman-Moll P, Kurol J. Root resorption after orthodontic treatment in high- and low-risk patients: analysis of allergy as a possible predisposing factor. European Journal of Orthodontics 2000;22(6) 657-663.

[58] Kjær I. Morphological characteristics of dentitions developing excessive root resorption during orthodontic treatment. European Journal of Orthodontics 1995;17(1) 25-34.

[59] Mirabella AD, Årtun J. Risk factors apical root resorption of maxillary anterior teeth in adult orthodontic patients. American Journal of Orthodontics and Dentofacial Orthopedics 1995;108(1) 48-55.

[60] Lee RY, Årtun J, Alonzo TA. Are dental anomalies risk factors for apical root resorption in orthodontic patients? American Journal of Orthodontics and Dentofacial Orthopedics 1999;116(2) 187-195.

[61] Costopoulos G, Nanda R. An evaluation of root resorption incident to orthodontic intrusion. American Journal of Orthodontics and Dentofacial Orthopedics 1996;109(5) 543-548.

[62] Herszberg B, Ramos-Barbon D, Tamaoka M, Martin JG, Lavoie JP. Heaves, an asthma-like equine disease, involves airway smooth muscle remodelling. Journal of Allergy and Clinical Immunology. 2006;118(2) 382-388.

[63] Martin JG, Tamaoka M. Rat models of asthma and chronic obstructive lung disease. Pulmonary Pharmacology & Therapeutics 2006;19(6) 377-385.

[64] Xu KF, Vlahos R, Messina A, Bamford TL, Bertram JF, Stewart AG. Antigen-induced airway inflammation in the Brown Norway rat results in airway smooth muscle hyperplasia. Journal of Applied Physiology 2002;93(5) 1833-1840.

[65] Fujii Y, Takeuchi H, Sakuma S, Sengoku T, Takakura S. Characterization of a 2,4-dinitrochlorobenzene-induced chronic dermatitis model in rats. Skin Pharmacology and Physiology 2009;22(5) 240-247.

[66] De Jonge JD, Ezendam J, Knippels LM, Odink J, Pourier MS, Penninks AH, Pieters R, van Loveren H, Bis(tributyltin)oxide (TBTO) decreases the food allergic response against peanut and ovalbumin in Brown Norway rats. Toxicology 2007;239(1-2) 68-76.

[67] Jia XD, Li N, Wu YN, Yang XG. Studies on BN rats model to determine the potential allergenicity of proteins from genetically modified foods. World Journal of Gastroenterology 2005;11(34) 5381–5384.

[68] Bauer DC, Orwoll ES, Fox KM, Vogt TM, Lane NE, Hochberg MC, Stone K, Nevitt MC. Aspirin and NSAID use in older women: effect on bone mineral density and fracture risk, Study of Osteoporotic Fractures Research Group. Journal of Bone and Mineral Research 1996;11(1) 29-35.

[69] Carbone LD, Tylavsky FA, Cauley JA, Harris TB, Lang TF, Bauer DC, Barrow KD, Kritchevsky SB. Association between bone mineral density and the use of nonsteroidal anti-inflammatory drugs and aspirin: impact of cyclooxygenase selectivity. Journal of Bone and Mineral Research 2003;18(10) 1795-1802.

[70] Mavragani M, Brudvik P, Selvig KA. Orthodontically induced root and alveolar bone resorption: inhibitory effect of systemic doxycycline administration in rats. European Journal of Orthodontics 2005;27(3) 215-225.

[71] Wang B, Danjo A, Kajiya H, Okabe K, Kido MA. Oral epithelial cells are activated via TRP channels. Journal of Dental Research 2011;90(2) 163-167.

[72] Polzer K, Neubert K, Meister S, Frey B, Baum W, Distler JH, Gückel E, Schett G, Voll RE, Zwerina J. Proteasome inhibition aggravates TNF-mediated bone resorption. Arthritis &Rheumatology 2011;63(3) 670-680.

[73] Hallstrand TS, Henderson WR Jr. An update on the role of leukotrienes in asthma. Current Opinion and Allergy and Clinical Immunology 2010;10(1) 60-66.

[74] Davidson EM, Rae SA, Smith MJ. Leukotriene B4, a mediator of inflammation present in synovial fluid in rheumatoid arthritis, Annals of the Rheumatic Diseases 1983;42(6) 677-679.

[75] Emingil G, Cinarcik S, Baylas H, Coker I, Huseyinov. A Levels of leukotriene B4 in gingival crevicular fluid and gingival tissue in specific periodontal diseases. Journal of Periodontology 2001;72(8) 1025-1031.

[76] Traianedes K, Dallas MR, Garrett IR, Mundy GR, Bonewald LF. 5-Lipoxygenase metabolites inhibit bone formation in vitro. Endocrinology 1998;139(7) 3178-3184.

[77] Yamaza T, Miura Y, Bi Y, Liu Y, Akiyama K, Sonoyama W, Patel V, Gutkind S, Young M, Gronthos S, Le A, Wang CY, Chen W, Shi S. Pharmacologic stem cell based intervention as a new approach to osteoporosis treatment in rodents. PLoS One 2008;3(7) e2615.

5

Interceptive Orthodontics — Current Evidence

Maen H. Zreaqat

1. Introduction

From evidence found in human skulls, crooked teeth have been around since the time of Neanderthal man (about 50,000 BC), but it was not until about 3000 years ago that we had the first written record of attempts to correct crowded or protruding teeth. Long before braces, long before the word orthodontics" was coined, it was known that teeth moved in response to pressure. Primitive (and surprisingly well-designed) orthodontic appliances have been found with Greek and Etruscan artifacts. Archaeologists have discovered Egyptian mummies with crude metal bands wrapped around individual teeth. It is speculated that catgut was used to close the gaps [1]. The earliest description of irregularities of the teeth was given about 400 BC by Hippocrates (460-377 BC). The first treatment of an irregular tooth was recorded by Celsus (25 BC-50 AD), a Roman writer, who said, "If a second tooth should happen to grow in children before the first has fallen out, that which ought to be shed is to be drawn out and the new one daily pushed toward its place by means of the finger until it arrives at its just proportion." A clear mechanical treatment was advocated by Pliny the Elder (23-79 AD), who suggested filing elongated teeth to bring them into proper alignment. This method remained in practice until the 1800s [2].

Dentistry entered a period of marked decline during middle ages (5th to 15th centuries), as did all sciences. After the 16th century, considerable progress was made. Matthaeus Gottfried Purmann (1692) was the first to report taking wax impressions. In 1756, Phillip Pfaff used plaster of Paris impressions. Malocclusions were called "irregularities" of the teeth, and their correction was termed "regulating." It remained for the Enlightenment to reawaken the spirit of scientific thought necessary to advance dentistry and other disciplines. Beginning in the 18th century, Pierre Fauchard (1678-1761) was leading efforts in the field of dentistry. He has been called the "Father of Orthodontia." He was the first to remove dentistry from the bonds of empiricism and put it on a scientific foundation. In 1728, he published the first general work on dentistry, a 2-volume opus entitled "The Surgeon Dentist: A Treatise on the Teeth".

Fauchard described for first time the bandeau, an expansion arch consisting of a horseshoe-shaped strip of precious metal to which the teeth were ligated (Fig 1). This became the basis for Angle's E-arch, and even today its principles are used in unraveling a crowded dentition. He also "repositioned" teeth with a forceps, called a "pelican" because of its resemblance to the beak of that bird, and ligated the tooth to its neighbors until healing took place. At that time, little attention was paid to anything other than the alignment of teeth and then almost exclusively to the maxilla. moreover, he was the first to recommend serial extraction by extracting premolars to relieve crowding [3].

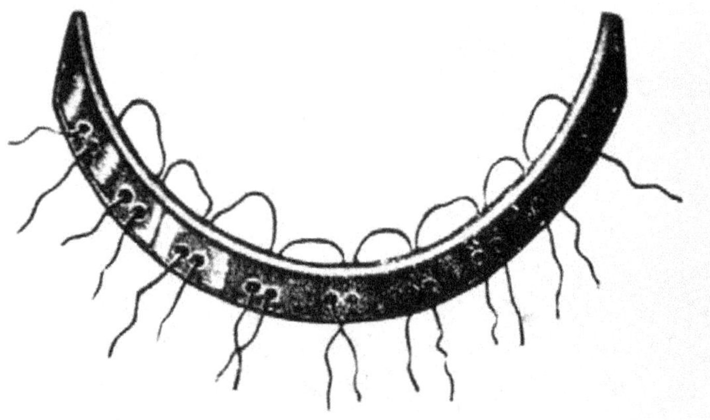

Figure 1. Fauchard's bandeau

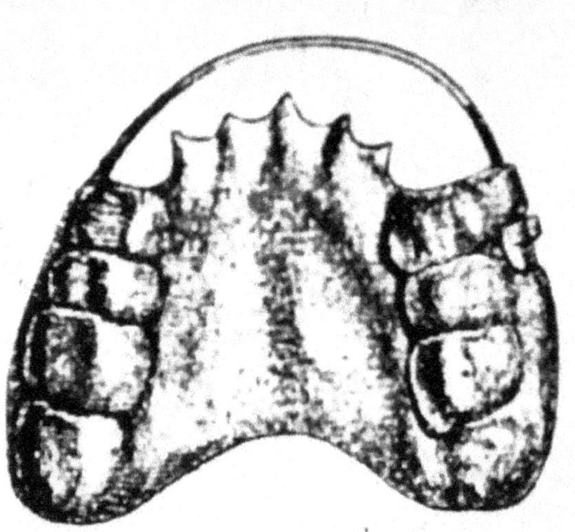

Figure 2. Removable "plate" used by Friedrich Christoph

Friedrich Christoph Kneisel (1797-1847), a German dentist, was the first to use plaster models to record malocclusion and removable appliance to fit prognathic teeth with a chin strap (Fig.

2). However, before the time of Edward Angle, the treatment of malocclusions was chaotic, with little understanding of normal occlusion and even less understanding of the development of the dentition. Appliances were primitive, not only in design but also in the metals and materials used. There was no rational basis for diagnosis and case analysis. It was Edward Hartley Angle (1855 –1930), early in the 20th century, who dominated the emergence of "orthodontia as a science and a specialty". He also created the first educational program to train specialists in orthodonticsand he developed the first prefabricated orthodontic appliance system. Angle is considered the father' of modern orthodontics [4].

2. The development of the occlusion of the teeth

The primary dentition begins to erupt at the age of about 6 months, and is normally completely in occlusion by about 3 years of age. Details of mean age of eruption and the range of variation have been reported by Van der Linden (1983) for Swedish children and by Sato and Ogiwara (1971) for Japanese children. There appear to be no significant differences between the sexes for the age of primary tooth eruption. The first teeth to erupt and to form occlusal contacts are the incisors, which ideally take up occlusal positions that are more vertical than the permanent incisors, with a deeper incisal overbite. The lower incisors in this condition will contact the cingulum area of the upper incisors in centric occlusion. Spaces are present between the primary incisor teeth. Following eruption of the incisors, the first primary molars erupt into occlusion. These teeth take up occlusal contacts so that the lower molars are slightly forward in relation to the upper molar. The last teeth to erupt into occlusion in the primary dentition are the second molars. These teeth erupt slightly spaced from the first molars, but the space quickly closes by forward movement of the second molars which take up a position so that the distal surfaces of the upper and lower second molars are in the same vertical plane in occlusion. Thus certain features of the 'ideal' occlusion of the primary dentition when fully erupted can be described as following:

1. Spacing of incisor teeth.
2. Anthropoid spaces mesial to upper canine and distal to lower canine, into which the opposing canine interdigitates.
3. Vertical position of incisor teeth, with lower incisor touching the cingulum of upper incisor.
4. The distal surfaces of the upper and lower second primary molars in the same vertical plane.

From the age of about 6 years onwards the primary dentition is replaced by the permanent dentition. The primary incisors, canines and molars are replaced by the permanent incisors, canines and premolars, and the permanent molars erupt as additional teeth. There is some difference in size between the primary teeth and the permanent teeth which directly replace them. The permanent incisors and canines are usually larger than the corresponding primary teeth, and the premolars are usually smaller than the corresponding primary molars. Studies reported by Van der Linden (1983), have shown that the overall difference in size between the two dentitions is not large, amounting on average to about 3 mm in the upper teeth and less than 1 mm in the lower teeth. There is, however, not a strong correlation between the sizes of the primary dentition and the permanent teeth. The relationship of the jaws to each other will have a large influence on the relationship of the dental arches. The relationship of the jaws to each other can also vary in all three planes of space, and variation in any plane can affect the occlusion of the teeth. The antero-posterior positional relationship of the basal parts of the upper and lower jaws to each other, with the teeth in occlusion, is known as the skeletal relationship. This is sometimes called the dental base relationship, or the skeletal pattern. A classification of the skeletal relationship is in common use, namely:

1. Skeletal Class 1—in which the jaws are in their ideal antero-posterior relationship in occlusion.
2. Skeletal Class 2—in which the lower jaw in occlusion is positioned further back in relation to the upper jaw than in skeletal Class 1.
3. Skeletal Class 3—in which the lower jaw in occlusion is positioned further forward than in skeletal Class 1.

In addition, the teeth erupt into an environment of functional activity governed by the muscles of mastication, of the tongue and of the face. The muscles of the tongue, lips and cheeks are of particular importance in guiding the teeth into their final position, and variation in muscle form and function can affect the position and occlusion of the teeth. Moreover, some dental and local factors can affect the development of occlusion. These include: alterations in size of the dentition in relation to jaw size, crossbite, aberrant developmental position of individual teeth, presence of supernumerary teeth, developmental hypodontia, labial frenum, thumb or finger sucking. Early interference and modification of these basic etiological features can help to avoid malocclusion or reduce the need for treatment in some cases. Consequently interceptive orthodontic treatment has been set as an important aspect of orthodontic care [5].

3. Interceptive orthodontics: Definition of the concept

The concept and the necessity of interceptive orthodontic treatment, so called early, have been controversial. Some define it as removable or fixed appliance intervention in the deciduous, early mixed, or midmixed dentition. Others place it in the late mixed dentition stage of development (before emergence of the second premolars and the permanent maxillary canines). The American Association of Orthodontists' Council of Orthodontic Education defines interceptive orthodontics as "that phase of the science and art of orthodontics employed to recognize and eliminate potential irregularities and malpositions in the developing dentofacial complex." [6]. While some profession's leaders advocate that early treatment is always desirable because tissue tolerance and their power of adjustment are at or near their maximum, others warn that there is no assurance that the results of early treatment will be sustained, and that several-phased treatment will always lengthen overall treatment time.

Early treatment not only may do some damage or prolong therapy, it may exhaust the child's spirit of cooperation and compliance [7]. Joseph Fox (1776-1816, English), in his "Natural History of the Human Teeth" (London, 1803), recommended that treatment be started "before 13 or 14 years of age, and as much earlier as possible." Angle advocated the institution of orthodontic treatment "as near the beginning of the variation from the normal in the process of the development of the dental apparatus as possible". Although Nance advocated that "active treatment in the mixed dentition period is desirable only in Class III cases, crossbites, and Class II cases wherein facial appearance is markedly affected," he freed orthodontists from their hesitancy to treat patients before the development of the adult dentition [8].

4. Orthodontic interceptive measures during primary and mixed dentition

4.1. Space maintainers

The primary dentition plays a very important role in the child's growth and development, not only in terms of speech, chewing, appearance and the prevention of bad habits but also in the guidance and eruption of permanent teeth. Exfoliation of primary teeth and eruption of permanent teeth is a normal physiological process. When this normal process is disrupted, due to factors like premature loss of primary teeth, proximal carious lesions etc, it may lead to mesial migration of teeth resulting in loss of the arch length which may manifest as malocclusion in permanent dentition in the form of crowding, impaction of permanent teeth, supraeruption of opposing teeth etc. The best way to avoid these problems is to preserve the primary teeth in the arch till their normal time of exfoliation is attained. Hence it is rightly quoted that primary teeth serve as best space maintainers for permanent dentition. However, if premature extraction or loss of tooth is unavoidable due to extensive caries or other reasons, the safest option to maintain arch space is by placing a space maintainer. The fixed space maintainers are usually indicated to maintain the space created by unilateral/bilateral premature loss of primary teeth in either of the arches. Of the various fixed space maintainers, Band and Loop type of space maintainers are one of the most frequently used appliances with good high success rates [9]. Cemented lower lingual bars, transpalatal arches, crowns with distal extensions are other forms of space maintainers utilizing similar mechanisms (Fig. 3) Nevertheless, disintegration of cement, solder failure, caries formation along the margins of the band and long construction time are some of the disadvantages associated with them [10].

Considering this, there has been many pilot studies that explain the use of newer adhesive directly bonded splints. They are glass fiber reinforced composite resins (e.g. Ribbond, Everstick) as fixed space maintainers [11, 12]. Ribbond is a biocompatible esthetic material made from high strength polyethylene fibers (Fig. 4). The various advantages of this material includes its ease of adhesion to the dental contours, fast technique of application and good strength, well tolerated by the patient [13]. However there is limited literature is available in terms of efficacy and longevity [14].

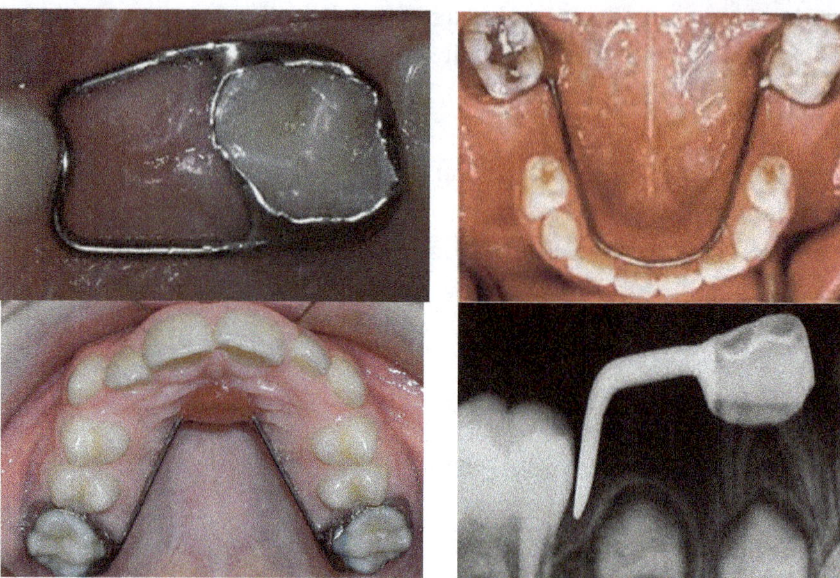

Figure 3. Various space maintainers

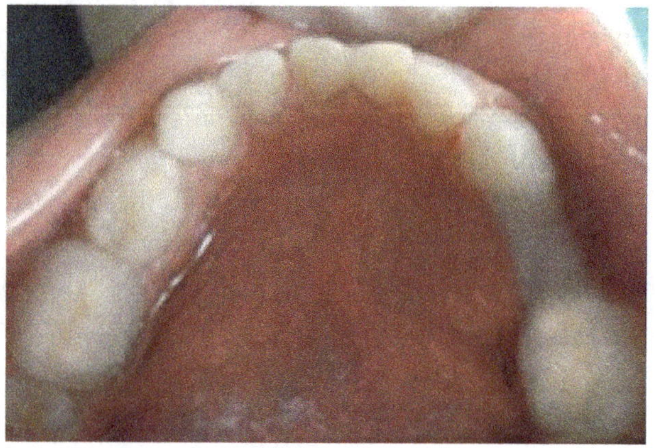

Figure 4. Ribbond space maintainer

5. Elimination of oral habits

Oral habits are learned patterns of muscle contraction and have a very complex nature. They are associated with anger, hunger, sleep, tooth eruption and fear. Some children even display oral habits for release of mental tension. These habits might be non-nutritive sucking (thumb, finger, pacifier and/or tongue), lip biting and bruxism events. These habits can result in damage to dentoalveolar structure; hence, dentists play a crucial role in giving necessary information to parents. This information includes relevant changes in the dentoalveolar structure and the method to stop oral habits. Also, a dentist is required to treat the ensuring malocclusion. The prevalence of oral habits in high school girls and primary school students has been reported to be 87.9 and 30%, respectively [15].

Oral habits could be divided into 2 main groups:

1. Acquired oral habits: Include those behaviors which are learned and could be stopped easily and when the child grows up, he or she can give up that behavior and start another one.

2. Compulsive oral habits: Consist of those behaviors which are fixed in child and when emotional pressures are intolerable for the child, he or she can feel safety with this habit, and preventing the child from these habits make him or her anxious and worried.

5.1. Thumb sucking

Thumb sucking is the most common oral habit and it is reported that its prevalence is between 13 to 60% in some societies [16]. Basically, sucking is one of an infant's natural reflexes. They begin to suck on their thumbs or other fingers while they are in the womb. Infants and young children may suck on thumbs, other fingers, pacifiers or other objects. It makes them feel secure and happy, and it helps them learn about their world. The prevalence of this habit is decreased as age increases, and mostly, it is stopped by 4 years of age. There is a relationship between the level of education in parents, the child nutrition and the sucking habit [17]. If the child chooses this habit in the first year of his or her life, the parents should move away his or her thumb smoothly and attract the child's attention to other things such as toys. After the second years of age, thumb sucking will decrease and will be appear just in child's bed or when he/she is tired. Some of children who do not stop this habit, will give it up when their permanent teeth erupt, but there is a tendency for continuing the sucking habit even until adult life. According to a study in 1973, millions of kids do not give up this habit before the eruption of teeth [18]. Nowadays, the level of stress is higher than the time of that study, and as stress is a powerful stimulus in sucking habit, it is probable to find more kids with long-term sucking habit if we do a research exactly like the one which was done in 1973.

Thumb sucking has 2 types:

1. Active: In this type, there is a heavy force by the muscles during the sucking and if this habit continues for a long period, the position of permanent teeth and the shape of mandible will be affected.

2. Passive: In this type, the child puts his/her finger in mouth, but because there is no force on teeth and mandible, so this habit is not associated with skeletal changes.

In the case of active thumb sucking habit, it is better for a child not to be blamed, teased, offended, humiliated and punished, because these methods will increase the anxiety and consequently increase the incidence of the habit. Long-term finger sucking habit has harmful effects on dentition and speech. In 1870s decade, Camble and Jander reported for the first time that long-term finger sucking has harmful effects on dentition [19].

The side effects of finger sucking are: Anterior open bite, increased overjet, lingual inclination lower incisor and labial inclination upper incisor, posterior cross bite, compensatory tongue thrust, deep palate, speech defect, and finger defects (Eczema of the finger due to alternate dryness and moisture that occurs and even angulations of the finger). The severity of changes in dentition due to finger sucking is related to the duration and times of doing the habit. Also, the position of finger in mouth, dental arches relation and child's health affect the severity of changes [20].

Dental changes due to finger sucking do not need any treatment if the habit stopped before the 5 years of age and as soon as giving up the habit, dental changes will be corrected spontaneously [21]. At the time of permanent anterior teeth eruption and if the child is motivated to stop the sucking habit, it is time to start the treatment as follows:

1. Direct interview with child if he/she is mature enough to understand
2. Encouragement: This can give the child more pride and self-confidence
3. Reward system
4. Reminder therapy
5. Orthodontic appliance: The final stage in treatment is the use of orthodontic appliance whether fixed or removable, which can play the role of reminder and can reduce the willing of finger sucking. For long-term habits or unwilling patient, the fixed intra oral appliance is the most effective inhibitor. In the case of using fixed or removable appliance, we should alarm the parents about potential problems in speaking or eating during the first 24 to 48 h, which are usual and self correcting. After active phase of treatment, the appliance should remain in place for more 3 to 6 month to minimize the relapse potential [22, 23].

5.2. Use of pacifier

The use of pacifier is common in most countries and it will not cause permanent changes in dentition if it is stopped at the age of 2 or 3 years. After that, the use of pacifier has harmful effects on dentition development, and if it is used more than 5 years old, these effects would be more severe [24]. The children who use pacifier are not willing to suck their fingers. pacifier has the following negative effects:

1. Anterior open bite
2. Shallow palate
3. Increased width of lower arch
4. Posterior cross bite.
5. Median otitis

It is suggested that pacifier should be replaced in children who have the habit of finger sucking, because the harmful effects of sucking pacifier are less than finger. In comparison between different pacifiers, despite the claims, it has been shown that there is no significant advantage for physiologic pacifiers over conventional ones [25].

5.3. Nail biting or onychophagia

Nail biting is a common and untreated medical problem among children. This habit starts after 3 to 4 years of age and is in its peak in 10 years of age. Its rate increases in adolescency, while it declines later. This problem is not gender dependent in children less than 10 years of age, but its incidence in boys is more than girls among adolescents [26]. This problem is a reaction in response to psychological disorders and some children will shift their habits from thumb sucking to nail biting. Complications caused by nail biting include malocclusion of the anterior teeth, teeth root resorption, bacterial infection and alveolar destruction. Moreover, about one forth of patients with temporo-mandibular joint pain and dysfunction have been shown to suffer from nail biting habit [27]. It is seen in clinic that boys with nail biting have a kind of psychological disorder especially attention deficient hyperactivity disorder (ADHD) more than girls. This habit in higher ages will be replaced with some habits such as lip chewing, gum chewing or smoking (Finn, 1998). Children with nail biting should be evaluated for emotional problems. In addition, putting nail polish or distasteful liquids on nails may be a therapeutic choice.

5.4. Tongue thrust

Tongue Thrust refers to a swallowing pattern in which the tongue is placed in the front of the mouth to begin the swallow (Fig. 5). Forward position of the tongue may also be seen at rest (mouth breathers). Normal swallowing patterns after infancy involve a coordinated smooth movement of the tongue toward the back of the mouth. This consistent forward movement of the tongue may cause speech errors and misaligned teeth. Forward positioning of the tongue during rest has the most influence on misaligning the teeth due to duration of the pressure. The speech disorder most commonly associated with tongue thrust is a frontal lisp, in which the tongue is place between the teeth for the sounds s and z, and sometimes for sh, ch, j, and soft g.

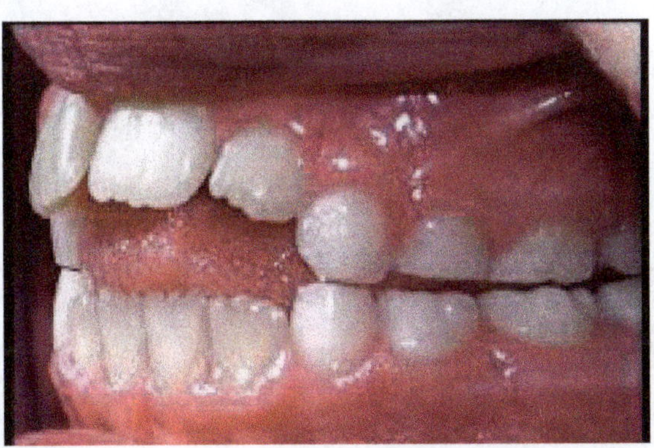

Figure 5. Tongue thrust

The line of treatment for these habits includes removal of the etiology, retraining exercises, and use of mechanical restraining appliances. Tongue bead appliances are commonly used as retraining exercise devices. In severe tongue thrusting cases and in cases with anterior open bite, a bead appliance alone may not be effective in restricting the habit. Tongue crib appliances (Fig. 6) are extremely effective in breaking the tongue thrust habit [28]. They create a mechanical barrier and prevent the tongue from thrusting between the incisors. In most of the cases with severe thumb/digit sucking habit, an anterior open bite develops. This will result in the development of a secondary tongue thrust habit. Hence, in cases with severe prolonged thumb or digit sucking, an appliance which can eliminate both of these habits. The Hybrid Habit Correcting Appliance (HHCA) can be used to effectively restrain and correct tongue thrusting as well as thumb sucking habit (Fig.7). HHCA incorporates a tongue bead, a palatal crib and a U-loop which is attached to the molar bands on either sides. The tongue bead consists of a spinnable acrylic bead of 3mm diameter. The appliance is designed to position the acrylic bead over the posterior one-third of the incisive papilla. The bead acts as a tongue retrainer. The patient is asked to constantly pull the bead towards the posterior region of the mouth. The palatal crib and the U-loop are made of 0.9mm stainless steel wire. Three to four spurs are bent on either sides of the bead, starting from the canine region on one side, running anteriorly as a smooth curve (in conventional crib appliances, the cribs run obliquely from one canine to the other side canine) and lying 1mm lingual to the cervical margin of the maxillary anterior teeth. In the region of the incisive papilla, the acrylic bead is incorporated in such a way that it lies over the posterior one-third of the incisive papilla. The tip of the crib should be almost in line with the incisor tip of the maxillary central incisor or 2 mm longer without interfering with the lower incisors when in occlusion. In cases with anterior open bite, the crib should be longer and can be up to 3/4th of the interincisal distance between the upper and lower central incisors. This is to avoid the tongue from thrusting over the tip of the crib. The palatal crib acts as a barrier against the thrusting tongue and works as a mechanical restrainer. The U-loop is incorporated in the second premolar region and it helps to reposition the appliance posteriorly during the retraction phase, when it is used along with fixed orthodontic appliances.

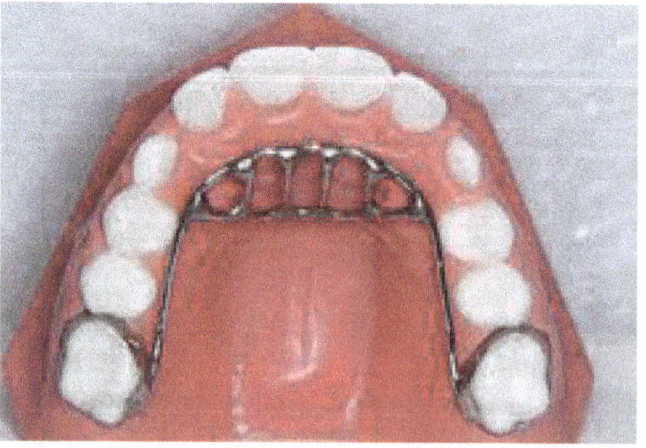

Figure 6. Tongue crib appliances

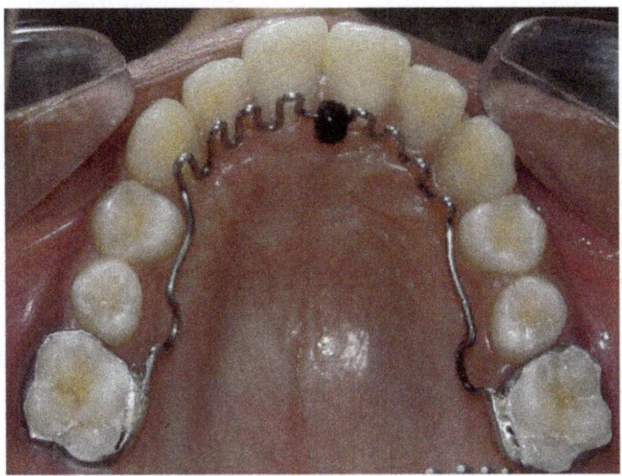

Figure 7. Hybrid Habit Correcting Appliance (HHCA).

5.5. Bruxism

The actions of masticatory system are divided into 2 groups. Functional actions such as mastication, speaking and swallowing, and parafunctional actions such as teeth impacting (clenching) and bruxism.

Functional activities are controllable and occurred daily. Parafunctional actions may be conscious or unconscious and are normally without sound. However, bruxism in nights is unconscious and mostly it is with sound production. Sleep bruxism occurs during stages first and second of non rapid eye movement (REM) sleep and REM sleep. These people do not have any complaint about bruxism, and it would not affect their quality of sleep. But in the old and people with sleep apnea, bruxism can reduce the quality of sleep [29]. Sleep bruxism has 2 types: Primary or idiopathic and secondary or iatrogenic. The first type is without any medical reason and the secondary type is whether with use of drug or without the use of drug. Risk factors are as follows: Genetics: 20 to 50% of patients with sleep bruxism have positive family history [30]; age: The prevalence of this habit decrease with age; cigarette smoking: The prevalence of sleep bruxism in smokers is 1.9 times more than non-smokers; use of alcohol and caffeine [31]; tension and stresses. Clinical findings of sleep bruxism include; report of grinding or impacting sounds of teeth; erosion of the teeth occlusal surfaces and breakdown of repairs; hypertrophy of masticatory muscles; hypersensitivity of teeth to cold air, and joint sounds. The treatment includes no special recommended regimen, but increasing awareness of the patient, intra oral appliances, behavioral treatment and drugs like diazepam and clonazepam have been reported to be effective [32,33].

6. Anterior cross bite correction

Anterior crossbite is defined as a malocclusion resulting from the lingual positioning of the maxillary anterior teeth in relationship to the mandibular anterior teeth. An anterior crossbite is present when one or more of the upper incisors are in linguo-occlusion (reverse over jet). This may involve just a single tooth or could include all four upper incisors. Anterior dental crossbite has a reported incidence of 4-5% and usually becomes evident during the early mixed-dentition phase [34]. Anterior crossbite correction in early mixed dentition is highly recommended as this kind of malocclusion does not diminish with age. Uncorrected anterior crossbite may lead to abnormal wear of the lower incisors, dental compensation of mandibular incisors leading to thinning of labial alveolar plate and/or gingival recession. However early treatment does not always eliminates orthodontic treatment need in permanent occlusion. The aim of early treatment of this type of malocclusion is to correct anterior crossbite, as otherwise often can lead to very serious Class III mallocclusion which would be possible to treat only with combined orthodontic and orthognatic method.

A variety of factors has been reported to cause anterior dental crossbite, including a palatal eruption path of the maxillary anterior incisors; trauma to the primary incisor resulting in lingual displacement of the permanent tooth germ; supernumerary anterior teeth; an over-retained necrotic or pulpless deciduous tooth or root; odontomas; crowding in the incisor region; inadequate arch length; and a habit of biting the upper lip. Various treatment methods have been proposed to correct anterior dental crossbite, such as tongue blades, reversed stainless steel crowns, fixed acrylic planes, bonded resin-composite slopes, and removable acrylic appliances with finger springs.

Bayraka and Tunca, 2008, described the use of bonded resin-composite slopes for the management of anterior crossbite in children in early mixed dentition. Dental crossbite was corrected by applying a 3-4 mm bonded resin-composite slope to the incisal edge of the mandibular incisor with an angle 45° to the longitudinal axis of the tooth (Fig. 8). Correction was achieved within 1-2 weeks with no damage to either the tooth or the marginal periodontal tissue. The procedure was a simple and effective method for treating anterior dental crossbite [35].

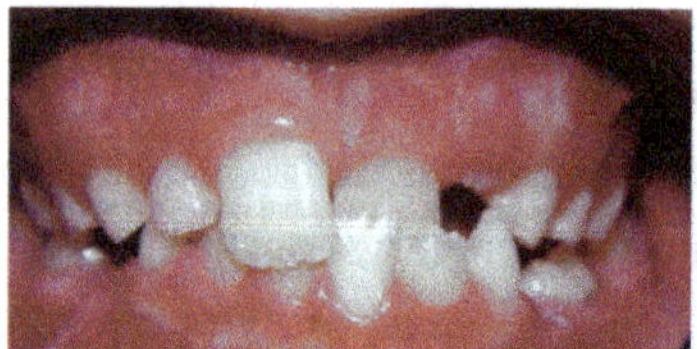
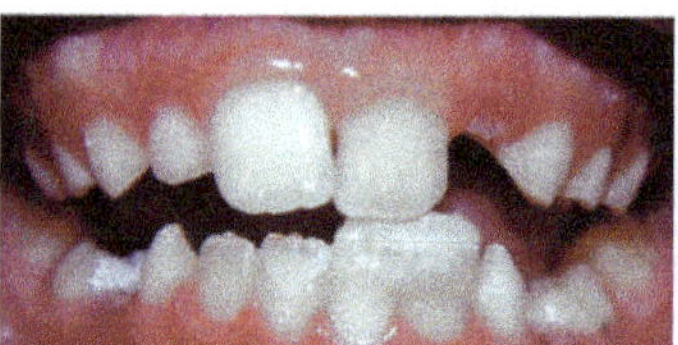
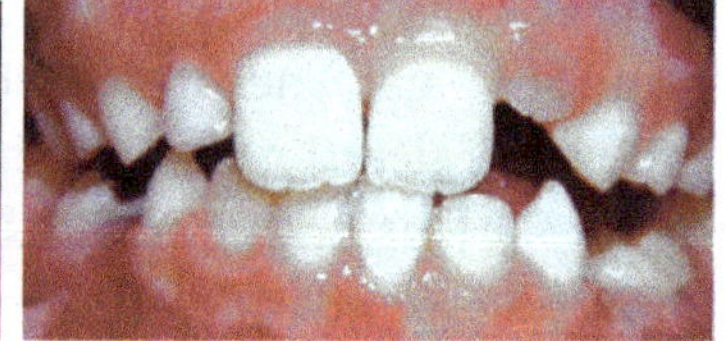

Figure 8. Anterior crossbite correction with bonded resin-composite slope

Some authors believe that removable appliances are not preferred in anterior crossbite correction as they tend to get displaced as the turning frequency decreases following activation. Moreover, poor patient compliance with removable appliance can cause relapse of the case and poor success rate. Therefore, a fixed appliance was proposed as a more sound therapy. Yaseen and Acharya, 2012, described the use of hexa helix, a modified version of quad helix for the management of anterior crossbite and bilateral posterior crossbite in early mixed dentition (Fig. 9). Correction was achieved within 15 weeks with no damage to the tooth or the marginal periodontal tissue. The procedure is a simple and effective method for treating anterior and bilateral posterior crossbite simultaneously. it provides advantages such as minimal discomfort, reduces need for patient cooperation, and better control of tooth movements [36].

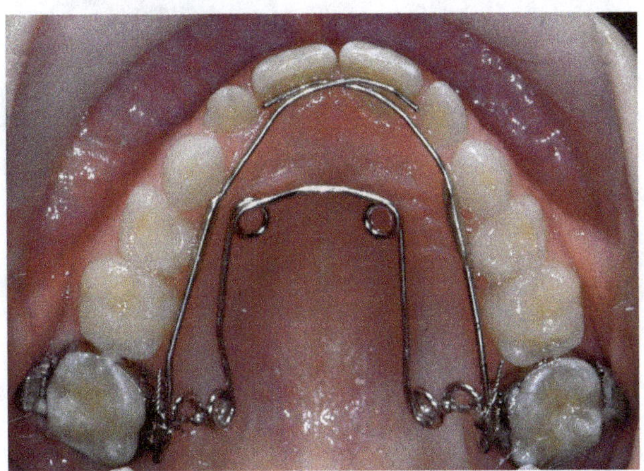

Figure 9. Hexa helix appliance.

In a recent study, Wiedel and Bondemark, 2014, evaluated and compared the stability of correction of anterior crossbite in the mixed dentition by fixed or removable appliance therapy. The study comprised 64 consecutive patients who met the following inclusion criteria: early to late mixed dentition, anterior crossbite affecting one or more incisors, no inherent skeletal Class III discrepancy, moderate space deficiency, a nonextraction treatment plan, and no previous orthodontic treatment. The study was designed as a randomized controlled trial with two parallel arms. The patients were randomized for treatment with a removable appliance with protruding springs or with a fixed appliance with multi-brackets. The outcome measures were success rates for crossbite correction, overjet, overbite, and arch length. Measurements were made on study casts before treatment (TO), at the end of the retention period (T1), and 2 years after retention (T2). Results showed that at T1 the anterior crossbite had been corrected in all patients in the fixed appliance group and all except one in the removable appliance group. At T2, almost all treatment results remained stable and equal in both groups. From T0 to T1, minor differences were observed between the fixed and removable appliance groups with respect to changes in overjet, overbite, and arch length measurements. These changes had no clinical implications and remained unaltered at T2. It was concluded that in the mixed dentition, anterior crossbite affecting one or more incisors can be successfully corrected by either fixed or removable appliances with similar long-term stability [37].

7. Anterior diastema and abnormal labial fraenum

Angle described the midline diastema as a common form of incomplete occlusion characterized by a space between the maxillary and, less frequently, mandibular central incisors. In his classical article, Andrews stated that interdental diastemas should not exist and all contacts should be tight so that the patient has 'straight and attractive teeth as well as a correct overall dental occlusion'.

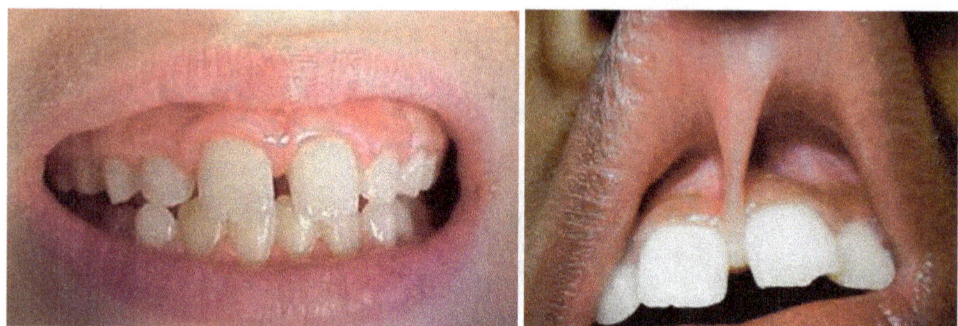

Figure 10. Midline diastema

Sanin et al., developed a method that could predict whether the space would close spontaneously in the developing dentition. This method is based on millimeter measurements in the early mixed dentition and is claimed to have an accuracy of 88%. As the size of the diastema increases the possibility of space closure without treatment reduces. Sanin's prediction is as follows:

- For a 1 mm space in the early mixed dentition the possibility of spontaneous space closure is 99%.
- For a 1.5 mm space the possibility is 85%.
- For a 1.85 mm diastema it is 50%.
- For a 2.7 mm space the possibility of closure without treatment is only 1%.

The measurement should be made after the eruption of the lateral incisors. Hence it is advisable to intervene early if the midline diastema is more than 1.85 mm after the eruption of the permanent lateral incisors [38].

To treat the midline diastema effectively, an accurate diagnosis of the etiology and an intervention relevant to the specific etiology is necessary. Timing of the treatment is important to achieve satisfactory results. Most of the researchers do not recommend tooth movement until the eruption of the permanent canines, but in certain cases, where very large diastemas exist, treatment can be initiated early [39].

Nainar and Gnanasundaram noted in their study of midline diastemas on 9774 Southern Indian individuals, that there was a relatively increased frequency of familial occurrence and hence proposed the presence of a genetic factor in the expression of midline diastema. Treatment methods include orthodontic correction with a fixed or removable appliance and prosthetic correction with composites and crowns. If the diastema is large, it is advisable to close the space using orthodontic appliances. In most cases, simple removable appliances incorporating finger springs or a split labial bow can give good results [40].

A hypertrophic labial frenum may be considered as a major etiological factor for midline diastema. In a thick and fleshy labial frenum, the fibro-elastic band crosses the alveolus and inserts into the incisive papilli, preventing the approximation of the maxillary central incisors. The blanching test is a simple diagnostic test to predict whether a normal tight contact between the central incisors. Most of the researchers, like Angle, Sicher, and Edwards, [41-43] are of the opinion that superior labial frenum causes midline diastema. Some researchers, like Popovich et al, believe that there is an inverse relationship between high frenal attachment and midline diastema. According to them, labial frenum persists owing to the existing diastema and, as the dentition applies little or no pressure on the tissues, here is little or no atrophy of the frenum [44]. However, most of the researchers agree that removal of the high bulbous labial frenum is important for the stability after the closure of the midline diastema.

Excessive anterior overbite is another major contributing factor for midline diastema. As a result of trauma to the maxillary anterior teeth from the mandibular incisors, the maxillary incisors procline. This results in an increase of the upper arch circumference, leading to a diastema. Practitioners should not fail to identify deep bite as an aetiology for the diastema. Any attempt to close the midline spacing without correcting the deep bite and anterior traumatic bite will lead to a speedy relapse of the condition.

Oral habits such as tongue thrusting and finger sucking can be other etiological factors for the appearance of the midline diastema. According to Proffit and Fields, tongue position at rest may have a greater impact on tooth position than tongue pressure, as the tongue only briefly contacts the lingual surface of the anterior teeth during thrusting [45]. The tongue pushes the anterior teeth to a forward position, increasing the circumference which results in spacing. An abnormal habit of the tongue can be detected by the tip of the tongue popping out through the anterior spacing when the patient is asked to swallow. In cases of anterior open bite, the tongue may be seen thrusting between incisal edges of the maxillary and mandibular incisors. Patients with tongue thrust often produce a snap sound on swallowing and also have hyperactivity of the orbicularis oris muscle.Deleterious habits have to be corrected by using habit-breaking appliances and by psychological approaches. The use of fixed tongue cribs are found to be effective in breaking the tongue-thrusting habit.

Peg-shaped laterals Supernumerary teeth/mesiodens, missing teeth, pathologic migration of teeth Tooth size, arch size discrepancy, angulation of teeth, odontomas occurring in the maxillary midline, developmental cysts in the orofacial midline, and flaccid lips are other proposed etiological factors leading to midline diastema. Relapse is a major concern in the correction of midline diastema. However, exact diagnosis and removal of the etiology is the key to obtaining a stable result. Long-term use of retainers or even permanent bonded lingual retainers are advocated, especially in cases with large diastema. Large pretreatment diastema presence of at least one family member with a similar condition increases the risk of relapse [46,47].

8. Serial extraction

The term serial extraction describes an orthodontic treatment procedure that involves the orderly removal of selected deciduous and permanent teeth in a predetermined sequence (Dewel, 1969). Serial extraction can be defined as the correctly timed, planned removal of certain deciduous and permanent teeth in mixed dentition cases with dento-alveolar disproportion in order to: Alleviate crowding of incisor teeth and to allow unerupted teeth to guide themselves into improved positions (canines in particular), and to lessen (or eliminate) the period of active appliance therapy. Thus, it is one of the positive interceptive orthodontic procedure generally applied in most discrepancy cases where supporting bone is less than the total tooth material [48].

Serial extraction has been of interest to dentist for many years. Throughout the history of dentistry it has been recognized that the removal of one or more irregular teeth would improve the appearance of the reminder. Nance presented clinics on his technique of progressive extraction in 1940 and has been called as the father of serial extraction philosophy in the United States. Kjellgren in 1940 termed this extraction procedure as planned or progressive extraction procedure of teeth. Hotz, 1970, named the same procedure on "Guidance of eruption". According to him the term guidance of eruption is comprehensive and encompasses all measures available for influencing tooth eruption [49]. Widespread adoption of serial extraction as a corrective treatment procedure continues to be a source of concern to all pedodontists who are aware of its limitations as well as of its possibilities. The principle reason is that its application involves growth prediction. Every serial extraction diagnosis is based on the promise that future growth will be inadequate to accommodate all of the teeth in a normal alignment.

If primary teeth are extracted prematurely, this will influence the eruption rate and position of the permanent successors. In general, the eruption will be delayed if the primary tooth overlying the permanent tooth is extracted 1 ½ years or more from the time the primary tooth would normally exfoliate. Conversely, the eruption rate can be accelerated if the primary tooth overlying the permanent tooth is extracted less than a year before the primary tooth would normally exfoliate. Biologic variation in eruption rates will affect these time tables, as will periapical inflammation of the primary tooth. Another useful principle is that crowded teeth adjacent to an extraction site tend to align themselves [50].

Normal dental, skeletal and profile development – influences the rationale for serial extraction. The work of Moorrees et al on arch dimensions and serial extractions indicates that there is minimal increase in mandibular intercanine width between 8 and 18 years, occurring usually around the time the permanent mandibular canines erupt. The maxillary intercanine width increases slightly more and over a longer time. The dental arch perimeter from the distal of the mandibular primary second molar to its antimere is less in the permanent dentition than in the primary. Also the principles of leeway space, interrelationship of overjet, overbite, axial inclinations, and mesial shift, and arch-length analysis must be considered in determining whether to institute a serial extraction procedure. The skeletal and profile factors that influence serial extractions are the another-posterior, vertical, and transverse relationships as well as the developmental pattern. Specifically the relation of the maxilla to the mandible and of the both to the cranial base must be determined to identify protrusions, retrusions, hyperdivergences, hypodivergences, crossbites, and asymmetries. Also rotational, vertical, and transverse growth patterns need to be integrated into the decision-making process [51].

The idea of serial extraction started when Pedodontist sees a child 5 or 6 years of age with all the deciduous teeth present in a slightly crowded state or with no spaces between them, he can predict, with a fair degree of certainly, that there will not be enough space in the jaws to accommodate all the permanent teeth in their proper alignment. As Nance (1940), Dewel (1954), and others have pointed out, after the eruption of the first permanent molars at 6 years of age, there is probably no increase in the distance from the mesial aspect of the first molar on one side around the arch to the mesial aspect of the first molar on the opposite side. If there is any change, it may be an actual reduction of the molar-to-molar arch length, as the "leeway" space is lost through the mesial migration of the first permanent molars during the tooth-exchange process and correction of the flush terminal plane relationship. At that time, a list of possible clinical clues for serial extraction were proposed: Premature loss of deciduous teeth, arch-length deficiency and tooth size discrepancies, lingual eruption of lateral incisors, unilateral deciduous canine loss and shift to the same side, mesial eruption of canines overlateral incisors, mesial drift of buccal segments, abnormal eruption direction and eruption sequence, flaring of incisors, ectopic eruption of mandibular first deciduous molar, abnormal resorption of II deciduous molar, ankylosis, labial stripping, and gingival recession, usually of lower incisor. However, a number of contraindications for serial extractions were addressed: Congenital absence of teeth providing space, mild to moderate crowding, deep or open bites, severe Class II, III of dental/skeletal origin, cleft lip and palate, spaced dentition, anodontia / oligodontia, Midline diastemia, dilacerations extensive caries, disportion between arc length and tooth material.

9. Considerations in serial extraction

1. Extracting primary canines will produce maximum amounts of self improvement in crowding with greatest inter-ception of lingual cross bite.

2. Extracting primary first molars produces earliest eruption of first premolars but reduces speed and amount of improvement in permanent central and lateral incisors crowding and position due to retention of C that it has limited application.

3. Extracting primary canines and first molars is a compromise between rapid improvement in and desired early eruption of permanent central and lateral incisors due to simultaneous eruption of first premolars with this extraction sequence.

There is no single technique for Serial Extraction. It is a long-range guidance program and it may be necessary to reevaluate and change tentative decisions several times. Usually the child is 7-8 years of age when he/she brought to the pedodontist. At this time the maxillary and mandibular central incisors are usually erupted, but there is inadequate space in anterior segments to allow normal eruption and positioning of lateral incisors. In some cases, mandibular lateral incisors have already erupted but they are usually lingually positioned and rotated. The same is with the maxillary lateral incisors.

9.1. Dewel's method

There are 3 stages in Serial Extraction Therapy:

First: Removal of deciduous canines : to permit eruption and optimal alignment of lateral incisors. There is some amount of improvement in position of central incisors also.

Second: Removal of first deciduous molars: to accelerate eruption of first premolars ahead of canine if possible.

Third: Removal of erupting first premolars: Before the first premolars are extracted, all the diagnostic criteria must again be evaluated. The status of developing third molars must be evaluated, because if the third molars are congenitally missing then extraction of 1st premolars would be unnecessary because there would be enough space. So in short, Dewel's method is:

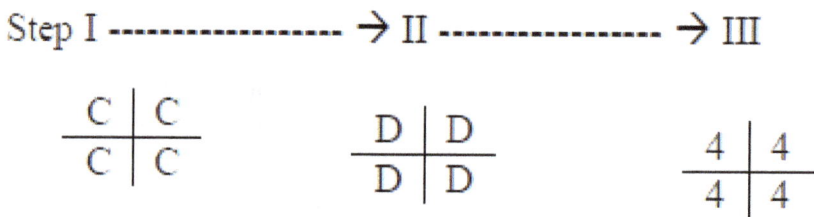

Step I ----------------- → II ---------------- → III

Step I		Step II		Step III	
C	C	D	D	4	4
C	C	D	D	4	4

9.2. Tweed's method

According to Tweed, if diagnosis shows the discrepancy exists between teeth and basal bone structures and if patient is between 7 ½ to 8 ½ years, Serial Extraction program is should be carried out. Sequence is:

First: At approximately 8 years all deciduous molars are extracted. It is preferable to maintain in deciduous canines to retard eruption of permanent canines.

Second: extract of first premolar and deciduous canines should he done 4-6 months prior to eruption of permanent canines when they erupt they migrate posteriorly into good position. Any irregularities in mandibular incisors if not too severe, get corrected themselves and they are also tipped lingually due to normal muscular forces.

9.3. Moyers method

Proposed when crowding seen in central incisor region. Fairly eruption of lateral incisors.

Stage I (Extraction of all deciduous lateral incisors). It helps in alignment of central incisors.

Stage II (Extraction of all deciduous canines after 7-8 months). It helps in alignment of lateral incisors and provides space for lateral incisors.

Stage III (Extraction of all deciduous first molars). It stimulates eruption of all first premolars.

Stage IV (Extraction of all first premolars after 7-8 months). It provides space for canines and stimulates eruption of canines.

Step I ----------- → II ----------- → III ------------ → IV

B | B	C | C	D | D	4 | 4
B | B	C | C	D | D	4 | 4

The technique of serial extraction was biologically sound proven, and was not considered a compromise. with continuous observation and study, the sight has changed. conventional orthodontic therapy is required to complete the alignment of teeth, to parallel the roots on either side, of the extraction space, to eliminate overbite, and to effect residual space closure. With advances in fixed orthodontics, less damage and more stable results are obtained. Moreover, it must be remembered that, once teeth have been extracted, they cannot be replaced if an error in judgment must be made, it is more expedient to error in a conservative manner without extraction as teeth can always be extracted at a later date. To summarize the limitations a and side effects of serial extraction:

First: Tendency of bite to close following loss of posterior teeth. A normal overbite depends on adequate vertical growth and Serial Extraction involves removal of strategically located deciduous and permanent teeth. Vertical and horizontal growth depends great part on normal proximal and occlusal function in maintaining arch length and normal overjet and overbite.

Second: Failure of premolars that fail to reach their normal occlusal level. In normally developing dentition, the premolars are ready to emerge soon after the loss of the deciduous molars and then proceed occlusally with no delay. But in Serial Extraction cases the premolars have to travel a long way before penetrating the gingival tissues. Prolonged absence of teeth in the posterior segment of arches permits the tongue to flow into remaining spaces and this may remain as a tongue thrusting habit. This in turn prevents premolars from attaining full eruption.

Third: Effect of serial extraction on facial esthetics. Most of us over emphasize on straight profile which has led to extraction of teeth in mixed dentition because the lips appear to be prominent. Its normal for lip line to have greater convexity during early transitional stages than it will have in mature dentition. Lip fullness is not a reliable criterion for extraction in early mixed dentition. The straight profile must be viewed with greater concern because early removal of premolars is likely to cause a concave profile.

Fourth: Nasal development is another unpredictable hazard. The nose is one structure that continues to grow long after other facial parts have reached maturity. Unrestrained extraction will accentuate its prominence by reducing skeletal development in dental area. Moreover growth of chin is unpredictable. If growth in nose and chin exceeds normal range a concave profile is obtained.

In conclusion, one team of clinicians and practioners demonstrate that undertaking a serial extraction protocol can afforded an improvement of the patient's self-esteem, resulting in a positive social impact due to esthetic enhancement. Furthermore, the low cost of this protocol permits the use of this therapy in underprivileged communities provided the diagnosis is certain and the post extraction movement of teeth is controlled by mechanical means. The other team suggest that serial extraction is counter-productive. The early extraction of primary cuspids will invariably result in crowding of the permanent cuspids region. In reality, they adopt the idea that the problem is maintained and the crowding shifts to involve the permanent cuspids. They remind us with the most basic canon of the health profession which is "first do no harm" [52].

10. Interceptive functional therapy

There is little doubt that functional appliances produce tooth movement and in many cases can correct occlusal discrepancies. The controversy over their use relates mainly to their mode of action, and in particular to two aspects. The first is the question of modification of growth of the basal parts of the jaws. Many authorities believe that basal jaw growth can be altered by functional means. The temporo-mandibular joint area has been thought to be a reactive growth site, i.e. any prolonged change in the position of the mandible during the growth period, such as is induced by wearing the appliance, results in bone apposition on the mandibular and temporal surfaces of the enlarged joint cavity. Baume, (1969) quotes histological evidence to support this concept, and ample clinical evidence has been produced in attempts to show that the use of functional appliances can alter the skeletal relationship of the jaws [53]. On the other hand, this clinical evidence does not always take into account the effects of normal growth. As functional appliances are normally used during the mixed dentition stage a considerable amount of normal growth must occur which could alter jaw size and relationships. Several investigators have failed to find evidence of altered growth with functional appliances, but instead have found the main effects to be tipping of the incisors and an opening rotation of the mandible [54,55].

The first practitioner to use functional jaw orthopedics to treat a malocclusion was Pierre Robin (1902).

His appliance influenced muscular activity by changing the spatial relationship of the jaws. Robin's monoloc was actually a modification of Kingsley's maxillary plate. It extended all along the lingual surfaces of the mandibular teeth, but it had sharp lingual imprints of the crown surfaces of both maxillary and mandibular teeth. It incorporated an expansion screw in the palate to expand the dental arches. In 1909, Viggo Andresen, a Danish dentist, used lingual horseshoe flange that guides the mandible forward to eliminate Class II malocclusion cases. The original Andresen activator was a tooth-borne, loosely fitting passive appliance consisting of a block of plastic covering the palate and the teeth of both arches, designed to advance the mandible several millimeters for Class II correction and open the bite 3 to 4 mm. The original design had facets incorporated into the body of the appliance to direct erupting posterior teeth mesially or distally, so, despite the simple design, dental relationships in all 3 planes of space could be changed.

The Herbst appliance (Dentaurum, Newtown, Pa) is suitable for slightly older children whose cooperation might not be dependable, because it is a fixed appliance worn 24 hours a day. The Herbst was introduced in 1905 by Emil Herbst, but his findings were not published until 1935. Little more was published on the appliance until the late 1970s, when Hans Pancherz, recognizing its possibilities for mandibular growth stimulation, revived interest. The typical Herbst consists of a telescoping mechanism connected to the maxillary first molars at one end and a cantilevered arm attached to the mandibular first molars at the other end; it forces the mandible forward (Fig. 11).

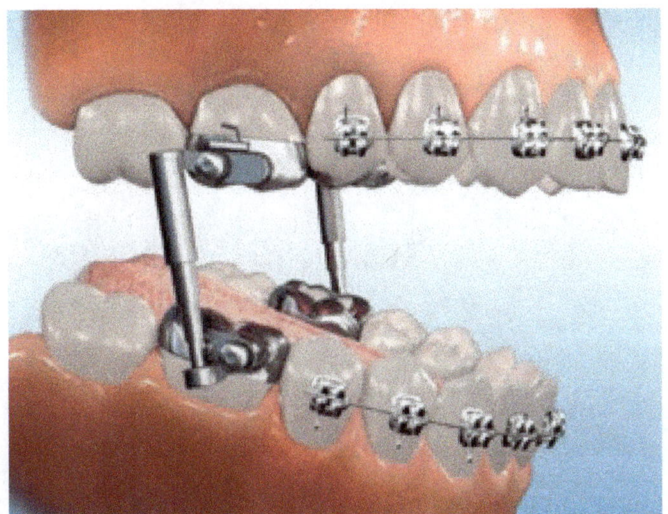

Figure 11. Herbst Appliance

In 1950, Wilhelm Balters (1893-1973), in an effort to treat Class II malocclusions characterized by deficient mandibles, began to modify Andresen's activator. He gave it the name bionator. It is indicated for patients with favorable facial growth patterns and is designed to produce forward positioning of the mandible. As with the function regulator, the bionator is available in 3 designs. Consisting of 2 halves connected by a Coffin spring, it is less restrictive of speech than Andresen's appliance. However, the treatment also highly depends on patient compliance, especially with regard to exercising

The Clark twin-block (Clark 1988) consists of separate upper and lower removable appliances, each with a 45° posterior bite plane designed to induce a mandibular posture of the desired amount and direction (Fig. 12) One or both sections may incorporate a mid-line screw to effect arch expansion(Fig. 13), and there is provision for the addition of extraoral traction.

Many clinical studies have been done on skeletal and dentoalveolar changes associated with functional appliances therapy in Class II malocclusions, but the scientific data are still controversial. Concerning skeletal effects induced by the functional appliances some authors

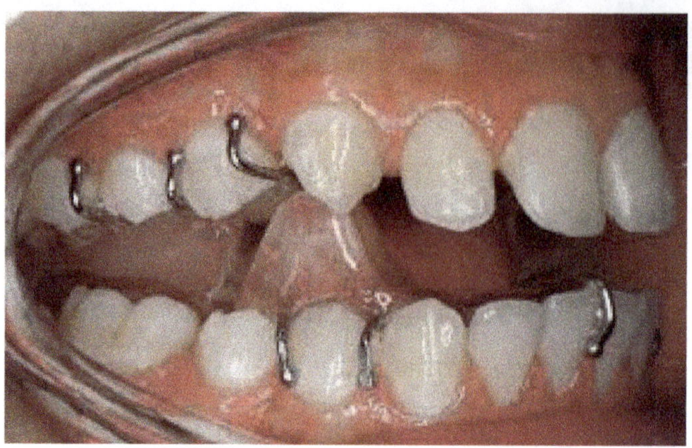

Figure 12. Twin-block appliance

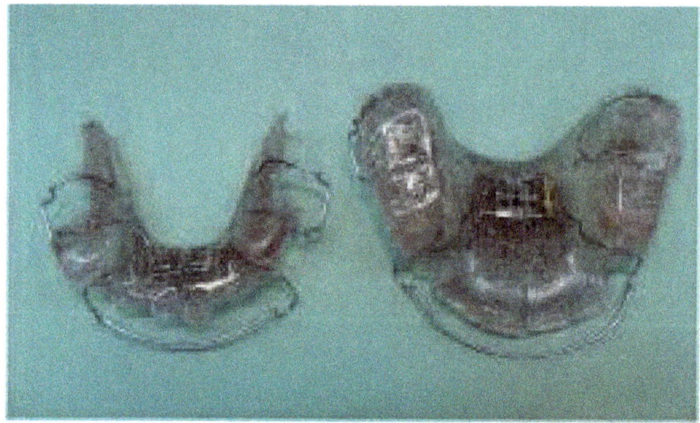

Figure 13. Expansion screw within Twin block appliance

demonstrate significant influences on mandibular growth [56], the others claim that it may be induced only small skeletal changes by this type of treatment [57]. The latter group of researchers found that the main changes occurred with functional appliance therapy were dentoalveolar distalization of the buccal and retroclination of the frontal upper teeth, along with mesial movement of the lower buccal segments and proclination of the lower labial segments[58]. Such diversity of results on skeletal changes might be related first of all to difficulties in applying treatment at the maximum growth spurt time. Another reason for the inconsistence in assessment of treatment results might be the use of not reliable reference lines and/or structures for cephalometric analysis before and after treatment. This makes difficult to assess real contribution of skeletal and dental components to occlusal changes [59]. A new paradigm for successful treatment presents a philosophical challenge to combine the benefits of orthodontic and orthopedic techniques to extend our horizons in the treatment of malocclusion that requires dental and skeletal correction.

The prefabricated myofunctional appliances are a series of prefabricated appliances produced by myoresearch company, Queensland, Australia. These appliances were also called "Trainers™" which include T4K™ and T4F™ appliances (Fig.14,15). The idea of prefabricated functional appliances was recently introduced to the orthodontic field and it becomes more practical with the new customizable functional appliance T4F™. The T4F™ appliance is a prefabricated re-mouldable appliance when immersed in very hot water so it can be customized to accommodate the patient's dentition in the mouth and increase the retention. This new functional appliance has the advantage of the immediate issuing and the direct fitting of the appliance in the patient's mouth and it is also a better choice in terms of the cost for the private practitioners. The prefabricated appliances were claimed to be effective for class II Div.1 management but there was no evidence except for T4K™ type which is designed for young children.

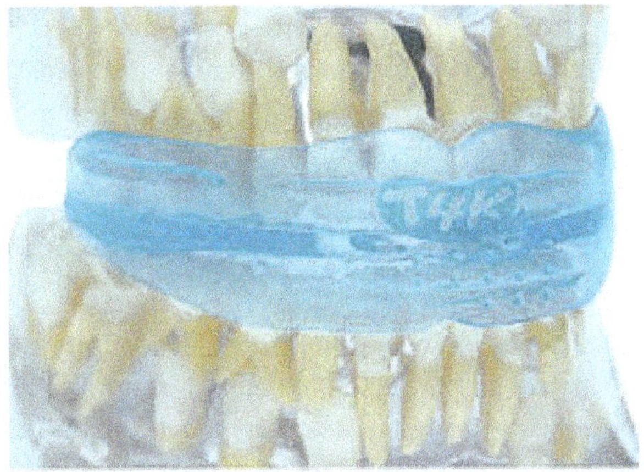

Figure 14. T4K™ The Pre-Orthodontic Trainer

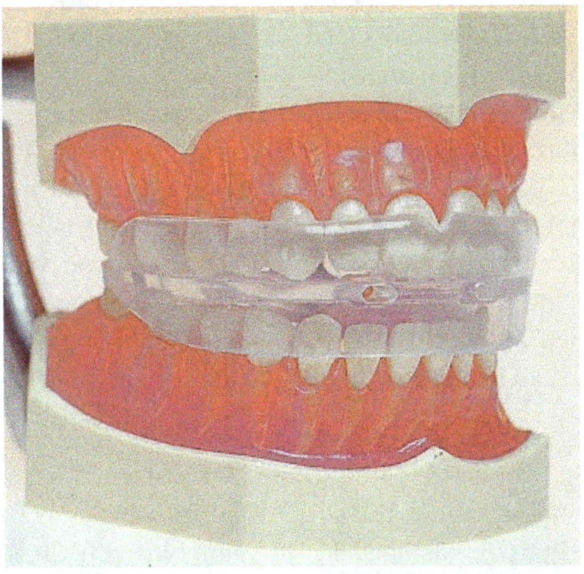

Figure 15. T4F™ The Pre-Orthodontic Trainer

Uysal et al., 2012, evaluated the effects of Pre-Orthodontic Trainer (T4F™) appliance on the anterior temporal, mental, orbicularis oris, and masseter muscles through electromyography (EMG) evaluations in subjects with Class II division 1 malocclusion and incompetent lips. Twenty patients (mean age: 9.8 ± 2.2 years) with a Class II division 1 malocclusion were treated with T4F™ (Myofunctional Research Co., Queensland, Australia). A group of 15 subjects (mean age: 9.2 ± 0.9 years) with untreated Class II division 1 malocclusions was used as a control. EMG recordings of treatment group were taken at the beginning and at the end of the T4F™ therapy (mean treatment period: 7.43 ± 1.06 months). Follow-up records of the control group were taken after 8 months of the first records. Recordings were taken during different oral functions: clenching, sucking, and swallowing. Statistical analyses were undertaken with Wilcoxon and Mann-Whitney U-tests. During the T4F™ treatment, activity of anterior temporal, mental, and masseter muscles was decreased and orbicularis oris activity was increased during clenching and these differences were found statistically significant when compared to control. Orbicularis oris activity during sucking was increased in the treatment group ($P < 0.05$). In the control group, significant changes were determined for anterior temporal ($P < 0.05$) and masseter ($P < 0.01$) muscle at clenching and orbicularis oris muscle at swallowing during observation period ($P< 0.05$). Findings indicated that treatment with T4F™ appliance showed a positive influence on the masticatory and perioral musculature [60].

Usumez et al., 2004, evaluated the dentoskeletal treatment effects induced by a preorthodontic trainer appliance (T4K™) treatment on Class II, division 1 cases. Twenty patients (10 girls and 10 boys, mean age 9.6+/-1.3 years) with a Class II, division 1 malocclusion were treated with T4K™ (Myofunctional Research Co., Queensland, Australia). The patients were instructed to use the trainer every day for one hour and overnight while they slept. A control group of 20 patients (mean age 10.2+/-0.8 years) with untreated Class II, division 1 malocclusions was used to eliminate possible growth effects. Lateral cephalograms were taken at the start and end of treatment. Final cephalograms were taken 13.1+/-1.8 months after trainer application, compared with a mean of 11.2+/-2.4 months later for the control group. The mean and standard deviations for cephalometric measurements were analyzed by paired-samples t-test and independent-samples t-tests. At the end of the study period, the trainer group subjects showed significant changes including anterior rotation and sagittal growth of the mandible, increased SNB and facial height, reduced ANB, increased lower incisor proclination, retroclination of upper incisors, and overjet reduction. However, only total facial height increase, lower incisor proclination, and overjet reduction were significantly higher when compared with the changes observed in the control group. This study was the first that demonstrated that the preorthodontic trainer application induces basically dentoalveolar changes that result in significant reduction of overjet and can be used with appropriate patient selection [61].

In a very recent study, Dr. Hanoun and his colleagues evaluated the effectiveness of the prefabricated myofunctional appliance T4F™ (compared to Twin Block appliance) in the treatment of Class II Div.1 malocclusion. The study was a prospective randomized clinical trial. All subjects were growing patients aged 11 -14 years old with Class II Div.1 malocclusion based on Class II skeletal relationship with overjet of 7 mm or more. Those subjects who had anterior open bite or previous orthodontic therapy or craniofacial anomalies or history of facial trauma were all excluded from the trial. The overjet was reduced more favourably in the Twin Block group than in the T4F™ group with a mean difference between the two groups of 2.14 mm (p <0.01). Moreover, there was a significant difference between both groups in terms of horizontal skeletal linear dimensions of the mandible with more favourable increase in the Twin Block group ($p < 0.05$).

11. Conclusion

Interceptive orthodontics is employed to recognize and eliminate potential irregularities and malposition in the developing dentofacial complex. These procedures are directed to lessen or to eliminate the severity of developing malocclusion. The early assessment of the child, followed by regular review, and treatment at the appropriate time if necessary, will do much to reduce malocclusion to the basic non-preventable level. The key to prevention of this kind is awareness. This part examines the key areas relating to interceptive orthodontics with the available evidence to support the clinical management of common problems presenting in the mixed dentition.

Acknowledgements

I offer my sincerest gratitude to my wife, Mrs. Huda Zurigat who has supported me throughout my project with a lot of patience and enthusiasm. Her assistance in typing and organizing words and figures in this article was indispensible.

Author details

Maen H. Zreaqat*

Address all correspondence to: maenzreqat@yahoo.com

Al-Ogaly Medical Group, Saudi Arabia

References

[1] Weinberger BW. Historical résumé of the evolution and growth of orthodontia. J Am Dent Assoc 1934;21:201-221.

[2] Asbell MB. A brief history of orthodontics. Am J Orthod Dentofacial Orthop 1990;98:176-83.

[3] Casto FM. A historical sketch of orthodontia. Dent Cosmos 1934;76:111-35.

[4] Brodie AG. Orthodontic history and what it teaches. Angle Orthod 1934;4:85-97.

[5] Irurita J, Alemán I, López-Lázaro S, Viciano J, Botella MC. Chronology of the development of the deciduous dentition in Mediterranean population. Forensic Sci Int. 2014;240:95-103.

[6] Borrie F, Bonetti D, Bearn D. What influences the implementation of interceptive orthodontics in primary care? Br Dent J. 2014;216(12):687-91.

[7] Kerosuo H1, Väkiparta M, Nyström M, Heikinheimo K. The seven-year outcome of an early orthodontic treatment strategy. J Dent Res. 2008;87(6):584-8.

[8] Norman W. Orthodontics in 3 millennia. Chapter 12: Two controversies: Early treatment and occlusion Am J Orthod Dentofacial Orthop. 2006;130(6):799-804.

[9] Baroni C; Franchini A; Rimondini L: Survival of different types of space maintainers. Pediatr Dent. 1994;16:360-61.

[10] Kirzioglu Z, Ozay MS Z, Ozay MS. Success of reinforced fibre material space maintainers. J Dent Child. 2004;71;2:158-62.

[11] Kargul B, Caglar E, Kabalay U. Glass fibre reinforced composite resin as fixed space maintainer in children 12 month clinical follow up. J Dent Child. 2005; 72(3):109-12

[12] Kargul B, Çaglar E, Kabalay U. Glass fiber-reinforced composite resin space maintainer: case reports. J Dent Child. 2003;71:258-61.

[13] Goldberg AJ, Frelich MA. Tooth splinting and stabilisation Dent Clin North Am. 1999; 43 (1) :127-33.

[14] Setia V, Pandit IK, Srivastava N, Gugnani N, Sekhon HK. Space maintainers in dentistry: past to present. J Clin Diagn Res. 2013;7(10):2402-5.

[15] Kharbanda O. P, Sidhu S. S, Sundaram K, Shukla D. K, "Oral habits in school going children of Delhi: a prevalence study," Journal of the Indian Society of Pedodontics and Preventive Dentistry. 2003; 21 (3): 120–124.

[16] Larson EF. The prevalence and etiology of prolonged dumy and finger sucking habit. Am. J. Orthod., 1985; 87(5):172-174.

[17] Farsi NM, Salama FS.. Sucking habits in Saudi children: prevalence, contributing factors and effects on the primary dentition. Pediatr. Dent. 1997; 19(1):28-33.

[18] N. L. Villa, "Changes in the dentition secondary to palatal crib therapy in digit-suckers: a preliminary study," Pediatric Dentistry, vol. 19, no. 5, pp. 323–326, 1997.

[19] B. S. Haskell and J. R. Mink, "An aid to stop thumb sucking: the "Bluegrass" appliance," Pediatric Dentistry. 1991; 13 (2): 83– 85.

[20] Van Norman RA (1997). Digit-sucking: A review of the literature, clinical observations and treatment recommendations. Int. J. Orofacial Myol., 23: 14-34

[21] Warren JJ, Bishara SE (2002). Duration of nutritive and nonnutritive sucking behavior and their effects on the dental arches in the primary dentition. Am. J. Orthod., 121: 347-356.

[22] Moimaz SA, Garbin AJ, Lima AM, Lolli LF, Saliba O, Garbin CA. Longitudinal study of habits leading to malocclusion development in childhood. BMC Oral Health. 2014;(4):14-96.

[23] Maia-Nader M, Silva de Araujo Figueiredo C, Pinheiro de Figueiredo F, Moura da Silva AA, Thomaz EB, Saraiva MC, Barbieri MA, Bettiol H. Factors associated with prolonged non-nutritive sucking habits in two cohorts of Brazilian children. BMC Public Health. 2014;14:14-17.

[24] Fleming PJ, Blaive PS Pacifier use an sudden infant death syndrome. Arch. Dis. Children. 1999; 81(2): 112-116.

[25] Lopes TS, Moura Lde F, Lima MC. Breastfeeding and sucking habits in children enrolled in a mother-child health program. BMC Res Notes. 2014;14(7): 23-38.

[26] Tanaka OM, Vitral RW, Tanaka GY, Guerrero AP, Camargo ES. (. Nailbiting, or onychophagia: A special habit. Am. J. Orthod. Dentofacial Orthop. 2008;134(2): 305-308.

[27] Saheeb D. Prevalence of oral and parafunctional habits in Nigerian patients suffering temporomandibular joint pain and dysfunftion. J. Med. Biomed. Res., (2005; 4(1): 59-64

[28] Feu D1, Menezes LM, Quintão AP, Quintão CC. A customized method for palatal crib fabrication. J Clin Orthod. 2013 Jul;47(7):406-12.

[29] Kato T, Thein NMR, Montplaisir JY, Lavigne GJ. Bruxism and orofacial movements during sleep. Dent. Clin. North Am. 2001;45(4):651-676.

[30] Hublin C, Kaprio J, Partinen M, Koskenvuo M. Sleep bruxism based on self – report in a nationwide twin cohort. Sleep Res. 1998;7(1): 61-68

[31] Dahan JS, Lelong BA, Celant S, Leysen V. Oral perception in tounge thrust and other oral habits. Am. J. Orthod. Dentofacial Orthop., 2000;118:385-91.

[32] Pierce CJ, Gale EN. A comparison of different treatments for nocturnal bruxism. J. Dent. Res., 1988;67: 597-601.

[33] Ferreira NM, Dos Santos JF, Dos Santos MB, Marchini L. Sleep bruxism associated with obstructive sleep apnea syndrome in children. Cranio. 2014 Sep [Epub ahead of print].

[34] Major PW, Glover K. Treatment of anterior cross-bites in the early mixed dentition. Journal of the Canadian Dental Association. 1992;58(7):574–578.

[35] Bayrak S1, Tunc ES. Treatment of anterior dental crossbite using bonded resin-composite slopes: case reports. Eur J Dent. 2008;2(4):303-6.

[36] Yaseen SM, Acharya R. Hexa Helix:Modified Quad Helix Appliance to Correct Anterior and Posterior Crossbites in Mixed Dentition. Case Reports in Dentistry. 2012: 1-5.

[37] Wiedel AP1, Bondemark L. Stability of anterior crossbite correction: A randomized controlled trial with a 2-year follow-up. Angle Orthod. 2014 Jul 8. [Epub ahead of print]

[38] Sanin C, Sekiguchi T, Savara BS. A clinical method for the prediction of closure of the central diastema. ASDC J Dent Child 1969; 36: 415–418.

[39] Baum AT. The midline diastema. J Oral Med 1966; 21: 30–39.

[40] Nainar SM, Gnanasundaram N. Incidence and etiology of midlinediastema in a population in southIndia (Madras). Angle Orthod 1989; 59: 277–282.

[41] Angle EH. Treatment of Malocclusion of the Teeth 7th edn. Philadelphia: SS White Dental Manufacturing Company, 1907: p167.

[42] Sicher H. Oral Anatomy 2nd edn. St Louis: CV Mosby Co, 1952: pp272–273.

[43] Edwards JG. The diastema, the frenum, the frenectomy: a clinical study. Am J Orthod 1977; 71:489–508.

[44] Popovich F, Thompson GW, Main PA. Persisting maxillary diastema: indications for treatment. Am JOrthod 1979; 75(4): 399–404.

[45] Proffit WR, Fields HW. Contemporary Orthodontics 2nd edn. St Louis: Mosby Yearbook, 1993: p467

[46] Shashua D, Artun J. Relapse afterorthodontic correction of maxillarymedian diastema: a follow-up evaluation of consecutive cases. Angle Orthod 1999; 69: 257–263.

[47] Nagalakshmi S, Sathish R, Priya K, Dhayanithi D. Changes in quality of life during orthodontic correction of midline diastema. J Pharm Bioallied Sci. 2014 (Suppl 1): 162-4

[48] Almeida RR, Almeida MR, Oltramari-Navarro PV, Conti AC, Navarro Rde L, Souza KR. Serial extraction: 20 years of follow-up. J Appl Oral Sci. 2012; 20(4):486-92.

[49] Hotz P.R. Guidance of eruption versus serial extraction. Am. J. Orthod, 1970; 58(1): 1-20.

[50] Nagalakshmi S, Sathish R, Priya K, Dhayanithi D. Changes in quality of life during orthodontic correction of midline diastema. J Pharm Bioallied Sci. 2014; 6 (Suppl 1):. [Epub ahead of print]

[51] Lee KP. The fallacy of serial extractions. Aust Orthod J. 2013;29(2):217-21.

[52] Almeida RR, Almeida MR, Oltramari-Navarro PV, Conti AC, Navarro Rde L, Souza KR. Serial extraction: 20 years of follow-up. J Appl Oral Sci. 2012 Jul-Aug;20(4): 486-92.

[53] Baume, L. J. Cephalo-facial growth patterns and the functional adaptation of the temporo-mandibular joint structures. Eur Orthod Soc Trans, 1969: 79—98.

[54] Calvert, F. J. () An assessment of Andresen therapy on Class II Division I malocclusion. Br J Orthodk 1982; 9: 149-153.

[55] Hamilton, S. D., Sinclair, P. M. & Hamilton, R. H. A cephalometric, tomographic and dental cast evaluation of Frankei therapy. Am J Orthod. 1987; 92: 427-434.

[56] Pancherz H. A cephalometric analysis of skeletal and dental changes contributing to Class II correction in activator treatment. Am J Orthod 1984;85:125-134

[57] Mills C, McCulloch K. Treatment effects of the Twin-block appliance: a cephalometric study. Am J Orthod 1998;114:15-24.

[58] Windmiller EC. Acrylic splint Herbst appliance: cephalometric evaluation. Am J Orthod Dentofac Orthop 1993;104:73-84.

[59] Baccetti T. et al. Treatment timing for Twin-block therapy. Am J Orthod dentofacial Orhop 2000;118:159-70.

[60] Usumez S, Uysal T, Sari Z, Basciftci FA, Karaman AI, Guray E. The effects of early preorthodontic trainer treatment on Class II, division 1 patients. Angle Orthod. 2004 Oct;74(5):605-9.

[61] Uysal T1, Yagci A, Kara S, Okkesim S. Influence of pre-orthodontic trainer treatment on the perioral and masticatory muscles in patients with Class II division 1 malocclusion. Eur J Orthod. 2012 34(1):96-101

[62] Hanoun AB, Khamis MF Mokhtar N. The effectiveness of the prefabricated myofunctional appliance T4FTM in comparison with Twin Block (TB) appliance in the treatment of Class II Div.1 malocclusion. A randomized clinical trial. Master thesis. School of Dental Sciences, University Science Malaysia, 2014.

6

3D Scanning, Imaging, and Printing in Orthodontics

Emilia Taneva, Budi Kusnoto and Carla A. Evans

1. Introduction

Evolving technology and integration of digital solutions in private practice have transformed diagnosis and treatment planning from a traditional two-dimensional (2D) approach into an advanced three-dimensional (3D) technique. The use of digital technology meets the demand of multiple-doctor practices, multiple practice locations, patient volume growth, and allows efficient and convenient storage, retrieval, and sharing of information. Orthodontics is rapidly embracing new materials and advanced technologies, making the fully equipped 3D orthodontic office a reality. Recent developments and introduction of intraoral and facial scanners, digital radiology, cone-beam computed tomography (CBCT), and additive manufacturing improved the efficiency, accuracy, consistency, and predictability of the treatment outcomes. All those daily advances also led to a rapid growth of digital educational components and teaching tools, 3D video presentations and patient communication.

Computer-aided design and computer-aided manufacturing (CAD/CAM) systems were first used in the dental field in the mid-1980s. CAD/CAM consists of three key components: 1) data acquisition and digitizing; 2) data processing and design; and 3) manufacturing [1]. As computer software and dental materials evolved over time, the CAD/CAM technology became increasingly popular resulting in chairside design and milling of high-quality complete crowns and multiple-unit ceramic restorations. The advent of digital intraoral impression devices allowed high-resolution 3D virtual models to be captured. Intraoral mapping based on different non-contact optical principles and technologies is now possible without the negative aspects of dental impressions such as discomfort for the patient, imprecision, and lab work. In-office chairside or send to the lab, the digital models give the flexible options for design and manufacture of a large range of dental restorations, implants, study models, and orthodontic appliances such as customized indirect brackets, arch wires, expanders, aligners, retainers, etc. (Figure 1). The highly-accurate open file formats are incorporated in the patient electronic health record which can be remotely stored, accessed, and managed through a secure, cloud-based digital hub from basically anywhere. Most digital intraoral scanners work in conjunction with cloud based technology where raw images once scanned can be securely transmitted to the cloud storage facility and further processed/refined for diagnostic purposes.

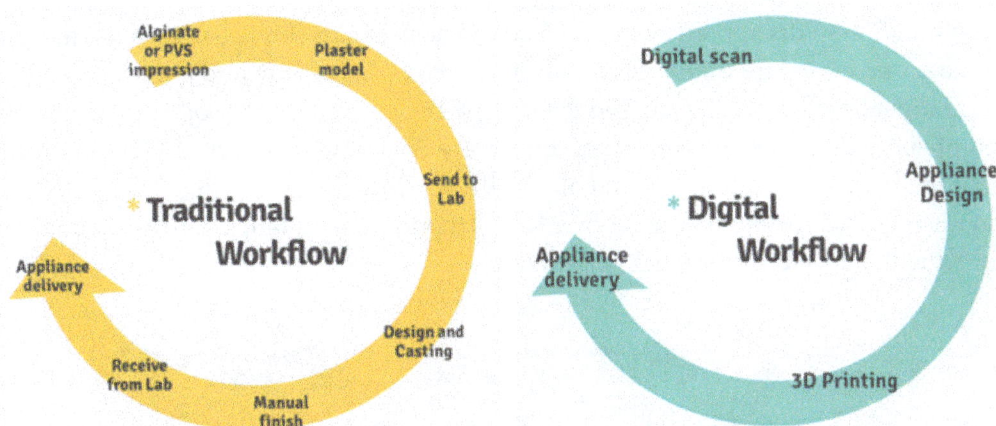

Figure 1. Traditional versus digital workflow in the orthodontic office

Cloud computing has significantly influenced the healthcare industry in the past years. The concept provides massive amounts of storage and computing power without requiring end-user special knowledge about the physical location and the configuration of the system [2]. The information technology enables convenient, on-demand access at a greater speed in less time to a shared pool of computer resources (network, server, database, software, storage, and applications). Hospitals, medical practices, insurance companies, and research facilities are now transitioning certain infrastructures to cloud services and mobile apps in order to improve the management and administration efficiency at a reduced cost. The cloud healthcare system, named hCloud, was specifically developed to address the requirements for highest level of availability, security, and privacy protection in healthcare [2]. Facilitated by hClouds, medical records and image archiving services can be synchronized and shared between healthcare organizations, medical professionals, clinics, and patients in real time on a daily basis. The file systems and employed structures are easily adaptable to since they are open, industry-standard formats instead of proprietary, closed formats.

2. Value of digital models

Plaster casts have a long and proven history as a routine dental record and have been the gold standard for dentition analysis for years. Nevertheless, plaster models have several disadvantages including labor-intensive work, demand on physical storage space, fragility, degradation, and problems of potential loss during transfer [3].

Digital study models offer a reliable alternative to traditional plaster models (Figure 2). Their advantages in orthodontic diagnosis and treatment planning include easy and fast electronic transfer of data, immediate access, and reduced storage requirement [4]. Digital models can be integrated into various patient management systems, digital records, along with the digital photographs, radiographs, and clinical notes. Digital models may be virtually manipulated to section and analyze specific teeth, arch form, amount of crowding or spacing, and type of malocclusion. Measurements such as overjet, overbite, tooth size, arch length, transverse distances, and Bolton discrepancy are achievable. The user can obtain a digital diagnostic set-up, simulate a proposed treatment plan, perform bracket placement, and indirect bonding [5]. CBCT and digital models can be merged to facilitate treatment planning of orthognathic cases, creation of surgical guides, placement of temporary anchorage devices (TADs), exposure of impacted teeth, or preparation for dental prostheses. Moreover, if a physical model of the dentition is required for the manufacture of an orthodontic appliance, digital models can be 3D printed with a rapid prototyping technology.

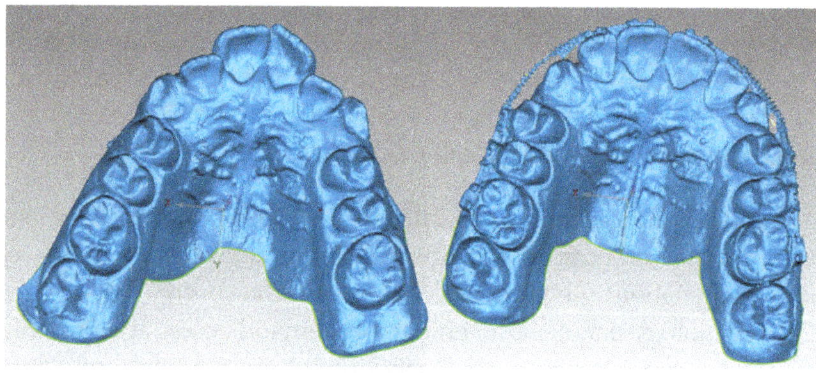

Figure 2. 3D digital models of the upper dental arch in Geomagic® (3D Systems, Cary, NC, USA). The software is an aid in the CAD/CAM process, able to repair errors in the mesh prior to 3D printing, edit the models, and design appliances.

Digital models were commercially introduced in 1999 by OrthoCAD™ (Cadent, Carlstadt, NJ). The results from a recent survey conducted by the Journal of Clinical Orthodontics demonstrated a significant increase in the use of digital models for pre-treatment diagnosis and treatment from 6.6% in 2002 to 18% in 2008 [6]. Today, many orthodontists acquire digital models through the use of proprietary services. Traditional impressions, plaster models, or intraoral scans are submitted to the selected company so that they can generate the digital models and made them available for download in proprietary or stereolithography (STL) file format. STL is an open, industry-standard file format that is supported by most intraoral scanners and widely used for rapid prototyping, computer-aided manufacturing, and across different 3D modeling interfaces. Another open file format is PLY, polygon file format (also known as Stanford triangle format), which is used when color and/or transparency information is needed.

Commercially available digital models may be obtained by a direct or an indirect method [5]. The direct method makes dental impressions redundant by using an intraoral scanner to capture directly in the patient's mouth. Indirectly, digital models can be produced by scanning alginate impressions and plaster models with a desktop scanner, intraoral scanner, or computed tomography imaging.

There are no universal standards for defining model accuracy. However, in orthodontics, it is generally accepted that measurement accuracy up to 0.1 mm is adequate for clinical purposes and does not compromise the diagnostic value of a model. Numerous studies have evaluated the reliability of stereolithographic models obtained by indirect methods by assessing the agreement of measurements on plaster and digital models [7-10]. It has been shown in the literature that digital models have clinically insignificant differences for reproducibility of orthodontic measurements. Tooth size has been found to be similar or slightly smaller in OrthoCAD™ compared to measurements made on plaster models. Overjet measurements were not significantly different in some studies however Quimby et al. (2004) found a significantly smaller overjet measurement when obtained with OrthoCAD™. Space available or arch length to be used in estimating crowding, demonstrated to be significantly different between OrthoCAD™ models and plaster models with differences ranging from 0.4 mm to 2.88 mm [9]. Laser-scanned models are suggested to be highly accurate in comparison to plaster models and CBCT scans and provide clinicians an alternative to physical models and CBCT reconstructions in diagnosis and treatment planning [10]. Both CBCT and intraoral scanning of alginate impressions were concluded to be valid and reliable methods to obtain measurements for orthodontic diagnostic purposes [11,12]. Furthermore, different digital model conversion techniques have shown no statistically mean differences when using 3D palatal rugae landmarks for comparison. 3D digital models are also proven as an effective tool in evaluating palatal rugae patterns for human verification and identification [13].

3. Intraoral scanners

3.1. Overview

Three-dimensional digital impressions were first introduced in 1987 by CEREC 1 (Siemens, Munich, Germany) using infrared camera and optical powder on the teeth to create a virtual model. Over the years, computer hardware and software developments have dramatically improved the technologies completely replacing traditional alginate and polyvinyl siloxane (PVS) impressions in a large number of dental and orthodontic offices. In most instances, production of precisely fitting final dental restorations no longer requires the use of a powder [14-16].

New intraoral scanners for acquisition of digital impressions are continuously entering the clinical practice all over the world. Improvements in the scanning technologies have resulted in truly portable cart-free systems with a single, forked USB cable that can be plugged into any workstation. Ergonomic design and reduction in wand size and weight have resulted in a more comfortable experience for both patients and staff. The optical scanners can be used to capture both in vivo images of the dentition and in vitro images of the physical models to create a 3D digital representation. Intraoral scanner devices offer numerous applications in orthodontics such as digital storage of study models and advanced software for cast analysis, landmark identification, arch width and length measurements, tooth segmentation, and evaluation of the occlusion [15]. The platforms allow clinicians to obtain a digital diagnostic set-up, perform indirect bonding, and export the digital scans into open source file formats. The electronic files are shared with third-party providers and imported into a variety of digital workflows for advanced treatment planning of surgical cases, implants, and superimposition with CBCT data.

3.2. Advantages

Traditional alginate and polyvinyl siloxane (PVS) impressions have been associated with numerous limitations which include complex workflow, lack of precise reproduction, lacerations on the margins, poor dimensional stability, limited working time, plaster pouring and solidification, and problems of transport and packaging. A general disadvantage of the conventional impressions is also the need to start over if an impression fails or take additional impressions (e.g. study models and appliance fabrication). In addition, the contact between the tray and the teeth could cause discomfort for the patient and trigger a bad gag reflex. Digital impressions eliminate all those negative aspects. They streamline and expedite the traditional workflow, reduce the number of patients' visits, and maximize the efficiency and cost savings in the orthodontic office [16]. Besides the better control and improved accuracy of the directly obtained digital models, scanners add the plug-and-play capability of an automatic exchange of patient information within the office or outside laboratories. Lost or broken appliances could easily be refabricated using the digital files from a database in the Cloud [2].

3.3. Optical scanning technologies

Several scanning technologies using different optical components and structured light sources are currently employed in orthodontics:

3.3.1. Confocal Laser Scanner Microscopy (CLSM)

Confocal laser scanning microscopy (CLSM or LSCM) is a technique for acquiring images with high-resolution and in-depth selectivity. Images are projected point-by-point, line-by-line, or multiple points at once and three-dimensionally reconstructed with a computer, rather than obtained through an eyepiece [18]. The key feature of confocal microscopy is its ability to produce optical slices of the objects at various depths with high resolution and contrast in the x, y, and z coordinates. Spatial filtering is employed to eliminate out-of-focus glare or light of background information. Change of display magnification and image spatial resolution, termed the zoom factor, is enabled by altering the scanning sampling period [17-19].

The basic principle of confocal microscopy was pioneered by Marvin Minsky in 1957 [17]. Advances in laser and computer technology coupled the new algorithms for digital manipulation of images in the late 1970s and 1980s, and led to an increasing interest in the technology which became a standard technique. Modern confocal microscopy systems integrate various components such as beam scanning mechanisms and wavelength selection devices which are often referred to as a video or digital imaging system [16]. It is now possible to employ these scanning technologies for multi-dimensional functional and structural analysis of molecules, living cells, and tissues.

3.3.2. Optical triangulation

Optical triangulation measures distance to objects without touching them with accuracy from a few millimeters to a few microns [20]. Triangulation sensors are particularly useful in acquiring high-speed data in inspecting delicate, soft, or wet materials where contacts are undesirable. The system uses a lens, a laser light source, and a linear light sensitive sensor [16]. The laser irradiates a point on a specimen forming a light spot image on the sensor surface. The distance from the sensor to the surface is then calculated by determining the position of the imaged spot and the baseline angles and length involved. The principle of triangulation has been used for centuries but practical sensors became available for industrial applications in 1971. Triangulation sensors are commonly used for monitoring vibrations, tire dimensions while rotating at high speed, and as a safety mechanism in automatic doors [20-22].

3.3.3. Optical Coherence Tomography (OCT)

Optical coherence tomography (OCT) is an interferometric technique that performs cross-sectional high-resolution imaging of the internal morphology of biological materials and tissues [23]. It is equivalent to ultrasound imaging, except that it uses light instead of sound. Micron-scale measurements of distance and microstructure are obtained from backscattered or backreflected light waves in real time and in vivo. Although OCT imaging depths are not as deep as with ultrasound, resolution of 1 to 15 μm can be achieved, 10 to 100 times higher than standard clinical ultrasound. The relatively long wavelength light is able to penetrate into the scattering medium up to 2-3 mm deep in most tissues [16,24]. OCT has become a well-established medical diagnostic technique after being first demonstrated in 1991. It is now widely used in ophthalmology, gastroenterology, and cardiology and can be successfully applied where standard excisional biopsy is not possible or hazardous [25].

3.3.4. Accordion Fringe Interferometry (AFI)

Accordion fringe interferometry (AFI) employs a revolutionary linear interferometry technology that traditionally projects to three dimensions [16]. AFI delivers the most precise laser fringe projection available which quickly digitizes the shapes of 3D objects with the highest accuracy of point cloud data. AFI employs laser beams from two point sources to illumine the objects and uses a charge-coupled device (CCD) camera to capture the curvature of the borders [26]. AFI is less sensitive to ambient light which gives the ability to capture and measure a wider variety of surface coatings, textures, and finishes than structured light. AFI is suitable for a wide range of applications that require high speed, portability, and infinite projector depth of field from a 3D digital system. The AFI approach has already been implemented in automotive and aviation industries, reverse engineering, tool inspection, analysis, and fabrication [27].

3.3.5. Active Wavefront Sampling (AWS)

Active wavefront sampling (AWS) uses a 3D surface imaging technique, which requires only one optical path of an AWS module and a single camera to acquire depth information [28]. The optical wavefront traversing a lens is sampled at two or more off-axis locations and a single image is recorded and measured at each position. Target feature image rotation can be used to calculate the feature's distance to the camera [29]. The aperture sampling can be implemented mechanically or electronically and different components can be modified for better performance. Aperture size, target illumination, and sampling plane position can be optimized in order to maximize the captured image quality. AWS reduces system cost by eliminating the need for expensive laser based target illuminators and multiple cameras to acquire 3D images [16]. That allows the technique to be applied in a wide range of currently available 2D systems such as cameras, endoscopes, and microscopes [30].

3.4. Scanning systems

Table 1 summarizes some of the characteristics of several intraoral scanning systems used in orthodontics.

3.4.1. iTero®, Align Technology

The iTero® digital impression scanner was developed by Cadent Ltd. in 2006, and acquired by Align Technology, Inc. (San Jose, CA) in 2011 [15]. iTero® employs confocal laser scanner microscopy technique. The device projects 100,000 parallel beams of red laser light which pass through a probing face and a focusing optics to reach the teeth. The reflected light is then transformed into digital data through the use of analog-to-digital converters. The system scanning capability does not require coating the teeth in powder thereby allowing the wand rest directly on the teeth during scanning. One disadvantage is that the iTero® camera needs a color wheel attached to the acquisition unit, which results in a larger and bulky scanner head in comparison to other systems.

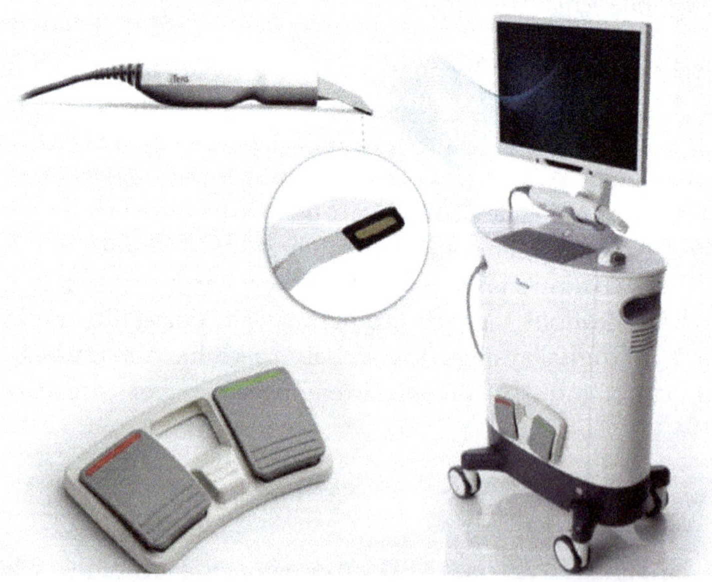

Figure 3. The iTero® Intraoral digital scanner [31]

iTero® comes as a mobile cart containing a central processing unit, large working surface with a touch screen display, a wireless mouse, a wireless foot pedal, a built-in keyboard, and a scanning wand (Figure 3) [31]. The intraoral scanner features continuous and click to capture scan mode; rendering in traditional stone color and true-color models; and optional voice guidance and visual commands. Digital images for orthodontic treatment are captured by proceeding through upper and lower quadrants [32]. Five different views of the scan area are required: buccal, occlusal, lingual, and the proximal surfaces between adjacent teeth. Overall, complete full mouth scan and a bite registration can take about 10 to 15 minutes. In a two-year study including 328 scans, it has been reported that the fastest intraoral scan can take 6 minutes and 22 seconds and the longest almost 18 minutes [33]. At the end of the scanning process, a line of diagnostic tools are available to assess and finalize the impression. Additional scans can be added to any areas of incomplete data. The final digital models are stored in the online MyAligntech database under the service provider profile and are available for export in the STL open file format.

3.4.2. True Definition, 3M ESPE

The 3M True Definition scanner was officially launched in 2013 as an updated version of the Lava™ chairside oral scanner which has been widely used in general and restorative dentistry since 2006 (Figure 4) [34]. The True Definition scanner captures 3D images using active wavefront sampling on the principle of structured light projection. 3M ESPE named this scanning technique "3D-in-motion video technology" [15]. The system employs a rotating aperture element placed off-axis in the optical apparatus either in the imaging or the illumination path which measures the defocus blur diameter. The user should first dry and lightly dust with powder the entire arch so the scanner can locate the reference points.

The True Definition features an ergonomic scanning wand and a rolling card with a HP® high-performance CPU computer unit with 22" touch screen monitor. The lightweight, stainless steel wand has a dental handpiece design with an on/off tap switch with no moving parts. Video imagery is captured at 20 frames per second and a complete full mouth scan with a bite registration take about 5 to 8 minutes. Upon completion, digital models are available immediately for 3D setup review, analysis, superimposition, enhanced measurements, and treatment planning. Unlimited patient scans can be stored in the Unitek™ treatment management portal allowing direct communication between the provider and the company customer service [34]. Open STL files are available for download, importing into a variety of digital workflows, and sharing with third-party providers.

3.4.3. Lythos™, Ormco Corporation

The Lythos™ Digital Impression System was introduced by Ormco Corporation (Orange, CA) in 2013. The intraoral scanner uses accordion fringe interferometry technology to capture and stitch together a 3D data in real time, acquiring high-definition details at all angulations of the tooth surface. Lythos™ provides 3D video imagery of 2.5 million points per second [35].

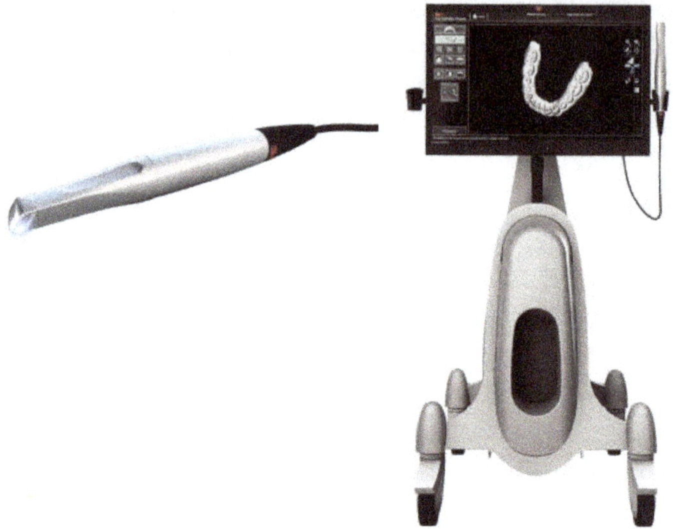

Figure 4. The 3M™ True Definition Scanner [34]

The Lythos™ scanner is portable, weighs around 13 kg, and can be positioned directly on the ground or on a chairside table (Figure 5). The device platform features an extendable touch screen monitor with wireless internet connectivity and a lightweight scanning wand.

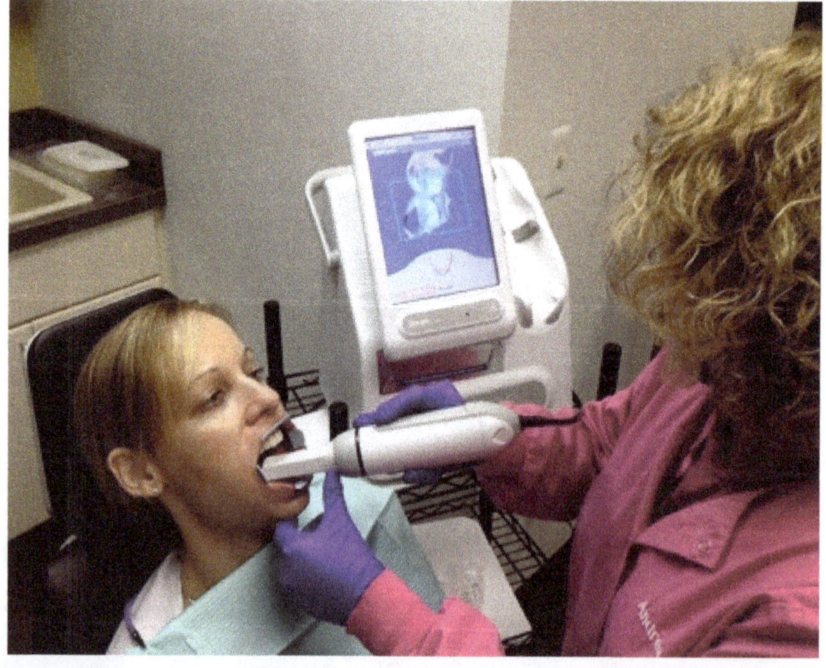

Figure 5. The Lythos™ Digital Impression System [36]

The touch screen helps in guiding the ward. First, the lower dental arch is scanned followed by the upper arch by pointing the tip of the wand on the occlusal surface and moving it from left to right [15]. The instantaneously displayed data are captured until missing regions are scanned or the results are satisfactory to the person who is scanning. The software also offers a capability to erase unwanted or accidently scanned regions. A dual-arch high-resolution scan can be completed in approximately 7 minutes. Ormco allows users to own and store the digital impressions on the company online portal, or send treatment scans to anyone that accepts STL files.

3.4.4. *CS 3500, Carestream*

Carestream Dental (Atlanta, GA) launched the portable digital impression system, CS 3500, at the end of 2013 (Figure 6). The scanner employs confocal laser scanner microscopy technique which allows capture of true-color 2D and high-angulation 3D scans of up to 45º with a depth of field of -2 to 13 mm [37]. The image resolution is 1024 x 728 pixels and the accuracy measures up to 30 microns. The system is trolley-free and uses a wand with a single, forked USB cable that can be plugged in any computer, eliminating the need for a dedicated workstation. Two scanning tip sizes are included to accommodate children and adults.

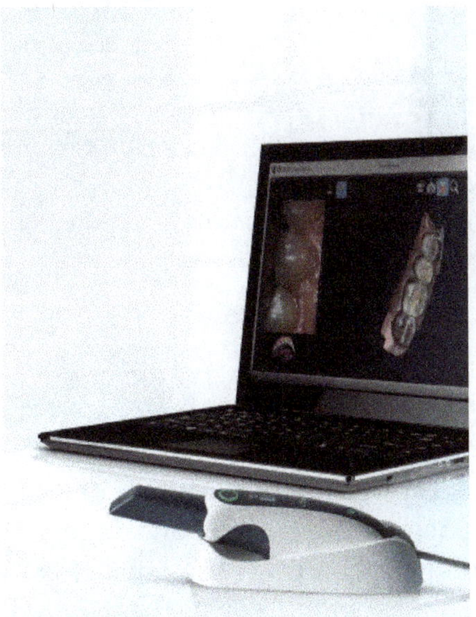

Figure 6. The CS 3500 Intraoral Scanner [37]

A built-in heater streamlines scanning by preventing mirror fogging. No external heater or powder is required. CS 3500 features a light system which guides the user during the data capture and the image acquisition process [15, 16]. The green light indicates a successful scan while the amber light shows that a rescanning of the area is needed. A full impression typically takes about 10 minutes. CS 3500 is compatible with open source software or it can work as part of the integrated Carestream CAD/CAM dental restorations system.

3.4.5. *TRIOS®, 3Shape*

3Shape (Copenhagen, Denmark) announced the TRIOS® intraoral scanning solution in December 2010 (Figure 7). The system operates by the principle of confocal microscopy, with a fast-scan rate [38]. Hundreds to thousands of 3D pictures, corresponding to different time instances and to respective different positions of the focus plane of the illumination pattern, are combined to create the final 3D digital impression. The high-definition camera features teeth shade measurement and provides scans in enhanced natural colors or in a standard noncolor pattern [16]. The scanning wand does not require the use of powder, has an autoclavable tip and an anti-fog heater. It takes approximately 5 minutes for a full mouth scan.

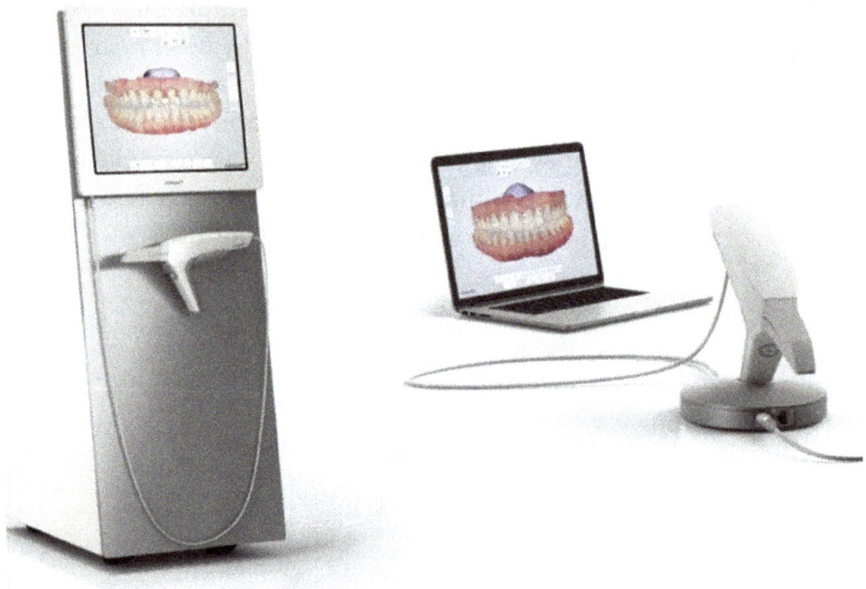

Figure 7. The 3Shape Intraoral Scanner is available as TRIOS® Cart or TRIOS® Pod configurations [38]

The 3Shape digital impression system is available as TRIOS® Cart, TRIOS® Chair integration, or TRIOS® Rod configuration. The TRIOS® Cart consists of a smart multi-touch screen which provides 3D visualization, video tutorials, Wi-Fi and Bluetooth connections, and technical support. The TRIOS® Rod configuration provides mobility by using USB connection to any computer or display. 3Shape offers Ortho Analyzer™ software for study model analysis and treatment planning which also stores cone-beam scans, patient photographs, panoramic x-rays, and cephalometric tracings [38]. TRIOS® saves the digital impression scans in the standard STL file format.

3.4.6. *FastScan®, IOS Technologies*

Glidewell Laboratories' IOS FastScan® intraoral camera and modelling system was commercialized in July 2010 (Figure 8). The digital impression system uses the principle of active triangulation with sheet of light projection [16]. Ego-motion technology is used to optimize image stabilization by having the camera moving automatically on a track within the housing wand. That built-in motion detection software eliminates hand-movement distortion, capturing high-resolution surface detail. The camera scans 40 mm per second throughout a depth of field that is greater than 15 mm [39]. An application of titanium dioxide powder is required.

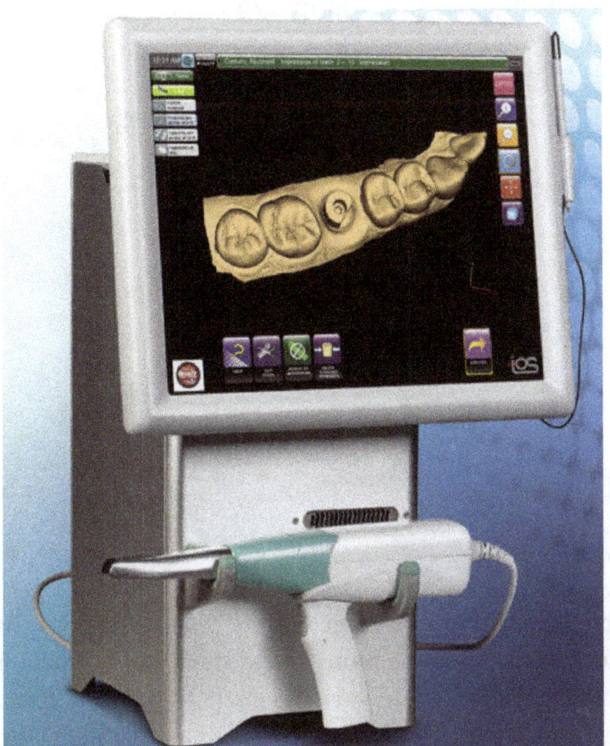

Figure 8. The FastScan® intraoral scanner [39]

FastScan® device is portable and consists of a touchscreen display and a large scanning area wand. A live 3D digital preview of the captured area is shown almost immediately. This feedback provides information about the wand positioning and orientation in relation to the patient's dentition and whether an adjustment is necessary. A full mouth scan and a bite registration can be obtained in about 4 minutes. The system is able to acquire color and translucent data along with the 3D anatomy of the dentition [39]. A single digital file combines the surface information, translucency, and color which can be stored or electronically sent to a CAD/CAM lab for an appliance fabrication. The output data is in the open source STL format which can be recognized, viewed, and manipulated by third party providers. *Unfortunately, FastScan® is no longer available on the market and the company is not planning to manufacture a replacement soon.*

3.4.7. 3D progress, MHT Optic research

The 3D Progress digital impression system is supplied by Medical Height Technology (MHT) company (Verona, Italy) and MHT Optic research (Zurich, Switzerland) (Figure 9). The technology beyond the product is a confocal scanning microscopy with a Moiré pattern detector [16]. A Smart pixel sensor supports precise and quick capture of up to 28 scans per second which are stitched in a single 3D image in less than one tenth of a second. 3D Progress allows a wide focus of acquisition, ranging between 0 to 18 mm depth of field [40]. The scanning process can be paused and re-started at any moment and parts of the scan can be modified or updated with new data acquisitions. A full mouth digital impression can be completed in approximately 4 minutes.

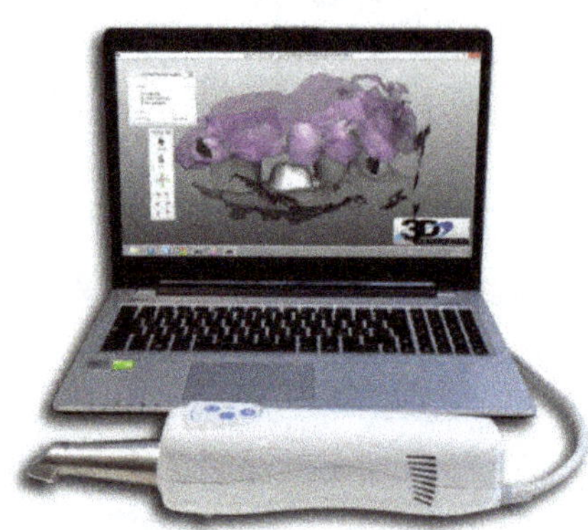

Figure 9. 3D Progress intraoral scanner [40]

3D Progress is portable, consisting of power supply and a light-weight wand which can be interfaced to a computer via USB connection. The system will not usually require powdering with exclusion of exceedingly reflective surfaces such as implant abutments [40]. Complete scans are generated as a point cloud which can be saved as digital 3D models in the usual STL open file format, compatible with all CAD systems.

3.4.8. Planmeca PlanScan®, E4D Technologies

Formerly known as the E4D NEVO scan and design system, the Planmeca PlanScan®, driven by E4D Technologies (Richardson, TX), is an intraoral scanner widely utilized in restorative dentistry (Figure 10). PlanScan® uses optical coherent tomography with blue laser technology [16]. Point-and-stitch image reconstruction occurs at video-rate scanning speed [41]. The single smaller wavelength of 450 nm is more reflective, capturing sharper images of various hard and soft tissue translucencies, and dental restorations. Adjustable field-of-view software optimizes the target window while scanning in order to avoid capture of extraneous data such as lips, cheeks, and tongue. Intraoral fogging is prevented by the use of actively heated mirrors on the scanning tip [15].

The PlanScan® intraoral scanner comes with three removable tips, a cradle, and a power cable. Planmeca CAD software is used for data process, analysis, and editing by utilizing Thunderbolt connectivity to any computer or workstation. Integration and collaboration with other systems and third-party providers for scanning review, completion, or appliance fabrication is enabled through the STL open file format.

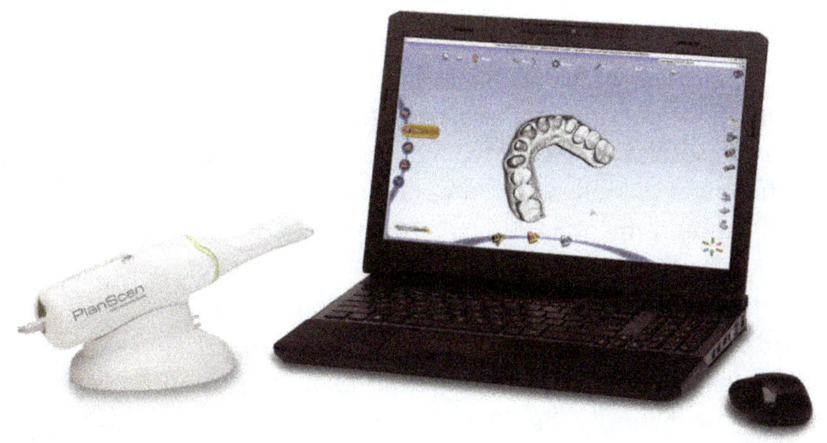

Figure 10. Planmeca PlanScan® intraoral scanner [41]

Features	iTero®	True Definition	Lythos™	CS 3500	TRIOS®	FastScan®	3D Progress	PlanScan®
Company	Align Technology, San Jose, CA	3M ESPE, Monrovia, CA	Ormco, Orange, CA	Carestream, Atlanta, GA	3Shape, Copenhagen, Denmark	IOS Technologies, San Diego, CA	Medical High Technologies and Optic Research, Verona, Italy	E4D Technologies, Richardson, TX
Optical Technology	Confocal Laser Microscopy	Active Wavefront Sampling	Accordion Fringe Interferometry	Confocal Laser Microscopy	Confocal Laser Microscopy	Optical Triangulation	Confocal Laser Microscopy	Optical Coherent Tomography
Year Launched	2006	May 2013/ updated version August 2014	May 2013	Nov 2013	Dec 2010	July 2010	2012	2008
Powder-Free	√		√	√	√		√	√
Scan Time	10-15 min	5-6 min	7 min	10 min	5 min	4 min	4 min	8-10 min
File Export	Open STL	Open STL	Open STL	Open STL	Open STL	Open STL	Open STL	Open STL
Trolley-Free				√	Cart and Pod-only versions available		√	√
Invisalign	Yes	Yes	No	No	No	No	No	No
SureSmile	Yes	No	No	No	Yes	No	No	No
Incognito	Yes	Yes	No	No	No	No	No	No
Insignia	Yes	No	Yes	No	No	No	No	No
Product Website	www.itero.com	http://solutions.3m.com	www.ormco.com	www.carestreamdental.com	www.3shapedental.com	www.ios3d.com	www.3dprogress.it	http://planmecacadcam.com

Table 1. Comparison of intraoral scanning systems

3.5. Assessment

Increased accuracy and time efficiency of the intraoral scanners have contributed to their growing popularity in dental offices. Published studies have found a comparable or better general accuracy of intraoral scans compared with conventional impressions [3-5,42]. Reported absolute mean differences in tooth-width measurements between digital and plaster models vary from 0 to 0.384 mm in the literature [10]. In 2013, Naidu and Freer analyzed the reproducibility of the iOC intraoral scanner (Cadent, Carlstand, NJ; later acquired by Align Technology, Inc.) by comparing plaster models and intraoral scans obtained from thirty subjects. Tooth widths were measured with a digital caliper from the physical models and with the OrthoCAD™ software (Align Technology, Inc., San Jose, CA) from the virtual models. Although there were statistically significant mean differences between tooth widths and Bolton rations, the bias of 0.024 mm was judged to be not clinically significant when the clinical threshold for a tooth-width discrepancy of 0.5 mm was applied [43]. The intraoral scans were suggested to be used for tooth-width measurements and Bolton ration calculations with clinically acceptable accuracy and excellent reliability [7-10]. Tooth-size arch-length measurements obtained in dry skulls from CBCT scans and iTero models provided interchangeable results with manual measurements, making both methods sufficient for orthodontic diagnosis and treatment planning [3]. In a study on the Lava chairside oral scanner, Cuperus et al. (2012) found that generally tooth-width measurements made on virtual models had the tendency to be greater than measurements made on physical stereolithographic models [10].

Orthodontic treatment with Invisalign requires intraoral scans or PVS impressions at several time points [32]. The rejection rate reported for 328 submitted cases with the iTero® intraoral scanner was less than 1% [33]. Intraoral scans demonstrated more accurate digital information in certain types of malocclusion compared to the conventional PVS impressions: severe anterior crowding, overlapping incisors, ectopically positioned teeth, missing teeth, planned extractions, severe deep bite, and late mixed dentition cases. The scanned distal surface of upper second molars in Class II cases showed adequate detailing, eliminating the need for retaking the frequently distorted PVS impressions in the time-consuming two-step impression technique. Intraoral scans submitted for Invisalign cases instead of PVS impressions showed no difference in terms of aligners' quality, durability, or function. However, it was noticed that orthodontists receive the first ClinCheck much sooner, sometimes within 24 hours of scanning, and consequently the aligners are manufactured sooner, allowing the treatment to start earlier [32,33].

Although an individual clinician's speed and effort have a substantial influence on the efficiency of the impression technique, procedure durations for digital and conventional approaches have been studied. The time efficiency for single implant restorations has been reported with a total treatment time of 24 minutes 42 seconds for the conventional approach and 12 minutes 29 seconds for the digital impression. Longer impression material preparation, working time, and retakes were necessary to complete an acceptable conventional impression. In 2014, Patzelt et al. investigated in vitro the working times of three intraoral scanners in three different prosthodontic scenarios. Compared with the conventional approach, digital impressions showed up to 23 minutes faster obtain rate and accelerated workflow in all tested scenarios of the study [45].

Digital scans were recognized as the most favored impression technique by inexperienced second year dental students [46]. The perceived level of difficulty for digital and conventional impression techniques showed that 60% of the participants favored the intraoral scans, 7% favored the conventional impressions, and 33% preferred either technique. The learning process for working with an intraoral scanner was suggested to be simpler, requiring less experience and proficiency than conventional impressions.

4. Desktop scanners

Various extraoral 3D scanners have been designed to capture 3D images of both impressions and physical casts for the acquisition of digital study models. The scanning technology employs a non-destructive laser beam and several digital cameras to reproduce high resolution images of the target's surfaces. Impressions, models, or bite registrations are positioned inside a chamber platform which is automatically rotated and inclined during scanning, ensuring complete multiple angle coverage of the model's geometry. The laser light is projected onto the object, and the cameras acquire its mirror image from the surface [47]. Upon scanning completion, a rendered stereolithographic model is created and plaster models, impressions, and bite registration can be discarded, eliminating the need for storage.

Ortho Insight 3D™ (Motion View Software, LLC, Chattanooga TN) was introduced in 2012, offering a high-resolution, robotic scan with an accuracy of 40-200 microns (Figure 11). The automated laser scanner is designed to capture full arch impressions, plaster models, and bite registrations, and create 3D digital models [47]. A single cast scan and virtual model reconstruction can be completed in approximately 5 to 7 minutes. The Ortho Insight 3D™ software offers digital storage of patient records, cast analysis, and treatment planning features. The software also allows measurements and automated functions such as landmark identification, arch length analysis, tooth segmentation, and evaluation of the occlusion. The optional software modules include indirect bonding and cephalometrics.

3Shape company (Copenhagen, Denmark) offers three desktop 3D scanners with the capability to digitize both plaster models and impressions with different resolutions and speeds (Figure 12). The R500 and R700 series use red light laser technology with two 1.3-megapixel digital cameras which ensure 20 microns accuracy [38]. The advertised R500 series scanning time is 2 minutes and 20 seconds for a plaster model and 6 minutes and 40 seconds for an impression. The advertised R700 series scanning time is 1 minute and 30 seconds for a plaster model and 7 minutes for an impression which makes the scanner suitable for medium-sized orthodontic offices and labs. The 3Shape R900 series scanner uses blue LED laser technology and employs four 5-megapixel cameras which ensure 15 microns scanning accuracy with color texture. The advertised R900 scanning time is 1 minute and 20 seconds for a plaster model and 2 minutes and 10 seconds for an impression which makes the scanner suitable for large high-volume, productive-orientated labs. Ortho Analyzer™ is the 3Shape imaging and digital model

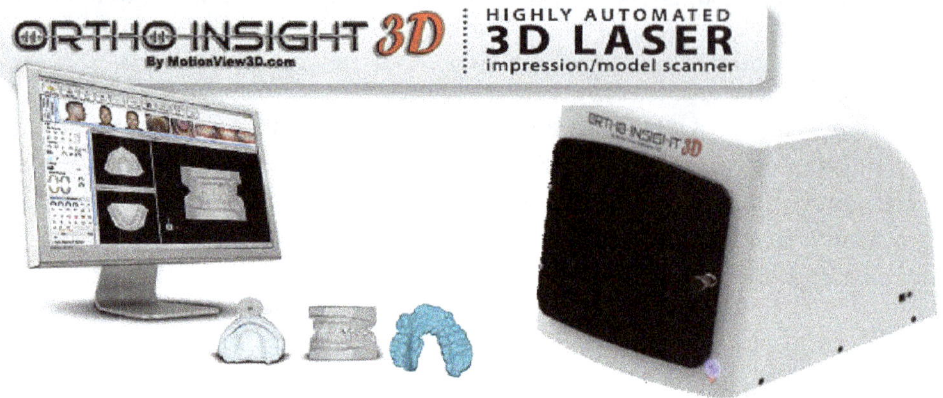

Figure 11. The Motion View 3D Desktop Model Scanner [48]

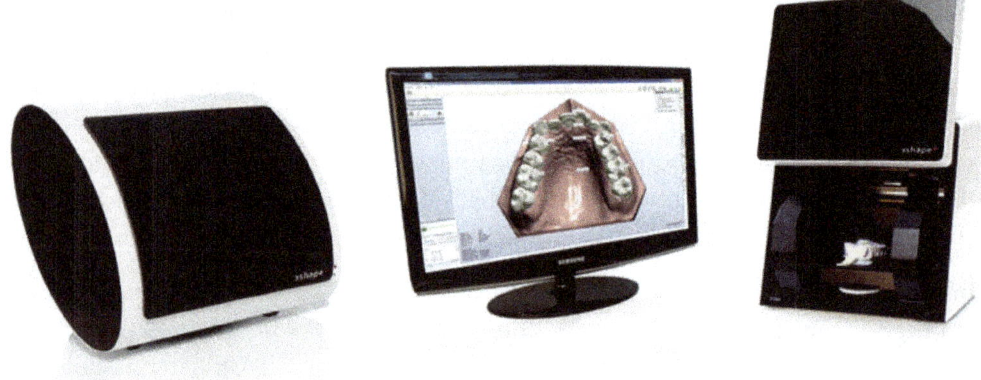

Figure 12. 3Shape's R500 and R7000 model scanners [38]

software package which features sculpt and rebase applications with collision control, tooth movement simulation, superimposition of study models with photographs or DICOM data originating from CBCT scanners, and digital manufacture of appliances or dental restorations.

Maestro 3D (AGE Solutions, Piza, Italy) is another desktop scanning device which allows digital conversion and storage of physical models and impressions (Figure 13). The scanner system has a LED projector with two digital cameras which capture scans with 0.07 mm resolution and 10 microns accuracy [49]. The Maestro 3D extraoral scanner comes with several modules: Easy Dental Scan software for inspection and editing; Ortho Studio software for tooth, arch, overjet, and overbite measurements, cross sectioning, and occlusion inspection; Virtual Setup module for tooth movement, distance and collision evaluation, attachment management, modeling, and export for 3D printing.

To date, the precision of 3D model scanners has been verified in several papers in the literature. A recent study evaluated the accuracy of Ortho Insight 3D™ plaster model scans for assessing

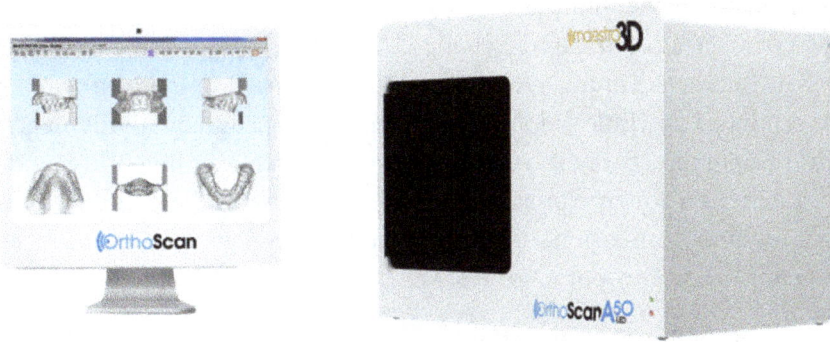

Figure 13. The Maestro OrthoScan A50 LED (AGE Solutions, Piza, Italy) [49]

tooth width, arch width, and arch length [11]. Significant differences were found in mesio-distal widths of maxillary molars, mandibular premolars and molars, arch widths of maxillary premolars, and arch lengths between Ortho Insight 3D™ and plaster model measurements however 90% of the mean differences were less than 0.20 mm. Similarly, the mean bias of Ortho Insight virtual models in comparison with caliper measurements (0.24 ± 0.67 mm) was found smaller than the mean biases of GeoDigm emodels and CBCT generated models [50]. In 2013, Hayashi et al. compared the in vitro reliability of three scanning systems (SureSmile OraScanner, Konica Minolta VIVID910, and 3Shape R700) to the gold standard SLP250 Laser Probe digital models. The authors found that the deviation values for each comparison were small (< 0.048 mm) and each scanning device generated sufficiently accurate digital models for use by clinicians [51]. Another study also documented slight, non-significant difference in the linear tooth size and arch length measurements between the 3Shape R700 digital models and plaster models [47]. With respect to intraoral scanners, certain desktop scanners demonstrated higher digitization precision in areas with strong changes of curvature and undercuts but lower accuracy in reproduction of interdental spaces [42].

5. Facial scanners

5.1. 3D surface imaging

Facial scanners provide three-dimensional topography of the facial surface anatomy, automatic facial landmark recognition, and analysis of the symmetry and proportions of the face. Practical applications further include quantitative and qualitative assessment of growth and development, ethnic variations, gender differences, and isolation of specific diagnostic traits in selected populations of patients with craniofacial anomalies [52,53]. In addition, facial phenotype associated with fetal alcohol syndrome, cleft lip and palate patients, and short- and long-term effects of nasoalveolar molding have been evaluated using three-dimensional surface imaging [54]. Volumetric results are also valuable clinical tools to assess primary palate reconstruction in infants with cleft lip and palate.

Clinical evaluation of facial morphology is still largely subjective and prevents accurate documentation of facial structure or the changes following various esthetic and reconstructive procedures [55]. Recent scanning technology innovations provided valuable methods for precise three-dimensional clinical documentation and objective qualitative and quantitative analysis of the human face. Several techniques such as laser scanning, ultrasound, computed tomography, magnetic resonance imaging, and electromagnetic digitization can analyze facial characteristics in three dimensions but stereophotogrammetric systems are becoming the instrument of choice in anthropometric research [54,56].

Stereophotogrammetry is a unique method which utilizes means of triangulation and camera pairs in stereo configuration to recover the 3D distance to features on the facial surface (Figure 15 and 16). As early as 1967 Burke and Beard discussed and introduced the concept [57]. 3D stereophotogrammetry has evolved and is now systematically used for anthropometric assessment instead of the direct sliding and spreading caliper-based measurements. Today, it is predominately used in plastic surgery, medical genetics, and research settings. 3D photogrammetry acquires a 180° high-resolution color representation of the human face from ear to ear without direct contact or risks to the patients [56]. A major advantage of the surface imaging system is a near-instantaneous image capture (on the order of 1.5 milliseconds) which reduces motion artifacts and makes it suitable for children, even babies. Upon acquisition, image quality can be immediately reviewed to determine whether repeat imaging is necessary due to blurring or absence of surface data. Furthermore, software tools are available to view and manipulate the image, facilitate landmark identification and calculate anthropometric linear, angular, and volumetric measurements. The disadvantages of 3D photogrammetry are its relative expense, limited availability, difficulties in recording shiny, shadowed, or transparent facial structures, and lack of ability to calculate interactive landmarks.

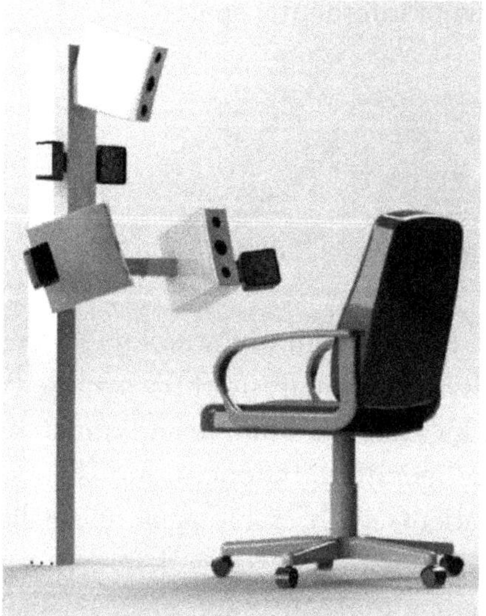

Figure 14. Facial Insight 3D Scanner [48]

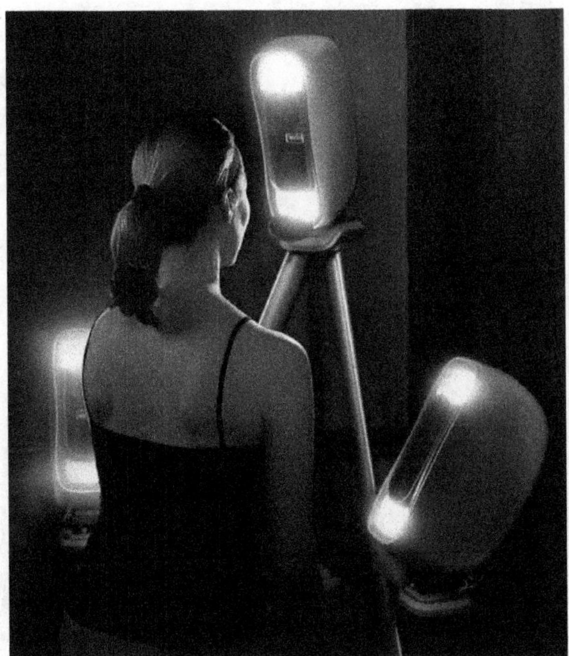

Figure 15. VECTRA M3 Imaging System [59]

Three-dimensional surface imaging enables assessment of the spatial position of soft-tissue facial landmarks by assigning coordinates to each point. It could be difficult to identify a substantial number of landmarks and place them accurately in the three planes of space to gain a comprehensive understanding of the facial structure (Figure 16) [58-63]. In a reproducibility study of 3D facial landmarks, Hajeer et al. (2002) used C3D facial scans before and after orthognathic surgery of five patients to identify 24 landmarks on each scan. In addition, they defined four new landmarks by utilizing the Farkas's anthropometric landmarks (1994) [63]. Three sessions of landmark digitization were performed within a week interval. Each landmark had x, y, and z coordinates given by the software and the mean differences were calculated from the three identification sessions by identifying the differences between the individual coordinate points. The results showed that 20 of the chosen landmarks had high reproducibility based on accepted 0.5 mm cut off point. The following landmarks whose localization depended on the underlying skeleton had problems of reproducibility: menton, left and right zygion, and left and right gonion (x-coordinate); left and right zygion, left and right gonion, left and right tragion, and glabelle (y-coordinate); menton, left and right otobasion inferius, left and right tragion, and left and right gonion (z-coordinate) [62]. In a different study, facial landmarks with distinct margins or borders also showed higher degree of consistent identification than those located on gently curved rounded surfaces. It is likely that digital measurements of the philtral length/upper prolabial width will require direct marking [64]. Several other studies also recommended direct labeling of certain landmarks in order to improve identification before image acquisition and/or direct measurements [54,65].

Several types of 3D photogrammetric imaging systems have been described and evaluated in the literature, e.g. 3dMDface System (3dMD, Atlanta, GA, USA), C3D Imaging System

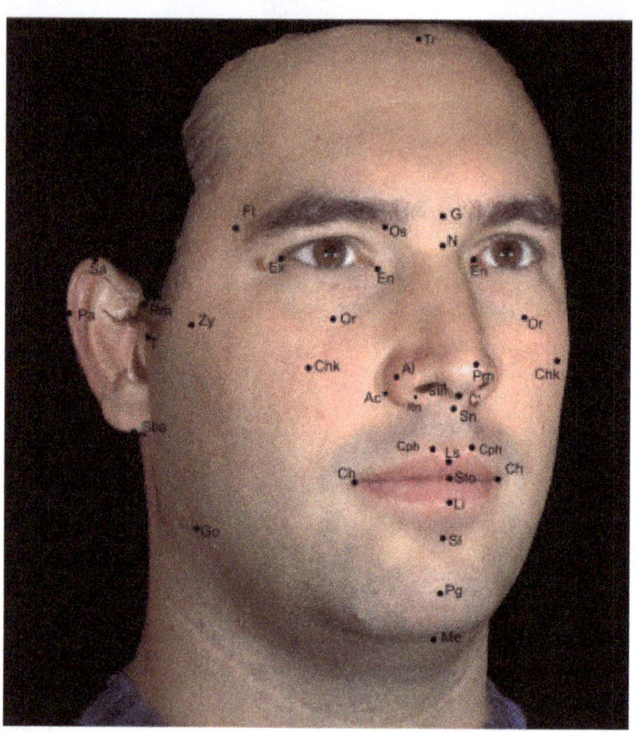

Figure 16. Digitized facial landmarks used in direct and indirect anthropometric measurements: *Tr*- trichion; *G*- glabella; *N*- nasion; *Prn*- pronasale; *C'*- columella; *Sn*- subnasale; *Ls*- labiale superius; *Sl*- sublabiale; *Pg*- pogonion; *Me*- menton; *Ex*- exocanthion; *En*- endocanthion; *Os*- orbitale superius; *Or*- orbitale; *Ft*- frontotemporale; *Zy*- zygion; *Chk*-cheek; *T*-tragion; *Pra*- preaurale; *Sa*- superaurale; *Pa*- postural; *Sba*- subaurale; *Al*- alare; *Ac*- nasal alar crest; *Itn*- inferior point of the nostril axis; *Stn*- superior point of the nostril axis; *Cph*- crista philtri; *Ch*- cheilion; *Go*-gonion [70].

(Ferranti, Birmingham, UK), Rainbow 3D Camera (Genex Technologies, Inc., Kensington, MD, USA), 3D Vectra (Canfield Imaging Systems, Fairfield, NJ, USA), and the Facial Insight 3D (Motion View Software, LLC, Chattanooga TN, USA) [57,65-68]. Aldridge et al. (2005) evaluated the precision and reproducibility of coordinate data and 190 distances on two sets of measurements made on 30 3dMDface images taken from 15 human subjects and found this system to be highly precise and reliable with a submillimeter average error in landmark placement. Weinberg et al. (2006) published a comparison of measurements of mannequin heads using two 3D surface imaging systems, 3dMDface and Rainbow 3D Camera, and direct anthropometry. These three techniques yielded a high degree of agreement among selected anthropometric variables, and the intraobserver precision was high for each method [65].

Manipulation of the scans and precise landmark identification requires proficiency with 3D computer software [53]. That's why, in order to improve reproducibility, it is necessary to become accustomed to the selected software implemented to capture and process the images (Figure 17). Facial models captured with Facial Insight 3D were found to be affected by the angles of the subject's face, hair interference, and head position, but in general, the precision of the digital images was within an acceptable range. It has been suggested that head position, projection, and stabilization should be consistently the same in order to achieve optimum standardized settings. Several internal module failures of the software while initiating a new series of scan, clearing the cache after scans, or modifying the location of already placed landmarks are still to be addressed by the manufacturer [69].

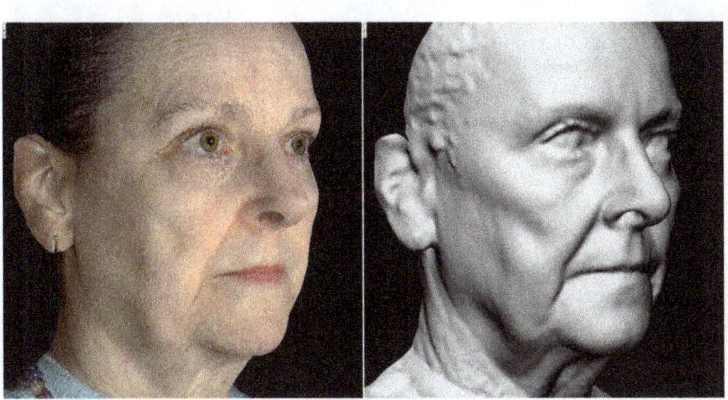

Figure 17. Virtual facial model [59]

Direct comparison of multiple faces is challenging due to the diverse size and orientation of each face. Facial average methods like the Generalized Procrustes Analysis (GPA) have been proposed where the scans are scaled and fitted into equal size reference frames [60]. This implies that transition and rotation are applied in order to eliminate size difference between facial scans and equilibrate the squared summed distances between corresponding facial landmarks. To obtain linear measurements, surface areas, and color mapping, a facial shells superimposition can be applied using the best-fitting alignment method or registration over relatively stable anatomical reference points and planes. A study evaluating 350 facial scans of children aged 15.5 years old identified the midendocanthion landmarks as the most stable facial structure for facial shell superimposition [52].

3D facial images easily integrate with study models, radiographs, and photographs and allow further simulations of orthodontic tooth movement and treatment results (Figure 18) [53, 70]. In order to validate and elaborate the correlation and matching process between facial images and dental casts, Rosati et al. (2010) merged dental digital models with 3D stereophotogrammetric open and closed lips images. The present anterior teeth in both facial and dental acquisitions were used as reference in the open-lips image superimpositions. In the closed lips image superimpositions the following facial soft-tissues landmarks were marked on the face before each acquisition and were used as fiducial points: Ftl, frontotemporale left; Ftr, frontotemporale right; and N, nasion. Seven linear measurements were virtually and directly performed between the facial landmarks and the occlusal plane on each subject. The results showed mean relative error smaller than 1.2%. The matching process was also found within a tolerable anthropometric and clinical context: the forehead mean distance in the open and closed lips image acquisitions was 0.4 mm, with a range between 0.04 mm and 1.1 mm [70].

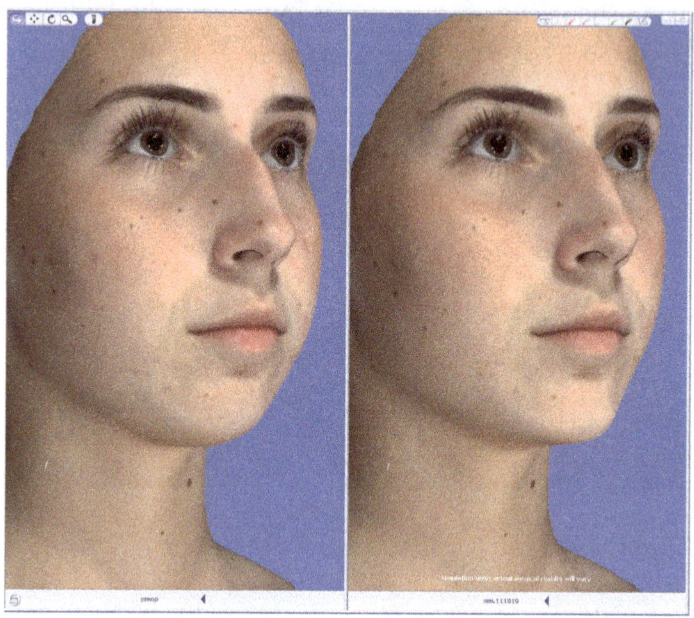

Figure 18. Virtual surgical planning with the 3D Vectra photosystem (Canfield Imaging Systems, Fairfield, NJ) [59]

Over the past 20 years, a number of 3D facial databases containing static and time sequence of images have been built with the purpose of aid in automatic face recognition and analysis algorithms. Several publicly available databases have facilitated the research for tracking and superimposition of 3D facial shells and feature extraction methodologies. However, most of the existing 3D expression datasets are of small size comprising of deliberately posed or exaggerated expressions mostly of the six universal emotions (e.g. happiness, surprise, anger, sadness, fear, and disgust), obtained under directed settings. Spontaneous behaviors have been suggested to vary in timing and appearance from acted ones. For instance, deliberate smiles have faster onset and offset and larger amplitude than the velocity and amplitude of genuine smiles [71]. Additional databases of recorded micro-expressions and dynamic 3D faces captured in wider range of contexts, unprompted behaviors, and affective states will have to be designed.

5.2. 4D facial dynamics

Production sequential 3D surface imaging systems (4D Facial Dynamics) are commercially available to provide a quantifiable understanding of soft tissue mobility, true anatomical motion, and facial expression [72]. The 4D systems are used to assess facial function in conjunction with natural head movements, functional progress and outcomes for patients undergoing dental treatment and surgical interventions. Human face is capable of making unique microexpressions which can be of very low intensity and last less than 0.04 seconds. Therefore, the dynamic systems continuously track frame by frame the facial surface movements in order to achieve accuracy in understanding the tracking motions. The 4D technology acquires exact 3D surface information at approximately 60 frames per second from various coordinated standpoints for up to a 10 minute acquisition high resolution cycle. The video sequence of the area of interest is recorded with grey-scale cameras record while the surface texture is captured with a color camera [73]. A unified point cloud continuous image is displayed from the viewpoints of two or more stereo cameras, reducing the errors from the stitching process of different datasets. Motion capture systems with automatic facial landmark recognition software have been found practical objective solutions for the soft tissue quantification movements.

Assessment of facial animation could be an essential part for orthodontic diagnosis and craniofacial abnormality, virtual surgical planning, and treatment outcomes. Furthermore, various surgical interventions could affect the function of nerves and associated musculature which could influence the magnitude and the speed of the soft tissue motions. Shujaat et al. (2014) evaluated the dynamics of four facial movements (maximum smile, grimace, cheek puff, and lip purse) pre- and post- lip split mandibulotomy, by using six facial landmarks. The similarity of the facial animation pattern before and after the surgery was calculated after eliminating the head motion and aligning the movement curves using the right and left endocanthion and pronasale as stable landmarks unaffected by the surgery. The results showed that the velocity of all landmarks was lower after the surgery; the smile animation difference was the least (-0.1 mm/s), whereas the largest changed was found for the grimace animation (-5.8 mm/s). Mouth width maximum change after the surgery was found to be for lip purse (3.4 mm), whereas grimace showed the least difference after the surgery. Lip purse animation similarity was highest (0.78) while grimace had lowest similarity (0.71). The 4D dynamic devices have also been employed for interlandmark and vector deviations, and shape and gender comparisons [74]. Virtual and sound animations have been incorporated in some of the recent system improvements [75].

6. 3D printing

Additive manufacturing or 3D printing was founded in 1990 by Wilfried Vancraen, CEO and Director of Materialise NV, the first Rapid Prototyping sector company in the Benelux region [1]. 3D printing technology allows the user to create or "print" 3D physical objects, prototypes, and production parts of any shape from a virtual model in a growing range of materials including plastic, cobalt, nickel, steel, aluminum, titanium, etc. [76,77]. Those materials are joined in successive layers one on top of the other through additive processes under automated computer control. The 3D printing process usually begins with a 3D model, virtually designed or obtained through scanning of a physical object. Slicing software automatically transforms the point cloud into a stereolithographic file which is sent to the additive manufacturing machine for building the object (Figure 19).

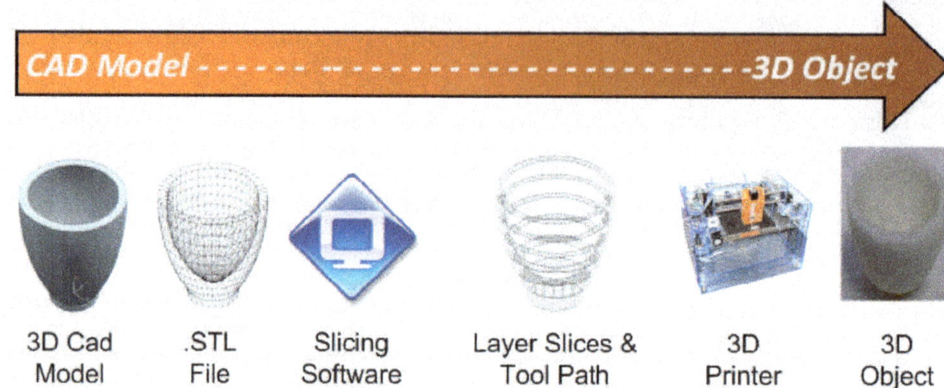

Figure 19. The 3D Printing process [79]

Today, 3D printing has grown to be competitive with the traditional model of manufacturing in terms of reliability, speed, price, and cost of use. In comparison with other technologies, additive manufacturing is more effective due its ability to use readily available supplies, recycle waste material, and has no requirements for costly tools, molds, or punches, scrap, milling, or sanding. 3D printing technology is used for distributed manufacturing, rapid manufacturing, mass customization, and rapid prototyping with applications in engineering, civil engineering, automotive, architecture, construction, aerospace, military, human tissue replacement, dental and medical industries, industrial design, jewelry, fashion, eyewear, geographic information, education, footwear, and many other fields (Figure 20) [78,80]. Additive manufacturing is likely to continue rapid growth in conjunction with intraoral scanning technology as a more effective system for orthodontic practices and laboratories for automatic fabrication of high-resolution study models, retainers, metal appliances, aligners, and indirect bonding, accelerating the production time and increasing the capability [15,77].

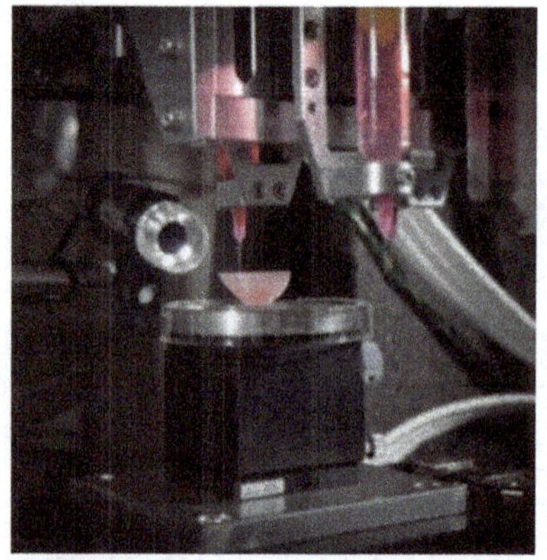
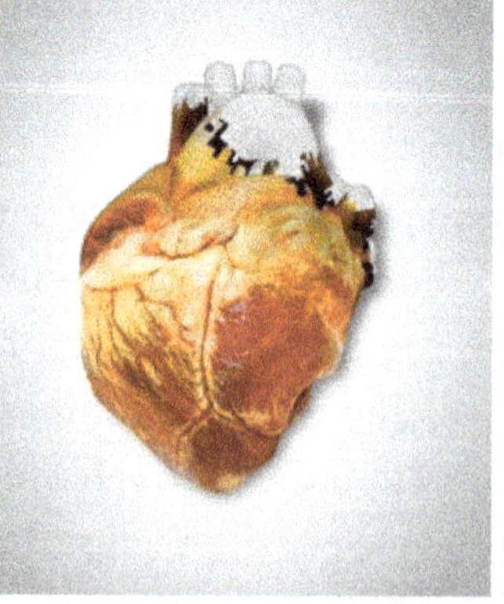
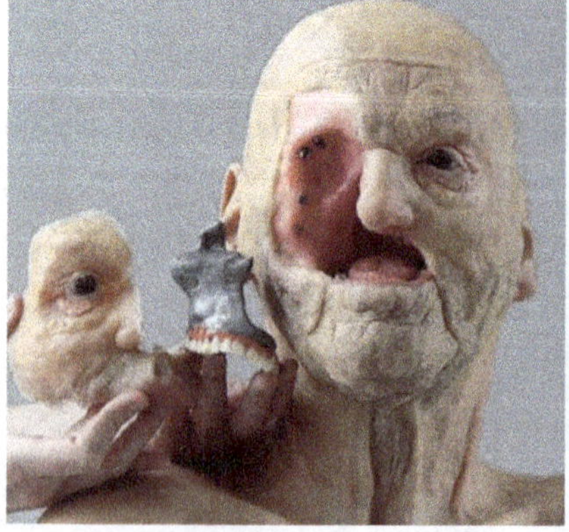

Figure 20. 3D Printing is revolutionizing medicine and dentistry by creating body parts: heart valves, ears, artificial bone, joints, soft tissue prostheses, and blood vessels [86-88]

6.1. Additive technologies

Currently, there is a huge selection of available 3D printing technologies suitable for orthodontic use:

6.1.1. Fused Deposition Modelling (FDM)

Fused depositing modelling (FDM) is frequently used for modelling, manufacture applications, and prototyping. The technology was introduced by S. Scott Crump towards the end of 1980s and was popularized by Stratasys, Ltd in 1990 [1]. FDM employs the "additive" method of laying down thermoplastic material in layers. In order to produce a part the material is supplied through a heated nozzle after a metal wire or a plastic filament wound in a coil are released. The melted material hardens immediately after extrusion, thus minimizing inaccuracies [81]. The nozzle can be directed in both vertical and horizontal lines by a numerically controlled software mechanism. Several materials such as acrylonitrile butadiene styrene (ABS) polymer, polyphenylsulfones and waxes, polycaprolactone, polycarbonates, polyamides, lignin, among many others, with diverse strength and thermal properties are available.

Another approach to produce a 3D structure is for the material to be supplied from a basin through a small nozzle such as in the case of the 3D Bioplotter (EnvisionTEC, Gladbeck, Germany). The device is mainly applied in prototyping porous scaffolds for medical tissue engineering and organ bio-printing [82]. With an accuracy of just a few micrometers, the bioplotter is able to build body parts with different microstructural patterns including blood vessels, bone, and soft tissue. FDM is the most widely used process of 3D printing today, although there are other almost identical technologies like MakerBot (Stratasys, Ltd., Eden Prairie, MN) known as Fused Filiment Fabrication (FFF).

6.1.2. Selective Laser Melting (SLM) and Selective Laser Sintering (SLS)

Laser based additive manufacturing, such as selective laser melting (SLM) and selective laser sintering (SLS), uses power in the form of a high energy laser beam directed by scanning mirrors to build three-dimensional objects by melting metallic powder and fusing the fine particles together [83]. The laser energy is strong enough to allow full welding/melting of the particles to create a solid part. The process which can include partial and full melting or liquid-phase sintering is recurring layer after layer until the object is completed. The technology is commonly utilized due to its ability to form parts with complex geometries with very thin walls and hidden channels or voids directly from digital CAD data. Compared to other types of 3D printing, SLM/SLS have very high productivity and can build objects from a relatively big selection of commercial powder materials [1]. These include polyamides, polycaprolactone, hydroxyapatite, ultra high molecular weight polyethylene, polyethylene, ceramic, glass, stainless steel, titanium, and Co/Cr alloys. Although most of the initial applications of the laser based technologies were for manufacture of lightweight aerospace parts, the SLM/SLS have found an acceptance for production of orthopedic and dental implants, dental crowns and bridges, partial denture frameworks, and bone analogs [84].

6.1.3. Electron Beam Melting (EBM)

Electron beam melting (EBM) is a type of additive manufacturing for laying down successive layers and creating near-net-shape or highly porous metal parts that are particularly strong, void-free, and fully dense. The EBM technology uses the energy source of an electron beam, as opposed to a laser [85]. Objects are manufactured layer by layer from fully melted metal powder utilizing a computer controlled electron beam in a high vacuum. The technology operates at higher temperatures of up to 1000 °C, which could result in differences of the phases formed through solidification. EBM is able to form extremely porous mesh or foam structures in a wide range of alloys including stainless steel, titanium, and copper. The technology is commonly used in orthopedic and oral and maxillofacial surgery for manufacturing customized implants. Their structure permits the ingrowth of bone, provides better fixation, and helps to prevent stress shielding [1].

6.1.4. Stereolithography (SLA)

The term "stereolithography" was first presented by Charles W. Hull in 1986 as a technique for producing solid items by consecutively printing thin layers material that is solidified by a concentrated ultraviolet laser light. SLA is the first so-called "rapid prototyping" process. The resolution of the built item is higher when more layers are used and the number of layers may range from 5 to 20 per millimeter [1, 77]. After being built, objects are immersed into a solvent bath for excess resin removal and are consequently placed in an UV oven to finish the curing process. Based on object complexity and size, stereolithography can take from a few hours to more than 24 hours to create a particular part.

Most of the SLA immediate use was in the automotive and aerospace industries, but medical and dental applications of this technology gradually emerged. SLA models are currently used for planning cranial, maxillofacial, and neurosurgical procedures and constructing highly accurate replicas of human anatomy, customized implants, cranioplasties, orbital floors, and onlays. Surgical guides for dental implant placement are routinely produced by stereolithography [80].

6.1.5. Inkjet 3D printing

The inkjet printing technology employs a nozzle which "prints" a pattern on a thin layer of powder substrate by propelling a liquid binding agent (Figure 21) [1,77]. The small ink droplets are forced through the orifice by pressure, heat, or vibrations. The object is built through a recurring process layer by layer with each layer of material adhered to the last. Phase transformation from liquid to solid occurs immediately after droplets are deposited upon the substrate by UV curing light, drying, chemical reaction, or heat transfer [86-88]. The polyjet printers allow volumetric color objects to be built in simultaneous incorporation of multiple materials with quite distinct physical properties. As of 2014, manufacturers were able to combine sand and calcium carbonate, ceramic powder and liquid binder, acrylic powder and cyanoacrylate, water and sugar (for making candies), etc.

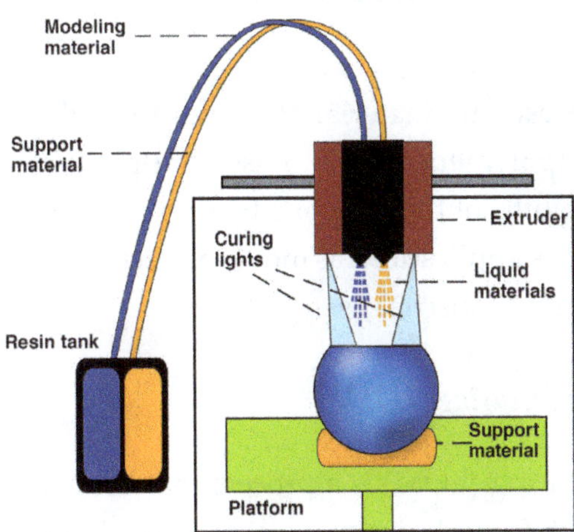

Figure 21. Representation of PolyJet photopolymer (PPP) 3D printing [77]

By combining rigid and rubberlike materials, it is possible to create a mouthguard with soft and hard regions in different colors. Further dental applications include reproduction of study models, surgical guides for implant placement, sleep apnea appliances, orthodontic bracket guides, and try-in veneers [87,89]. Extrusion rate, nozzle size, and droplet travelling speed are able to affect the dimensional accuracy of dental restorations [90]. Specially engineered dental materials for polyjet printing provide fine layers as thin as 16 microns, which render small features in great details with strength and durability. Biocompatible materials, which allow short-term mucosal membrane contact of up to 24 hours and prolong skin contact of more than 30 days, are used for manufacture of soft tissue prostheses and hearing aids.

In general, the inkjet printing technology is faster than other additive manufacturing processes such as fused depositing modelling. However, depending on the material and process, surface finish, object density, and accuracy may be inferior to stereolithography and selective laser sintering.

6.1.6. *Digital Light Processing (DLP)*

Digital Light Processing (DLP) is a type of nanotechnology that uses a digital micromirror device as a power source projector to cure liquid resin into solid 3D objects. DLP is similar to stereolithography as the method also employs light polymerization. One difference is that DLP creates a single layer as one digital image in tiny volumetric pixels as opposed to SLA's laser process which must scan the vat with a single point. DLP printing is faster and can build objects with a higher resolution, typically able to reach a layer thickness of fewer than 30 microns [91]. Furthermore, DLP can produce objects with a wide variety of properties such as high clarity, spngness, flexibility, water resistance, thermal resistance, and durability. The photopolymers have been designed to mimic ABS, polypropylene, and wax, blending layers together much more smoothly than plastic filament is able to. However, photopolymer prints can become brittle with increased light exposure over time. Objects may begin to show cracks and become more susceptible to breaking.

The DLP process can only use one material at a time since the object is built out of a vat containing a singular photopolymer solution. Post-print processing involves washing away the remaining resin and removal of the supports by snapping or cutting. DLP-based technologies are found in such diverse applications as movie projectors, cell phones, video wall, digital cinema, medical, security, and industrial uses [92].

6.1.7. Laminated Object Manufacturing (LOM)

Laminated object manufacturing (LOM) is a process that combines additive and subtractive techniques to build an object. It works by successively layering sheets of material one on top of another and binding them together using adhesive, pressure, and heat application. Once the process is complete, objects are cut to desired dimensions with a knife, a laser, or additionally modified by machine drilling. The technology is able to produce relatively large parts since no chemical reaction is necessary. The most common materials used in LOM are plastics, paper, ceramics, composites, and metals which are widely available and yield comparatively inexpensive 3D printing method. Materials can be mixed in various layers throughout the printing process giving more flexibility in the final outcome of the objects. Paper models have a wood-like texture and characteristics and can be finished accordingly. Surface accuracy is slightly inferior to stereolithography and selective laser sintering. LOM systems are used in sand casting, investment casting, ceramics processing, for concept modelling, and architectural applications [93].

6.2. 3D printers in orthodontics

The global additive manufacturing industry has been dominated by three large companies: Stratasys, Ltd. (Eden Prairie, MN), 3D Systems (Rock Hill, SC), and EnvisionTEC (Gladbeck, Germany), with market shares of 57%, 18%, and 11%, respectively [94]. As of January 2014, Stratasys sells 3D printing systems that range from $2,200 to $600,000 in price and are employed in several industries: aerospace, automotive, architecture, defense, medical and dental, among many others (Figure 22). MakerBot and Objet are the 3D printers recently acquired by Stratasys and currently used in dentistry and orthodontics. For example, ClearCorrect employs Objet in the aligner manufacture process while Invisalign uses the 3D Systems' SLA technology. Other companies like Concept Laser (Lichtenfels, Germany), Realizer (Borchen, Germany), and SLM Solutions (Lübeck, Germany) are also offering printing technologies and new materials to be used in dental 3D printing. Furthermore, a broad line of innovative professional 3D printers, orthodontic practical solutions, and price points exist for generating full-color parts, wax patterns, and investment castings. Table 2 summarizes some of the characteristics of several 3D printers used in orthodontics [86-88,95,96].

Features	Objet30 OrthoDesk	ProJet® 3510 MP	ULTRA® 3SP™ Ortho	Perfactory® Micro Ortho	MakerBot Replicator 2	FORMIGA P 110
Company	Stratasys, Ltd., Eden Prairie, MI	3D Systems, Rock Hill, SC	EnvisionTEC, Gladbeck, Germany	EnvisionTEC, Gladbeck, Germany	Stratasys, Ltd., Eden Prairie, MI	EOS, Munich, Germany
Technology	PolyJet Printing technology	PolyJet Printing technology	Digital Light Processing	Digital Light Processing	Fused Depositing Modelling	Selective Laser Sintering
Build Volume	300 x 200 x 100 mm	298 x 185 x 203 mm	266 x 177.8 x 76 mm	100 x 75 x 100 mm	285 X 153 X 155 mm	200 x 250 x 330 mm
Layer Thickness	0.0011 in	0.001-0.002 in	0.00098 in	0.0039 in, 0.002 in, 0.004 in	0.0039 - 0.0133 in	0.0024 in, 0.0039 in, 0.0047 in
Applications	High quality orthodontic models, surgical guides, temporary intraoral appliances and restorations	Drill guides, jaw models, orthodontic thermoforming model	High quality orthodontic appliances	High quality models for the fabrication of orthodontic appliances	Retainers and aligners with less esthetic appearance due to stair-stepping	High quality retainers and orthodontic appliances
Weight	93 kg	323 kg	90 Kg	13 kg	11.5 kg	600 kg
Product Website	www.stratasys.com	www. 3dsystems.com	http:// envisiontec.com	http:// envisiontec.com	www.makerbot.co m	www.eos.info

Table 2. Comparison of 3D printers currently used in orthodontics

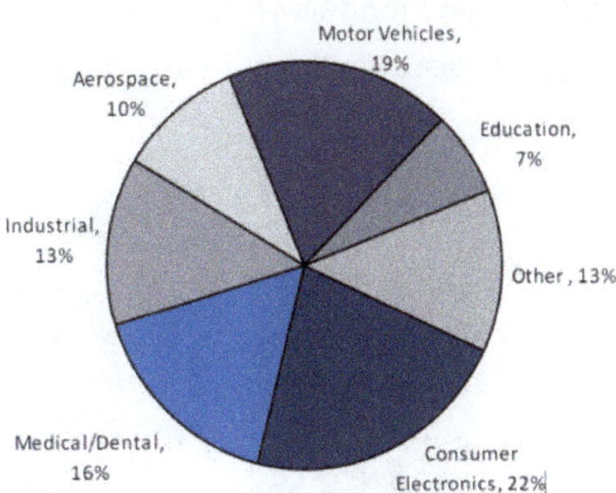

Figure 22. 3D Printing end markets [97]

Objet30 OrthoDesk (Stratasys, Ltd., Eden Prairie, MN) employs the PolyJet printing technology and is suitable for orthodontic offices and small- to medium-sized orthodontic labs (Figure 23). The 3D printer is able to fabricate durable orthodontic models with high feature detail and ultrafine layers of surface quality [77]. Every print run can create up to 20 models. Three dental materials, specially engineered for dentistry, come with the printer in sealed cartridges: VeroDentPlus (MED690), a dark beige, acrylic-based material prints layers as fine as 16 microns with accuracy as thin as 0.1mm used for most appliances; Clear biocompatible (MED610), a transparent material medically approved for temporary intraoral applications and surgical guides; and VeroGlaze (MED620), an acrylic-based material for veneer models or diagnostic wax-ups in A2-shade color match that can be used in the mouth as long as 24 hours [86].

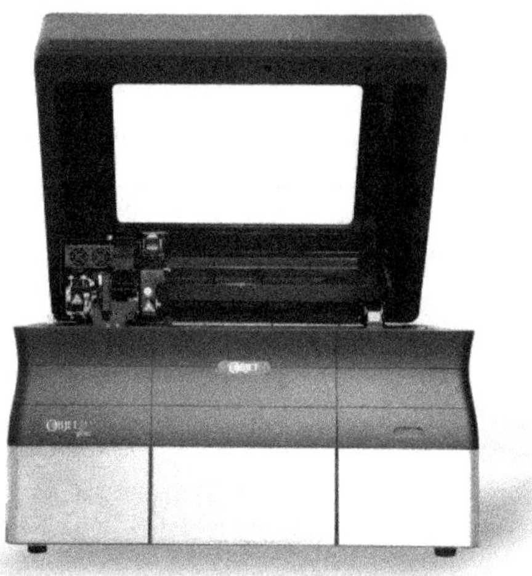

Figure 23. The Objet30 OrthoDesk (Stratasys, Ltd., Eden Prairie, MN) 3D printer [86]

ProJet® 3510 MP (3D Systems, Rock Hill, SC) is one of the several healthcare printing solutions, used for uniformly accurate thin wax-ups of crown, bridges, and partial dentures. The system can also produce any size dental or jaw models with a choice of two materials in smooth or matte printing mode. Up to 24 quad cases can be built at one time (Figure 24).

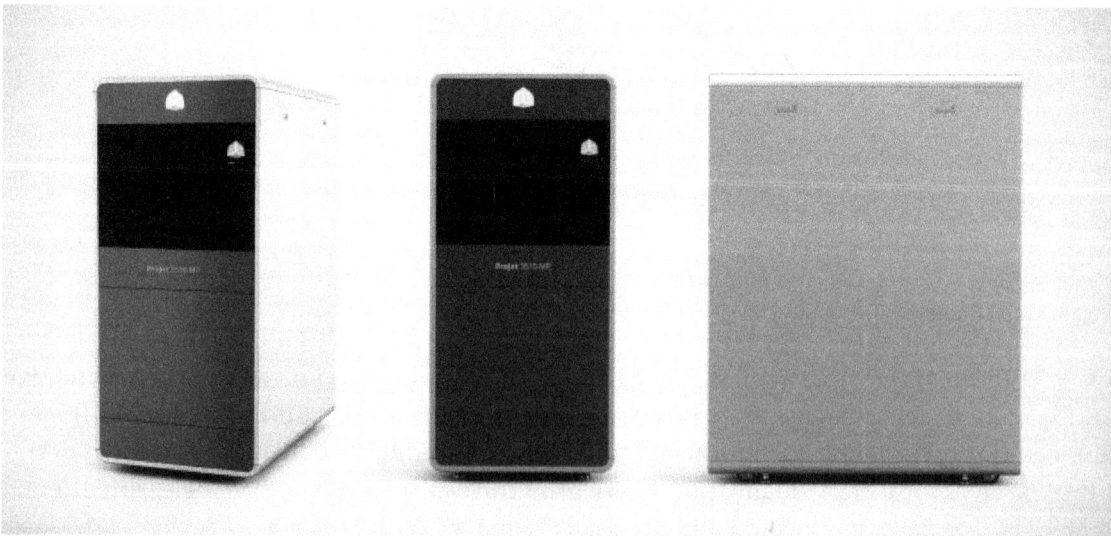

Figure 24. The ProJet® 3510 MP (3D Systems, Rock Hill, SC) 3D printer [88]

The 3D Systems professional printers support the VisiJet® line of materials, specially engineered to meet a wide range of applications. ProJet® 3510 series come with three UV curable acrylic materials: Dentcast, a dark-green, wax-up material, which burns out cleanly for ash-free castings (Figure 25); PearlStone, a while material with a solid stone appearance; and Stoneplast for transparent, clear or stone finish dental models. VisiJet® S300 is the fourth material which is a non-toxic white wax material for hands-free melt-away supports [88].

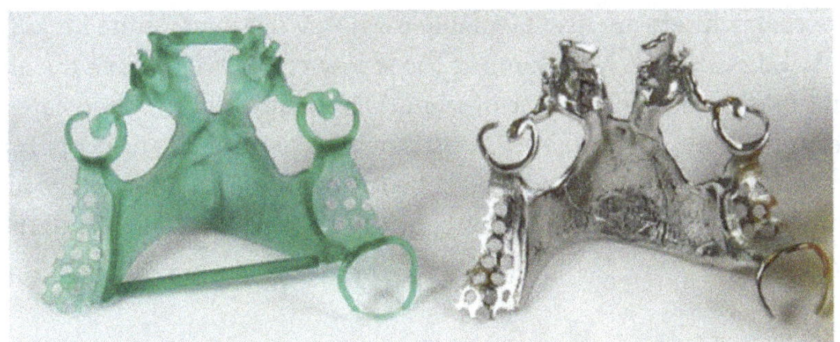

Figure 25. Dental wax-up and casting manufactured with ProJet® 3510 MP [88]

ULTRA® 3SP™ Ortho (EnvisionTEC, Gladbeck, Germany) employs the Scan, Spin, and Selectively Photocure (3SP™) technology, a DLP variant, which utilizes a laser diode with an orthogonal mirror spinning at 20,000 rpm (Figure 26). The printer is able to produce highly accurate and stable dental models that could be used for orthodontic appliance fabrication. The models are resistant to high temperature and have negligible water absorption.

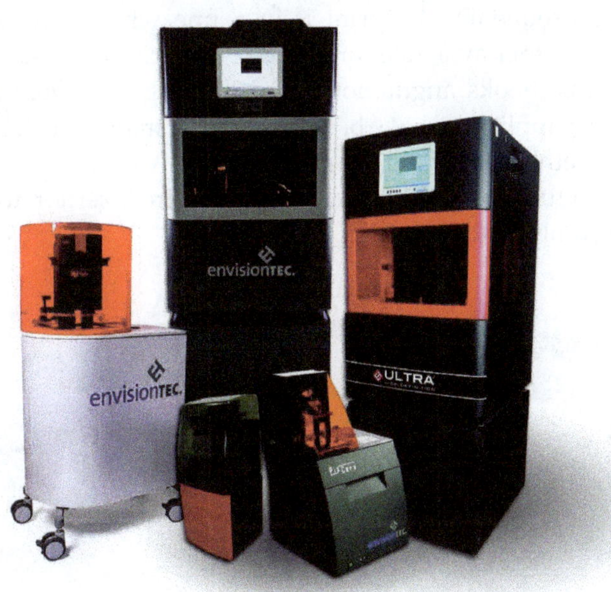

Figure 26. The EnvisionTEC (Gladbeck, Germany) 3D printers used in dentistry and orthodontics [87]

ULTRA® 3SP™ Ortho also comes with specially engineered photosensitive resins for dental and orthodontic applications: Press-E-Cast (WIC300), a wax-filled photopolymer for production of copings with extremely thin margins as well as up to 16 multiple unit bridge; E-Denstone (HTM140 Peach), a peach color material able to achieve the look and feel of traditional gypsum models with a high-accuracy detail; and D3 White, a fast-growing, tough material with similar characteristics to ABS plastic and the most common medium for dental model manufacturing for the production of orthodontic appliances [87].

A variety of low cost printers are also available for home use such as the MakerBot Replicator 2 (Stratasys, Ltd., Eden Prairie, MI). Some of those low cost devices have the ability to locally print objects in an astonishing number of materials, including ice, chocolate, rubber caulk, frosting, and ceramic clay. Low cost printers, however, still lack supports for overhanging geometry and their use in orthodontics could be problematic. The machines are often fragile with temperature, deposition, and position controls not accurate enough to make functional end-parts [95].

6.3. Application

3D printing solutions are capable to achieve various products with high level of precision. The use of the technology to build dental models, removable appliances, customized brackets and archwires, and occlusal splints has been attempted and reported in the orthodontic literature (Figure 27) [98-101]. Currently, the most common application of the 3D printers is for clear retainers and aligner fabrication [77]. Practitioners can virtually move the teeth to a final ideal position, print a sequence of physical models in the office, and use a thermoplastic material to fabricate aligner trays, working on similar premise to ClearCorrect and Invisalign. Skipping the step of 3D printing a physical model, researchers have also used the technology to digitally design a retainer and consequently 3D print it in a fine while polyamide material [99]. Sophisticated software is further available for shaping and trimming the dental model base, for design of bracket pads, hooks angulations, and guiding jigs. Digital titanium Herbst, Andresen, and sleep apnea appliances have been made with smooth surfaces, no sharp edges, and excellent fit on the teeth, palatal and gingival tissues. Additive manufacturing enables features such as hinge production, building threads, and wire insertion to be completed in a single build without assembly [102,104].

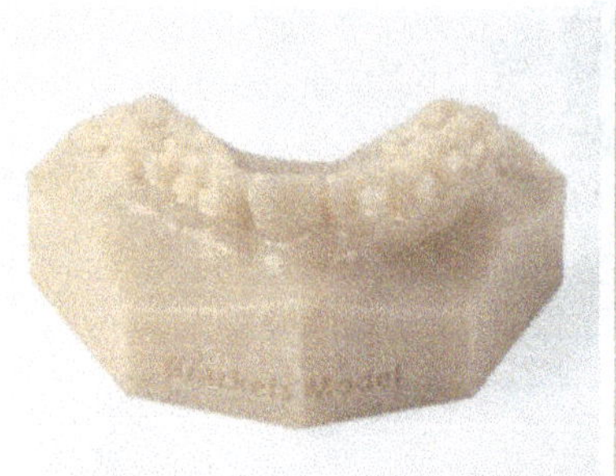

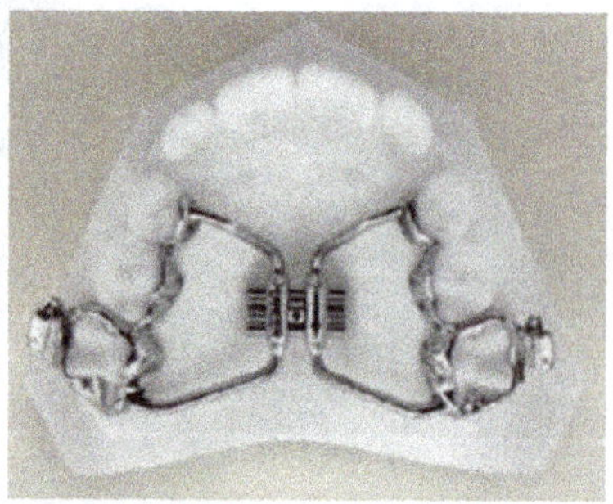

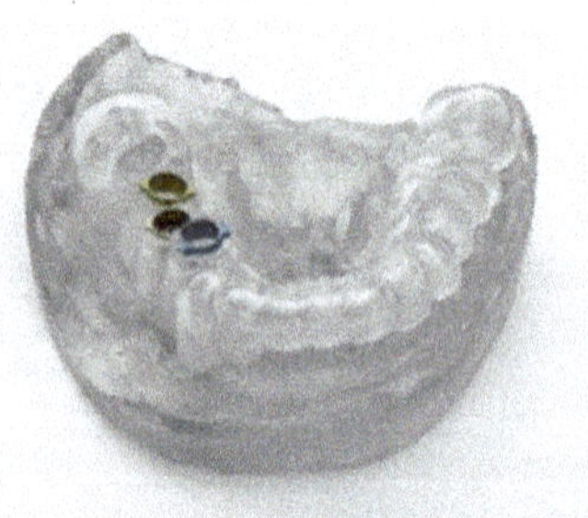

Figure 27. Dental model, RPE, and an implant surgical guide 3D printed from a STL generated file [38, 86]

Construction of metal dental frameworks of Co-Cr alloy, dental prosthesis wax patterns, facial prosthesis shells, and zirconia restorations using 3D printed technology have been successfully reproduced for use in prosthodontics [104-106]. In contrast, certain orthodontic appliances with soldered parts might require the use of a stone model since some 3D-printed models would deform or melt from the high temperature [77]. A broader range of materials with greater strength and resistance to moisture and heat should be specifically developed to suit the dental and orthodontic industries. Digitization of the manufacture process and standardization of the material ingredients are important steps for achieving consistent results.

7. Conclusion

With the rapid development and advanced research of diverse technologies and compatible materials, it is possible to obtain single scan digital impressions, virtually design, and 3D print different types of orthodontic appliances. 3D facial imaging further provides comprehensive analysis as an aid in orthodontics, maxillofacial, plastic, and esthetic surgery. Software integration of digital models, 3D facial scans, and CBCT facilitate treatment simulations and establish a meaningful communication with patients. Elimination of traditional impressions and dental-cast production stages enhance practice efficiency, patient and staff satisfaction for a fully integrated digital and streamlined workflow. Patient digital impressions are stored in a more convenient way and can be easily transferred to any lab or an in-office milling machine for a simpler, faster, and more predictable appliance fabrication. New companies, scanner and printer models are emerging daily which result in significant decline of systems cost and enhancement of material qualities. From imaging to product design and manufacture, technologies will offer more affordable and feasible diagnostic and treatment applications beyond the current methods.

Acknowledgements

This material is based on research sponsored by the Air Force Surgeon General's Office under agreement number FA7014-09-2-0003. The U.S. Government is authorized to reproduce and distribute reprints for Governmental purposes notwithstanding any copyright notation thereon. The views and conclusions contained herein are those of the authors and should not be interpreted as necessarily representing the official policies or endorsements, either expressed or implied, of the Air Force Surgeon General's Office or the U.S. Government. We thank the cited companies and journals for granting us permission to reproduce images included in this chapter. Figure 16 is reprinted from Rosati R, De Menezes M, Rossetti A, Sforza C, Ferrario VF. Digital dental cast placement in 3-dimensional, full-face reconstruction: a technical evaluation. Am J Orthod Dentofacial Orthop 2010;138(1): 84-8 with permission from Elsevier. Figure 21 is reprinted from Groth C, Kravitz ND, Jones PE, Graham JW, Redmond WR: Three-Dimensional Printing Technology. J Clin Orthod 2004;48: 475-485. Illustration by Nancy McCullick, reprinted with permission from JCO, Inc.

Author details

Emilia Taneva, Budi Kusnoto and Carla A. Evans

Department of Orthodontics, College of Dentistry, University of Illinois at Chicago, IL, USA

References

[1] van Noort R. The future of dental devices is digital. Dent Mater 2012;28(1): 3-12.

[2] Avula T, Nela M, Gudapati R, Velagapudi S. Efficient Use of Cloud Computing in Medical Science. Am J Comput Math 2012;2: 240-243.

[3] Akyalcin S, Cozad BE, English JD, Colville CD, Laman S. Diagnostic accuracy of impression-free digital models. Am J Orthod Dentofacial Orthop 2013;144(6): 916-22.

[4] Rheude BR, Sadowsky PL, Ferriera A, Jacobson A. An evaluation of the use of digital study models in orthodontic diagnosis and treatment planning. Angle Orthod 2005;75: 300–4.

[5] Fleming PS, Marinho V, Johal A. Orthodontic measurements on digital study models compared with plaster models: a systematic review. Orthod Craniofac Res 2011;14: 1–16.

[6] Keim RG, Gottlieb EL, Nelson AH, Vogels DS 3rd. 2008 JCO study of orthodontic diagnosis and treatment procedures, part 1: results and trends. J Clin Orthod 2008;42(11): 625-40.

[7] Okunami TR, Kusnoto B, BeGole E, Evans CA, Sadowsky C, Fadavi S. Assessing the American Board of Orthodontics objective grading system: digital vs plaster dental casts. Am J Orthod Dentofacial Orthop 2007; 31: 51-6.

[8] Santoro M, Galkin S, Teredesai M, Nicolay OF, Cangialosi TJ. Comparison of measurements made on digital and plaster models. Am J Orthod Dentofacial Orthop 2003;124(1): 101-5.

[9] Quimby ML, Vig KW, Rashid RG, Firestone AR. The accuracy and reliability of measurements made on computer-based digital models. Angle Orthod 2004;74(3): 298-303.

[10] Cuperus AM, Harms MC, Rangel FA, Bronkhorst EM, Schols JG, Breuning KH. Dental models made with an intraoral scanner: a validation study. Am J Orthod Dentofacial Orthop 2012;142(3): 308-13.

[11] Kim J, Heo G, Lagravère MO. Accuracy of laser-scanned models compared to plaster models and cone-beam computed tomography.

[12] Wiranto MG, Engelbrecht WP, Tutein Nolthenius HE, van der Meer WJ, Ren Y. Validity, reliability, and reproducibility of linear measurements on digital models obtained from intraoral and cone-beam computed tomography scans of alginate impressions. Am J Orthod Dentofacial Orthop 2013;143(1): 140-7.

[13] Taneva E, Johnson A, Viana G, Evans C. 3D evaluation of palatal rugae for human identification using digital study models. J Forensic Dent Sci (in press).

[14] Patzelt SBM, Emmanouilidi A, Stampf S, Strub JR, Wael A. Accuracy of full-arch scans using intraoral scanners. Clin Oral Investig 2014;18: 1687-94.

[15] Kravitz ND, Groth C, Jones PE, Graham JW, Redmond WR. Intraoral digital scanners. J Clin Orthod 2014;48: 337-47.

[16] Logozzo S, Zanetti EL, Franceschini G, Kilpelä AR, Mäkynen ANS. Recent advances in dental optics–Part I: 3D intraoral scanners for restorative dentistry. Opt Lasers Eng 2014;54: 203-221.

[17] Paddock SW, Eliceiri KW. Laser scanning confocal microscopy: history, applications, and related optical sectioning techniques. Methods Mol Biol 2014;1075: 9-47.

[18] Carlsson K, Danielsson PE, Lenz R, Liljeborg A, Majlöf L, Aslund N. Three-dimensional microscopy using a confocal laser scanning microscope. Opt Lett 1985;10(2): 53-5.

[19] Shotton, DM. Confocal scanning optical microscopy and its applications for biological specimens. Journal of Cell Science 1989;94 (2): 175-206.

[20] Ji Z, Leu MC. Design of optical triangulation devices. Opt Laser Technol 1989;21(5): 339-341.

[21] Costa, MFM. Surface inspection by an optical triangulation method. Opt Eng 1996;35(9): 2743-2747.

[22] Monks T, Robinson S. Optical triangulation sensor. US Patent 8,274,662; 2012.

[23] Podoleanu AG. Optical coherence tomography. J Microsc 2012;247(3): 209-19.

[24] Prati F, Regar E, Mintz GS, Arbustini E, Di Mario C, Jang IK, Akasaka T, Costa M, Guagliumi G, Grube E, Ozaki Y, Pinto F, Serruys PW; Expert's OCT Review Document. Expert review document on methodology, terminology, and clinical applications of optical coherence tomography: physical principles, methodology of image acquisition, and clinical application for assessment of coronary arteries and atherosclerosis. Eur Heart J 2010;31(4): 401-15.

[25] Fujimoto JG, Pitris C, Boppart SA, Brezinski ME. Optical coherence tomography: an emerging technology for biomedical imaging and optical biopsy. Neoplasia 2000;2(1-2): 9-25.

[26] Mermelstein MS, Feldkhun D, Shirley L. Video-rate surface profiling with acousto-optic accordion fringe interferometry. Opt Eng 2000;39(1): 106-113.

[27] Bloss R. Accordion fringe interferometry: a revolutionary new digital shape-scanning technology. Sens Rev 2008;28: 22-26.

[28] Frigerio F. Methods and apparatus for 3D surface imaging using active wave-front sampling. U.S. Patent No. 8,369,579. 5; 2013.

[29] Heber ST, Ranftl R, Pock TH. Variational Shape from Light Field. Energy Minimization Methods in Computer Vision and Pattern Recognition. Springer Berlin Heidelberg; 2013.

[30] Prakash H. The active wave-front sampling based 3D endoscope. Diss. Massachusetts Institute of Technology; 2007.

[31] iTero: Intra Oral Digital Scanner. http://itero.com/ (accessed 17 August 2014).

[32] Garino F, Garino B. The iOC intraoral scanner and Invisalign: a new paradigm. J Clin Orthod 2012;46(2): 115-21.

[33] Garino F, Garino GB, Castroflorio T. The iTero intraoral scanner in Invisalign treatment: a two-year report. J Clin Orthod 2014;48(2): 98-106.

[34] Digital Impressions: 3M™ True Definition Scanner. http://solutions.3m.com/wps/portal/3M/en_US/3M-ESPE-NA/dental-professionals/products/category/digital-materials/true-definition-scanner/ (accessed 22 August 2014).

[35] Lythos Digital Impression System. http://www.ormco.com/products/lythos/ (accessed 6 August 2014).

[36] Make a Digital Impression | Orthodontic Products. http://www.orthodonticproductsonline.com/2014/07/make-digital-impression/ (accessed 15 September 2014).

[37] CS 3500 | Intraoral Scanner from Carestream Dental. http://www.carestreamdental.com/us/en/scan/CS%203500#Features%20and%20Benefits/ (accessed 5 September 2014).

[38] 3Shape Orthodontics. http://www.3shapedental.com/orthodontics.aspx/ (accessed 5 September 2014).

[39] Dental Scanner – IOS FastScan – Handheld Laser Scanner. http://www.ios3d.com/dental-scanning/fastscan.aspx/ (accessed 5 September 2014).

[40] 3D Progress Digital Impression. http://www.3dprogress.it/ (accessed 5 September 2014).

[41] PLANSCAN COMPLETE SYSTEM | Planmeca CAD/CAM. http://planmecacadcam.com/planscan-complete-system/ (accessed 5 September 2014).

[42] Flügge TV, Schlager S, Nelson K, Nahles S, Metzger MC. Precision of intraoral digital dental impressions with iTero and extraoral digitization with the iTero and a model scanner. Am J Orthod Dentofacial Orthop 2013;144: 471-8.

[43] Naidu D, Freer TJ. Validity, reliability, and reproducibility of the iOC intraoral scanner: a comparison of tooth widths and Bolton ratios. Am J Orthod Dentofacial Orthop 2013;144(2): 304-10.

[44] Patzelt SB, Bishti S, Stampf S, Att W. Accuracy of computer-aided design/computer-aided manufacturing-generated dental casts based on intraoral scanner data. J Am Dent Assoc 2014;145(11): 1133-40.

[45] Patzelt SB, Lamprinos C, Stampf S, Att W. The time efficiency of intraoral scanners: an in vitro comparative study. J Am Dent Assoc 2014;145(6): 542-51.

[46] Lee SJ, Gallucci GO. Digital vs. conventional implant impressions: efficiency outcomes. Clin Oral Implants Res 2013;24(1): 111-5.

[47] Correia GD, Habib FA, Vogel CJ. Tooth-size discrepancy: A comparison between manual and digital methods. Dental Press J Orthod 2014;19(4): 107-13.

[48] Motion View Software, LLC. http://motionview3d.com/ (accessed 7 September 2014).

[49] 3D Professional Scanner – 3D Dental Scanner. http://www.maestro3d.com/ (accessed 7 September 2014).

[50] Akyalcin S, Dyer DJ, English JD, Sar C. Comparison of 3-dimensional dental models from different sources: diagnostic accuracy and surface registration analysis. Am J Orthod Dentofacial Orthop 2013;144(6): 831-7.

[51] Hayashi K, Sachdeva AU, Saitoh S, Lee SP, Kubota T, Mizoguchi I. Assessment of the accuracy and reliability of new 3-dimensional scanning devices. Am J Orthod Dentofacial Orthop 2013;144(4): 619-25.

[52] Zhurov A, Richmond S, Kau CH, Toma AR. Averaging Facial Images. In: (ed. Kau C, Richmond S. Three-Dimensional Imaging for Orthodontics and Maxillofacial Surgery. United Kingdom: Wiley Blackwell; 2010.

[53] Hajeer MY, Millett DT, Ayoub AF, Siebert JP. Applications of 3D imaging in orthodontics: part I. J Orthod 2004;31(1): 62-70.

[54] Wong JY, Oh AK, Ohta E, Hunt AT, Rogers GF, Mulliken JB, Deutsch CK. Validity and reliability of craniofacial anthropometric measurement of 3D digital photogrammetric images. Cleft Palate Craniofac J 2008;45(3): 232-9.

[55] Bush K, Antonyshyn O. Three-dimensional facial anthropometry using a laser surface scanner: validation of the technique. Plast Reconstr Surg 1996;98(2): 226-35.

[56] Jacobs RA. Plastic Surgery Educational Foundation DATA Committee. Three-dimensional photography. Plas Reconstr Surg 2000;107: 276-277.

[57] de Menezes M, Rosati R, Ferrario VF, Sforza C. Accuracy and reproducibility of a 3-dimensional stereophotogrammetric imaging system. J Oral Maxillofac Surg 2010;68(9): 2129-35.

[58] Aung SC, Ngim RC, Lee ST. Evaluation of the laser scanner as a surface measuring tool and its accuracy compared with direct facial anthropometric measurements. Br J Plast Surg 1995;48(8): 551-8.

[59] Canfield Scientific Inc. http://www.canfieldsci.com/ (accessed 7 September 2014).

[60] Souccar NM, Kau CH. Methods of Measuring the Three-Dimensional Face. Semin Orthod 2012;18(3): 187-192.

[61] Gwilliam JR, Cunningham SJ, Hutton T. Reproducibility of soft tissue landmarks on three-dimensional facial scans. Eur J Orthod 2006;28(5): 408-15.

[62] Hajeer MY, Ayoub AF, Millett DT, Bock M, Siebert JP. Three-dimensional imaging in orthognathic surgery: the clinical application of a new method. Int J Adult Orthodon Orthognath Surg 2002;17(4): 318-30.

[63] Farkas L. Anthropometry of the Head and Face. New York: Raven Press; 1994.

[64] Aynechi N, Larson BE, Leon-Salazar V, Beiraghi S. Accuracy and precision of a 3D anthropometric facial analysis with and without landmark labeling before image acquisition. Angle Orthod 2011;81(2): 245-52.

[65] Weinberg SM, Naidoo S, Govier DP, Martin RA, Kane AA, Marazita ML. Anthropometric precision and accuracy of digital three-dimensional photogrammetry: comparing the Genex and 3dMD imaging systems with one another and with direct anthropometry. J Craniofac Surg 2006;17(3): 477-83.

[66] Kimoto K, Garrett NR. Evaluation of a 3D digital photographic imaging system of the human face. J Oral Rehabil 2007;34(3): 201-5.

[67] Aldridge K, Boyadjiev SA, Capone GT, DeLeon VB, Richtsmeier JT. Precision and error of three-dimensional phenotypic measures acquired from 3dMD photogrammetric images. Am J Med Genet A 2005;138A(3): 247-53.

[68] Metzler P, Sun Y, Zemann W, Bartella A, Lehner M, Obwegeser JA, Kruse-Gujer AL, Lübbers HT. Validity of the 3D VECTRA photogrammetric surface imaging system for cranio-maxillofacial anthropometric measurements. Oral Maxillofac Surg 2014;18(3): 297-304.

[69] Evans C, Kusnoto B, Johnson T, Patra IP, Colvard M. Technical Report: Remote Sensing System/Software Test 1 Analysis. Chicago (IL): Univ. of Illinois at Chicago, 2014.

[70] Rosati R, De Menezes M, Rossetti A, Sforza C, Ferrario VF. Digital dental cast placement in 3-dimensional, full-face reconstruction: a technical evaluation. Am J Orthod Dentofacial Orthop 2010;138(1): 84-8.

[71] Sandbach G, Zafeiriou S, Pantic M, Yin, L. Static and dynamic 3D facial expression recognition: A comprehensive survey. Image Vis Comput 2012;30(10): 683-697.

[72] Shujaat S, Khambay BS, Ju X, Devine JC, McMahon JD, Wales C, Ayoub AF. The clinical application of three-dimensional motion capture (4D): a novel approach to quantify the dynamics of facial animations. Int J Oral Maxillofac Surg 2014;43(7): 907-16.

[73] Dynamic Surface Motion Caption (4D). http://www.3dmd.com/4d/ (accessed 14 September 2014).

[74] Weeden JC, Trotman CA, Faraway JJ. Three dimensional analysis of facial movement in normal adults: influence of sex and facial shape. Angle Orthod 2001;71(2): 132-40.

[75] Deng Z, Neumann U, Lewis JP, Kim TY, Bulut M, Narayanan S. Expressive facial animation synthesis by learning speech coarticulation and expression spaces. IEEE Trans Vis Comput Graph 2006;12(6): 1523-34.

[76] Berman B. 3-D printing: The new industrial revolution. Bus horiz 2012;55.2: 155-162.

[77] Groth C, Kravitz ND, Jones PE, Graham JW, Redmond WR. Three-dimensional printing technology. J Clin Orthod 2014;48(8): 475-85.

[78] Hieu L, Zlatov N, Vander Sloten J, Bohez E, Khanh L, Binh P, Oris P, Toshev Y. Medical rapid prototyping applications and methods. Assembly Autom 2005; 25(4): 284-292.

[79] Campbell T, Williams C, Ivanova O, Garrett B. Could 3D Printing Change the World?. Technologies, Potential, and Implications of Additive Manufacturing. Washington, DC: Atlantic Council of United States; 2011.

[80] Winder J, Bibb R. Medical rapid prototyping technologies: state of the art and current limitations for application in oral and maxillofacial surgery. J Oral Maxillofac Surg 2005;63(7): 1006-15.

[81] Zein I, Hutmacher DW, Tan KC, Teoh SH. Fused deposition modeling of novel scaffold architectures for tissue engineering applications. Biomaterials 2002;23(4): 1169-85.

[82] Chen M, Le DQ, Baatrup A, Nygaard JV, Hein S, Bjerre L, Kassem M, Zou X, Bünger C. Self-assembled composite matrix in a hierarchical 3-D scaffold for bone tissue engineering. Acta Biomater 2011;7(5): 2244-55.

[83] Rimell JT, Marquis PM. Selective laser sintering of ultra high molecular weight polyethylene for clinical applications. J Biomed Mater Res 2000;53(4): 414-20.

[84] Giacomo GD, Silva J, Martines R, Ajzen S. Computer-designed selective laser sintering surgical guide and immediate loading dental implants with definitive prosthesis in edentulous patient: A preliminary method. Eur J Dent 2014;8(1): 100-6.

[85] Ponader S, von Wilmowsky C, Widenmayer M, Lutz R, Heinl P, Körner C, Singer RF, Nkenke E, Neukam FW, Schlegel KA. In vivo performance of selective electron beam-melted Ti-6Al-4V structures. J Biomed Mater Res A 2010;92(1): 56-62.

[86] Professional 3D Printing I Stratasys. http://www.stratasys.com/ (assessed 21 September 2014).

[87] Professional Grade 3D Printers I EnvisionTEC. http://envisiontec.com/ (assessed 21 September 2014).

[88] Professional 3D Printers. http://www.3dsystems.com/3d-printers/professional/overview http://envisiontec.com/ (assessed 21 September 2014).

[89] Ebert J, Ozkol E, Zeichner A, Uibel K, Weiss O, Koops U, Telle R, Fischer H. Direct inkjet printing of dental prostheses made of zirconia. J Dent Res 2009;88(7): 673-6.

[90] Lin X, Shaw LL. Microstructure of dental porcelains in a laser-assisted rapid prototyping process. Dent Mater 2005;21: 336-346.

[91] Hornbeck LJ. Digital light processing update: status and future applications. Electronic Imaging. International Society for Optics and Photonics; 1999.

[92] 3D Printing Process – What is DLP?. https://thre3d.com/how-it-works/light-photopolymerization/digital-light-processing-dlp (accessed 25 September 2014).

[93] 3D Printing Process – What is Laminated Object Manufacturing (LOM)?. https://thre3d.com/how-it-works/sheet-lamination/laminated-object-manufacturing-lom/ (accessed 25 September 2014).

[94] Wong KV, Hernandez A. A review of additive manufacturing. ISRN Mechanical Engineering; 2012.

[95] MaketBot I 3D Printers I 3D Printing. http://www.makerbot.com/ (accessed 21 September 2014).

[96] FORMIGA P 110 – laser sintering 3D printer for rapid prototyping – EOS. http://www.eos.info/systems_solutions/plastic/systems_equipment/formiga_p_110/ (accessed 21 September 2014).

[97] Daryanan AM, Ackerman K, Steves M. 3D Printing: From Prototyping Evolution to Manufacturing Revolution. RBC Capital Markets, LLC; 2014.

[98] Hazeveld A, Huddleston Slater JJ, Ren Y. Accuracy and reproducibility of dental replica models reconstructed by different rapid prototyping techniques. Am J Orthod Dentofacial Orthop 2014;145(1): 108-15.

[99] Wiechmann D, Rummel V, Thalheim A, Simon JS, Wiechmann L. Customized brackets and archwires for lingual orthodontic treatment. Am J Orthod Dentofacial Orthop 2003;124(5): 593-9.

[100] Nasef AA, El-Beialy AR, Mostafa YA. Virtual techniques for designing and fabricating a retainer. Am J Orthod Dentofacial Orthop 2014;146(3): 394-8.

[101] Lauren M, McIntyre F. A new computer-assisted method for design and fabrication of occlusal splints. Am J Orthod Dentofacial Orthop 2008;133(4 Suppl): S130-5.

[102] Farronato G, Santamaria G, Cressoni P, Falzone D, Colombo M. The digital-titanium Herbst. J Clin Orthod 2011;45(5): 263-7.

[103] Wiechmann D, Schwestka-Polly R, Hohoff A. Herbst appliance in lingual orthodontics. Am J Orthod Dentofacial Orthop 2008;134(3): 439-46.

[104] Al Mortadi N, Eggbeer D, Lewis J, Williams RJ. CAD/CAM/AM applications in the manufacture of dental appliances. Am J Orthod Dentofacial Orthop 2012;142(5): 727-33.

[105] Sun J, Zhang FQ. The application of rapid prototyping in prosthodontics. J Prosthodont 2012;21(8): 641-4.

[106] Hems ED, Knott N. 3D printing in prosthodontics. Faculty Dental Journal 2014;5(4): 152-157.

7

Specificities of Adult Orthodontics

Mourad Sebbar, Nassiba Fatene, Asmaa El Mabrak, Narjisse Laslami, Zouhair Abidine and Zakaria Bentahar

1. Introduction

Adult orthodontics is becoming a larger proportion of many practices. Adult orthodontics is concerned with striking a balance between achieving optimal proximal and occlusal contact of the teeth, acceptable dentofacial esthetics, normal function, and reasonable stability. With the adult, it is more frequently concerned with physiological adaptation and is often symptom related, whereas with the child the dealing is with the signs. In the past three decades, a major reorientation of orthodontic thinking has occurred regarding adult patients [1].

Changed lifestyles and patient awareness have increased the demands for adult orthodontic treatment and multidisciplinary dental therapy has allowed better management of the more complicated and unique requirements of the adult patient population, thereby greatly improving the quality of care and treatment prognosis. In addition to goal clarification, adult patients desire treatment efficiency, convenience in appointment timings and good communication with other health care professionals. Almost 80% of the adult patients require interdisciplinary treatment planning and treatment execution. With the adult, consultation with another specialist isn't occasional. It is the rare adult whom one treats orthodontically without finding it necessary to collaborate with another specialist. This represents both the challenge and the excitement of adult orthodontics [2].

The objectives of adult orthodontics correspond to the general objectives of orthodontics i.e.: optimum occlusal function; improve the aesthetics of the face and teeth; contribute to the longevity of the stomatognathic system. However, a fourth objective can add in adults: realize a treatment of "aid" to the prosthesis.

The purpose of this chapter is to review, through clinical cases, the scope, effectiveness and limitations of orthodontic treatment in adult patients.

2. Psychological considerations

The demand for correction of malocclusion is often psychological and sociological rather than somatic. The relationship between psychology and orthodontics has been either ignored, or dealt with in mechanical ways. This is an area in which speculation and given work of irresponsible kind takes place [3].

Beauty is often more than skin deep because the psychological damage to a person who feels unattentive can be extreme. Orthodontic treatment provides a person a strong sense of feeling along with awareness, that he or she is not powerless, but that through proper co-operation can change and control outcomes.

Fundamental knowledge of psychology is necessary for modern orthodontics. The study of actions and reactions of individuals in social situations and the influence of such reactions on an individual is known as "dialectic psychology" [4].

Several authors have commented on the increase in the number of adults coming for orthodontic [5, 6]. This phenomenon has been attributed to various factors including the improved appearance of fixed appliances [7], increased awareness of the possibilities of orthodontic treatment, and the social acceptability of fixed appliances. Regardless of this, there is little information on this subgroup of patients; in particular, there is a lack of research on adults' motives for seeking orthodontic treatment. As early as 1971, Edgerton and Knorr [8] proposed the source of motivation to be the most crucial factor in determining and predicting patient satisfaction with treatment. This statement was made in relation to patients seeking esthetic surgery; however, it is likely that this hypothesis can be extrapolated to many types of treatment, including adult orthodontic treatment.

3. Biological considerations

The orthodontic treatment of adult patients differs from that of children in that there is no further appreciable skeletal growth in adult patients and the treatment is often multidisciplinary. There are, however, slow skeletal changes taking place in the facial bones during adulthood and the dentoalveolar compensation mechanism still occurs. The initially slower tissue response in adults compared with that in children does not significantly affect the total treatment time, since adult patients are general more co-operative than children, which seems to compensate for the slower tissue response [9].

- **Age changes in bone:** Cortical bone becomes denser and the spongy bone reduces with age. Marginal bone loss is more common in adults, which leads to apical shifting of the center of resistance of the involved tooth resulting in increased tipping moment produced by the applied force. This requires proper biomechanics utilizing adequate counter moment to achieve bodily movement of periodontally involved teeth [10].
- **Periodontal considerations:** A viable periodontal ligament is important for cell proliferation on application of mechanical force. There is a reduction in the periodontal ligament

vascularity with aging and insufficient source of preosteoblasts, which may explain the delayed response to orthodontic forces described in adults. It is mandatory to employ lighter force levels in adults as heavier forces result in vascular compression and necrosis of the blood vessels of the periodontal ligament. There is high-risk of iatrogenic damage to the periodontium with uncontrolled forces and it is important to keep the periodontal status under control during treatment [11, 12].

- **Vulnerability for root resorption:** Adults are more vulnerable to root resorption on application of orthodontic force. This is most commonly seen during intrusion of anterior and posterior teeth. Light continuous force must be employed to minimize the risk of root resorption and the patients must be informed of the potential risk before starting the treatment. It is mandatory to take periodical IOPA radiographs to evaluate for signs of root resorption. In case resorption is detected, active forces must be withdrawn for 7-8 weeks and further treatment can be continued after cessation of root resorption [13].

4. Diagnostic considerations

Careful diagnosis and treatment planning on a multidisciplinary approach is required to treat most adult patients. The adult, unlike the child, is usually a patient with high expectations from orthodontic treatment. He presents with minimal or no growth potential and meager accommodation to mechanics. In addition, the adult may exhibit a potential for such pathological changes as knife-edge ridges increased thickness of cortical plates, buried roots, impactions, gingival recession, periodontal breakdown, missing teeth, mesial tilting and extrusion of molars due to nonreplacement of extracted posterior teeth, TMJ problems, osteoporosis, osteomalacia and diabetes mellitus. These conditions, which obtain as a result of hormonal, vitamin or systemic disorders common to the adult, necessitate more careful and extensive diagnosis evaluations.

Orthodontic diagnosis involves development of a comprehensive database of pertinent information. The standard diagnostic aids such as case history, clinical examination and study casts, radiographs and photographs are mandatory [4].

Intraoral Periapical (IOPA), occlusal and TMJ films should be obtained routinely in addition to the panoramic radiograph and the cephalogram. The "problem oriented diagnostic approach" as described by Proffit and Ackerman, 1 is strongly recommended to ensure that no aspect of the patient need is neglected [14].

Additional diagnostic procedures that we should consider in an adult patient are:

- A full series intraoral periapical radiographs and TMJ X-rays.
- Diet evaluation
- Requirement of multidisciplinary approach towards treatment. Diagnostic steps involved in treating adult patients:
- Collection of accurate history and thorough patient examination

- Analyze the database
- Develop a problem list and priority
- Prepare tentative treatment plan according to the priorities
- Interact with other specialists involved. Acquire patient acceptance for the proposed treatment plan.

5. Therapeutic considerations

In the recent times, with the increasing expectations of the patients to an esthetically and functionally stable treatment result, the practice of dentistry is changing from a single specialist or general dentist practice to that of a team approach.

This enables the best utilization of the skills and expertise of clinicians of different specialties for the best possible treatment outcome of the patient. Such joint care of a patient's dental needs is defined as interdisciplinary treatment [15].

Interdisciplinary approach is indispensable for patients with mutilated dentition. Patients with congenital defects can be best treated with such a team work only. It is also of utmost importance in adult patients presenting with severe jaw discrepancies, abraded or worn teeth, old failing restorations, tipped teeth, multiple edentulous spaces from previous tooth extraction, periodontal breakdown, recession, and many other periodontal and restorative problems [16]

The role of orthodontist in such an interdisciplinary treatment approach can be primary or secondary. Primary as in a case wherein an orthodontic patient requires adjunctive other specialties treatment as prosthetic replacement of missing teeth, tooth build-up to match a Bolton discrepancy, periodontal rehabilitation, surgical exposure of an impacted tooth, etc. Secondary as in cases where the orthodontic treatment rendered is an adjunct to other treatment planned. Like in the case of space creation or tooth up righting to facilitate prosthetic replacement of a missing tooth, etc. [17].

Patient may have high expectations and hesitation in accepting visibility of orthodontic appliances. For esthetic reasons, patient may demand ceramic brackets or lingual orthodontics. Patient must be informed about the limitations of the treatment.

Closure of old extraction site may be difficult especially in molar region [18]. It may need uprighting to open the space mesially to receive prosthesis.

While bonding, special considerations may be required due to presence of restorations such as porcelains and metallic surfaces [19]. Excess adhesive around orthodontic attachments should be removed as surface roughness of adhesive attracts more plaque retention. Strict oral hygiene procedures must be reinforced as patients with periodontal problems may have various difficult areas to clean. All restorations must be properly polished to reduce the tendency of plaque retention. Stainless steel ligatures may be preferred to elastomeric modules due to less retentive to plaque [20].

Quantitative and qualitative changes in bone and compromised periodontal support and missing tooth may need special consideration to plan anchorage [21]. Headgears may not be acceptable to an adult due to esthetic reasons. Hence intraoral anchorage devices such as palatal arches and controlled forces are used. Microimplants can also be used to avoid dependence on teeth for anchorage.

Choice of extraction for orthodontic treatment may be affected by periorestorative problems or already extracted tooth. Occlusion achieved in adults, are stable in a healthy patient but compromised periodontal status may need permanent retention [22, 23].

5.1. Orthodontics-periodontics relationships

Under severe control against formation of dental biofilm and elimination or surveillance of periodontal pockets, patients who present susceptible or compromised periodontal status can be submitted to orthodontic treatment, like our patient who consulted for dental crowding which complicate hygiene measures (fig.1) [24, 25, 26]. Moreover, the orthodontic treatment allows that the stable periodontal status is maintained (fig 2).

Although there is no clear correlation between malocclusion and periodontal disease or between the effects of orthodontic treatments on periodontal improvement the literature describes clear interaction between Orthodontics and Periodontics [27].

Probable contributions of orthodontics in the periodontics field are:

1. It allows better oral hygiene by the patient, since it provides well shaped dental arches. Without dental crowding, malocclusion as a periodontal disease facilitator is eliminated (fig. 3)
2. It allows vertical occlusal impact parallels to the long axes of the teeth. Therefore, the applied muscle force is uniformly distributed all over the dental arch (fig. 4);
3. It contributes, along with prosthetic rehabilitations, for a normal vertical dimension;
4. In selected cases, it allows that the adequate dental crown-root relationship is achieved with induced orthodontic extrusion, with no bone loss;
5. It facilitates that bone vertical defects are corrected or improved with dental uprighting;
6. It improves the positioning of prosthetic pillars for fixed prostheses and of the next teeth of osteointegrated implants;
7. It decreases or eliminates effects of bruxism, as pain or muscle spasms, during the orthodontic therapy;
8. With the current available orthodontic technology and with correct planning and execution, it allows precise, light and efficient orthodontic movements.

Periodontal status is important and must be evaluated before contemplating orthodontic treatment in adult patients. If the periodontal disease is not treated and plaque control methods initiated before initiating orthodontic treatment, then the orthodontic tooth movement causes further periodontal destruction. This is particularly true if the teeth are moved in the direction of inflamed periodontal pockets that extend beyond the alveolar crest [28]. It is highly necessary to assess the patients' potential for bone loss and gingival recession during orthodontic tooth movement. The patient should be screened for the risk factors of periodontal disease.

Pre-treatment consultation with the periodontist should be routine and orthodontic objectives be altered according to his advice. Movement of teeth in the presence of periodontal inflammation will result in an increased loss of attachment and irreversible crestal bone loss.

Case n°1

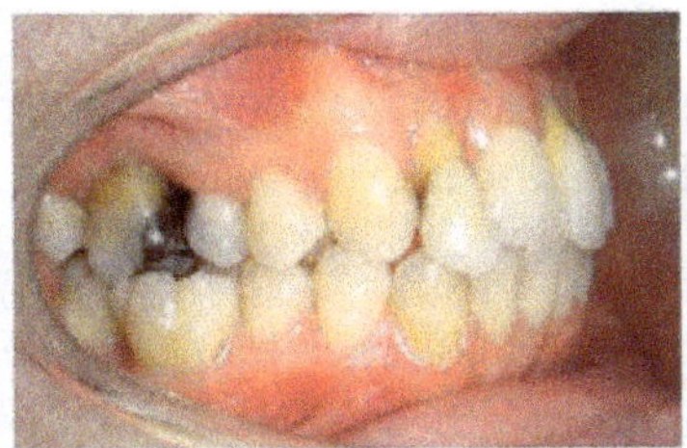
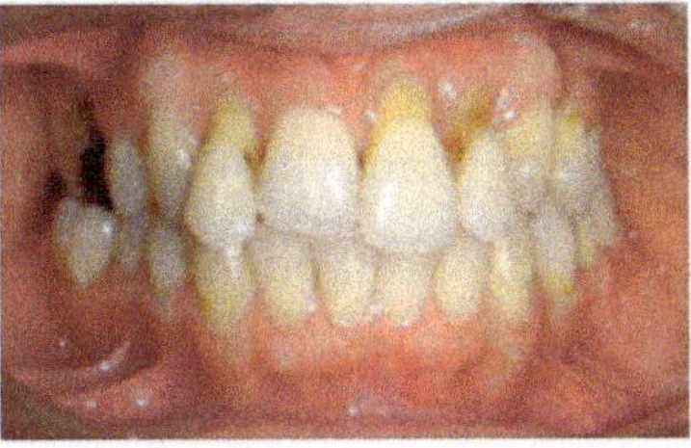
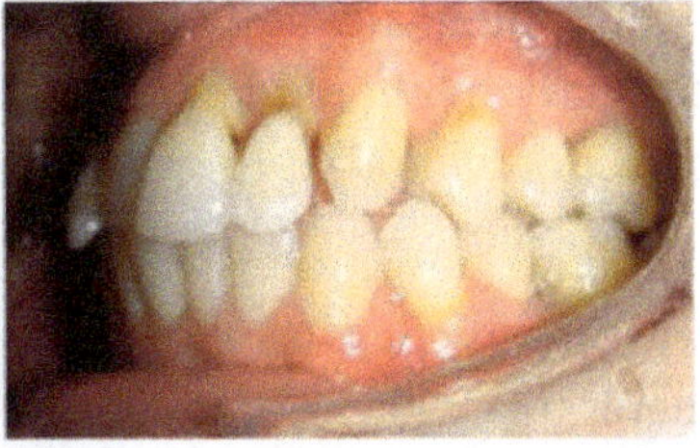

Figure 1. A young woman aged 20 years and the reason for consultation was gingival recession and dental crowding

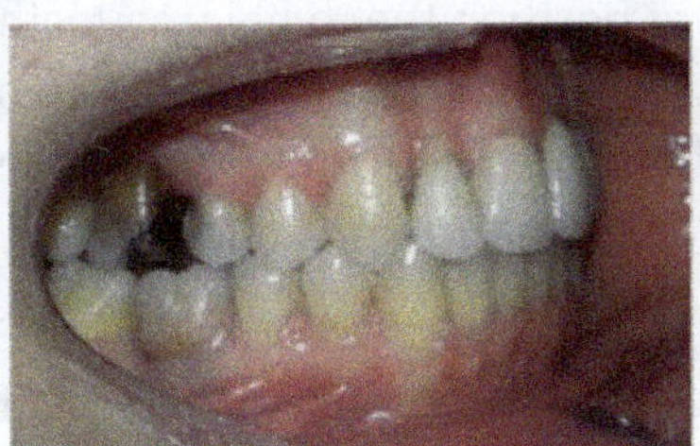
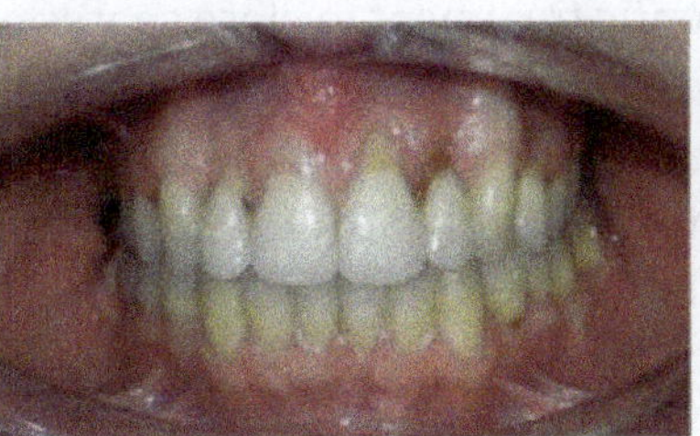
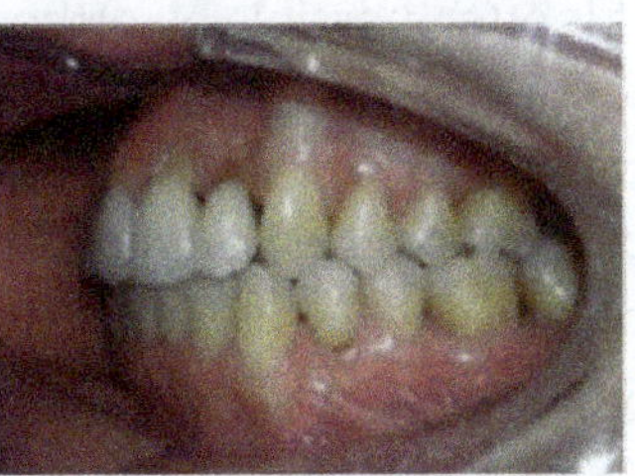

Figure 2. Orthodontic treatment consisted of an alignment and correction crowding, the patient was sent after removal of the orthodontic appliance to the periodontist for a gingival graft to cover gingival recession

Case n°2

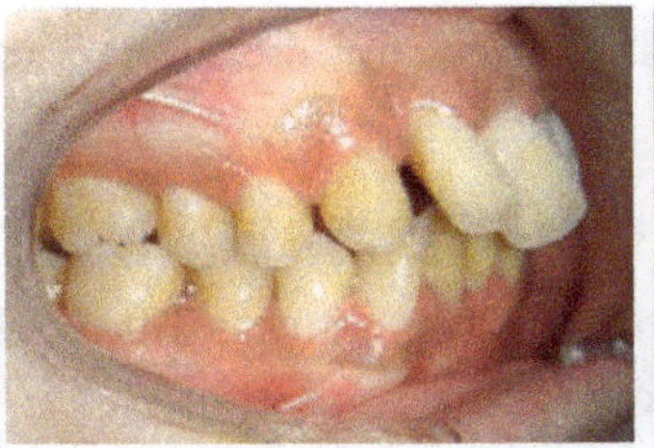
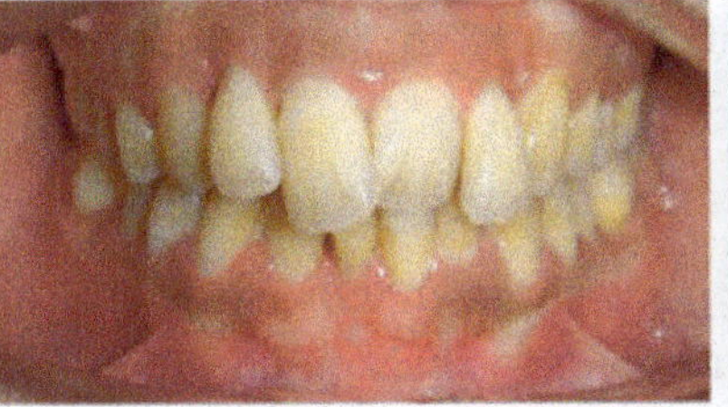
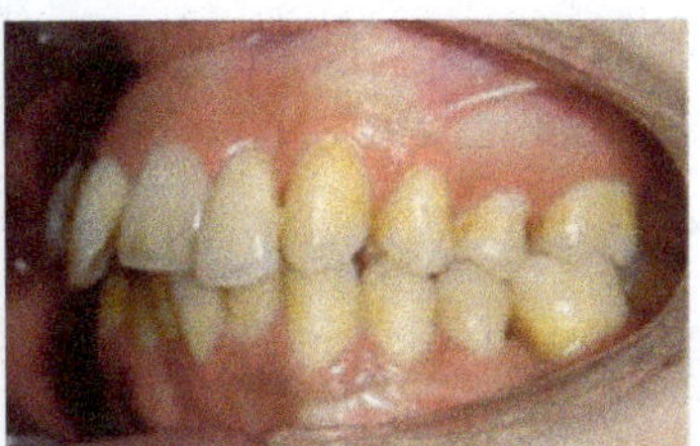

Figure 3. A patient who consults for malpositions and dental extrusions

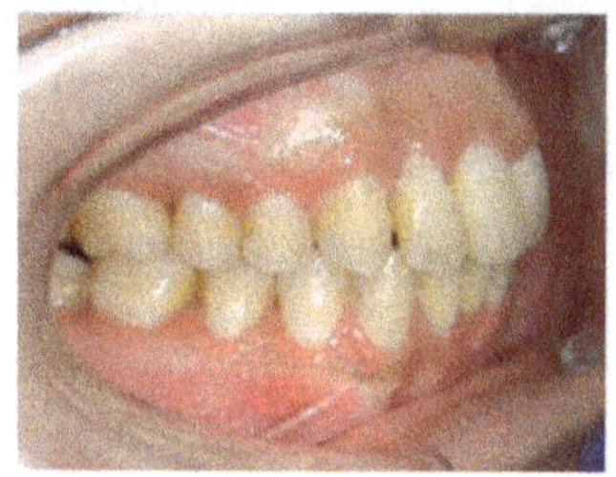
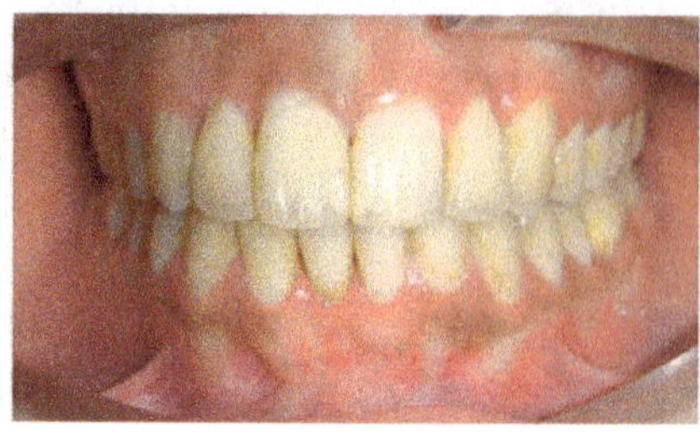
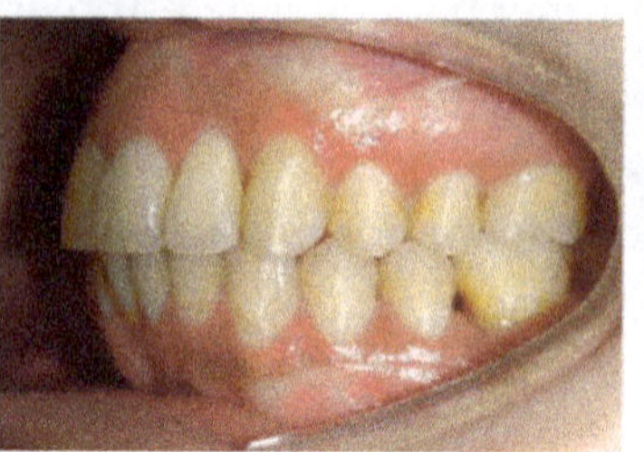

Figure 4. Orthodontic treatment was aimed at correcting dental malposition and regain proper alignment will facilitate the oral hygiene.

5.2. Orthodontic-prosthesis relationships

Adult patients usually require adjunctive and comprehensive treatment involving multidisciplinary treatment approach. Correcting the malocclusion helps in improving the quality of periodontal and restorative treatment outcomes besides providing esthetic benefits.

Adult are now more frequently referred for orthodontic treatment to improve the positioning and alignment of teeth prior to the replacement of missing teeth (fig. 5, 7). Such tooth movements may be undertaken to achieved parallel abutments of the teeth used to hold the prosthesis, to create space for a pontic (the false tooth in a bridge) or to make space for a dental implant (usually a titanium device that integrates with the jaw bone and can be used to support a crown or dental bridge). (fig. 6, 8)

It is often possible by orthodontic treatment to close spaces or re-position the remaining teeth following tooth loss. A good example of the usefulness of orthodontic treatment is when canines and premolars are moved posteriorly, eliminating either the need for a removable partial prosthesis to replace missing molars, or to allow insertion of a short-span fixed bridge, rather than the use a removable, partial prosthesis [9].

Adult patients have many preexisting conditions that are usually not present in adolescent patients. Hence, additional treatment objectives are established at the start of the treatment. Though acceptable esthetics is an integral part of treatment goal, but function, stability and health of dentition is given paramount importance. Additional treatment objectives are determined to facilitate and improve effectiveness of periorestorative treatment by [29]:

- Improving axial inclination of teeth, thereby improving root positioning with sufficient bone between roots for good vascular supply and proper contact area;
- Achieving parallelism of abutment teeth to minimize tooth cutting for fabrication of prosthesis;
- Most favorable distribution of abutment teeth to receive prosthesis for better stability;
- Uprighting and extrusion of posterior teeth with occlusal equilibration sometimes followed by endodontic treatment to improve vertical osseous defects and crown root ratio;
- Forced extrusion of teeth damaged up to one third of cervical line to provide better support at the margin of the prosthesis;

- To restore functional occlusion keeping in mind existing skeletal relationship rather than aiming for Andrew's six keys to normal occlusion;
- Achieving better lip support for flaccid & long upper lip by maintaining anterior teeth in slight procumbent position with correction of overjet by proclining & maintaining lower incisors in more procumbent position than normal position to avert wrinkles around the lips; & restoring vertical dimension with bite plate before placing prosthesis in bite collapse.

Case n°3

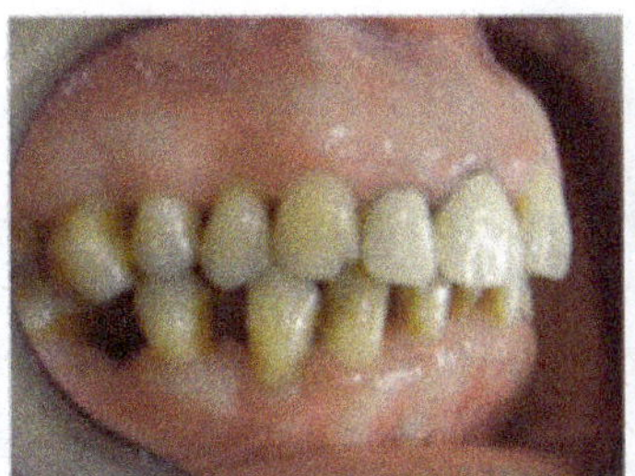
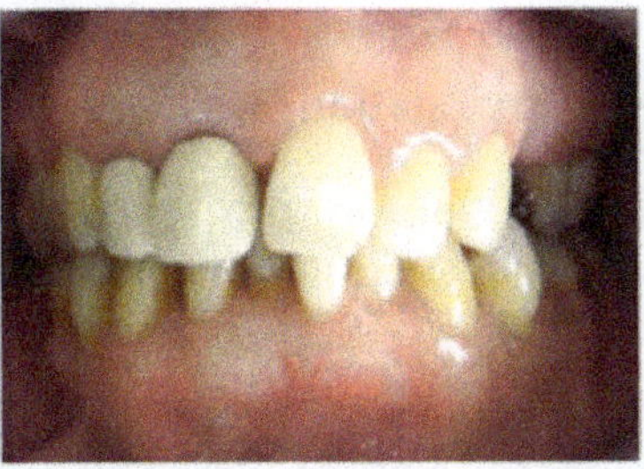
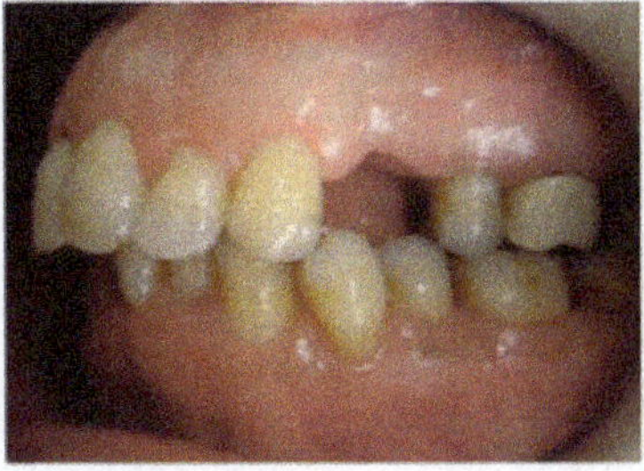

Figure 5. Clinical examination in this patient showed defective prostheses with poor periodontal status.

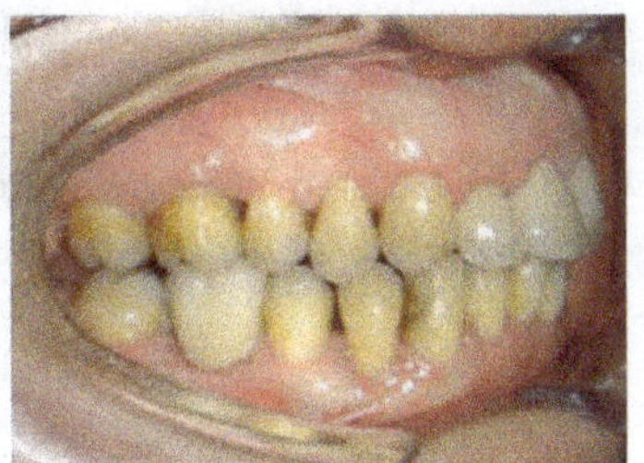
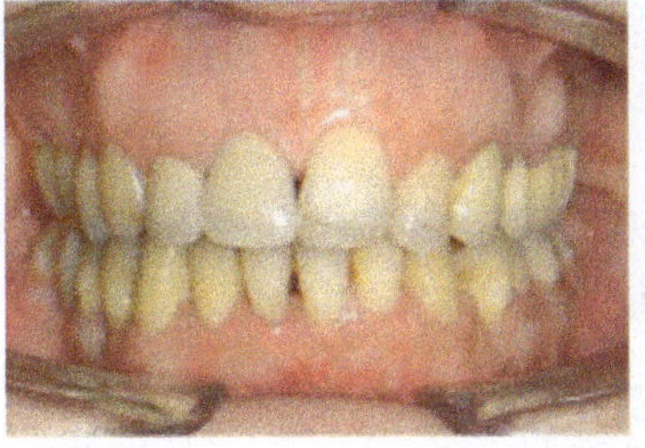
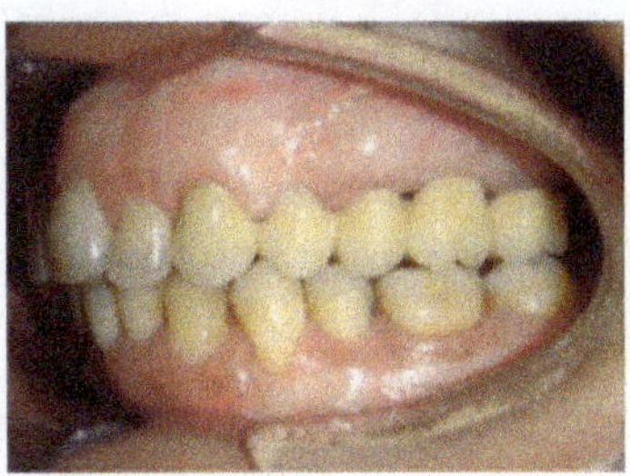

Figure 6. Orthodontic treatment was performed to correct the malocclusion. The patient also received a prosthetic rehabilitation.

Case n°4

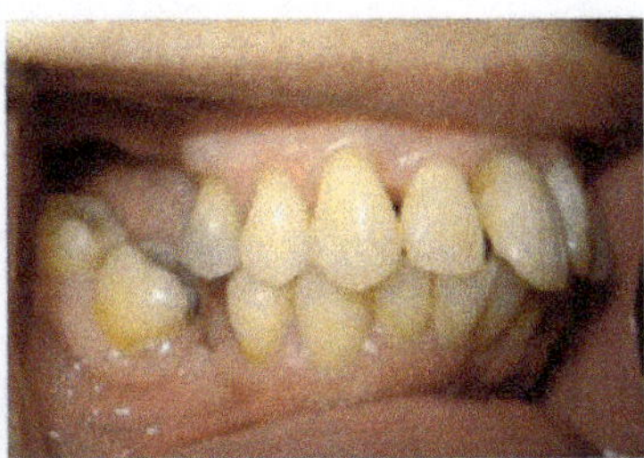
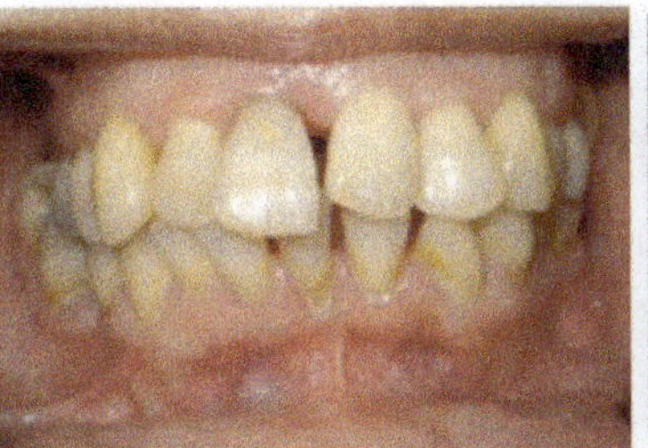
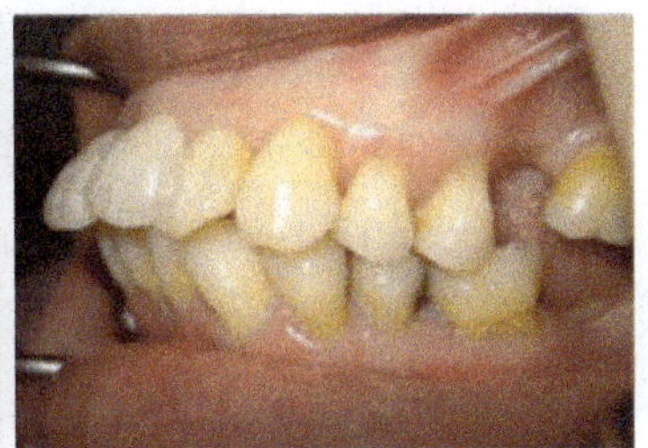

Figure 7. A patient aged 50years addressed for orthodontic treatment for future prosthetic rehabilitation.

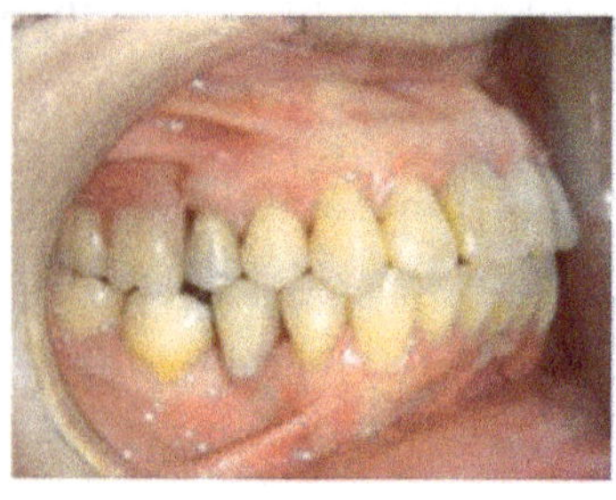 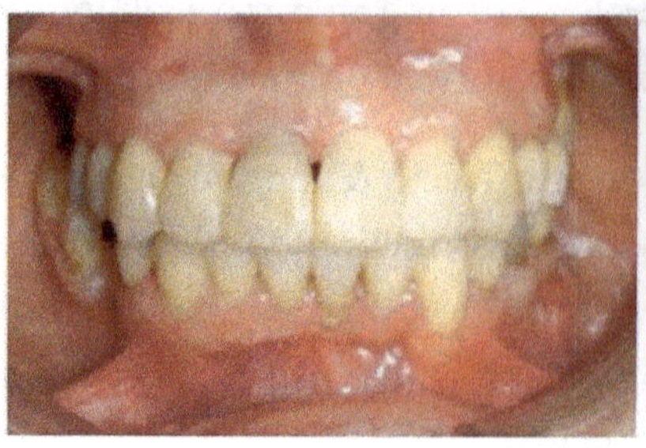 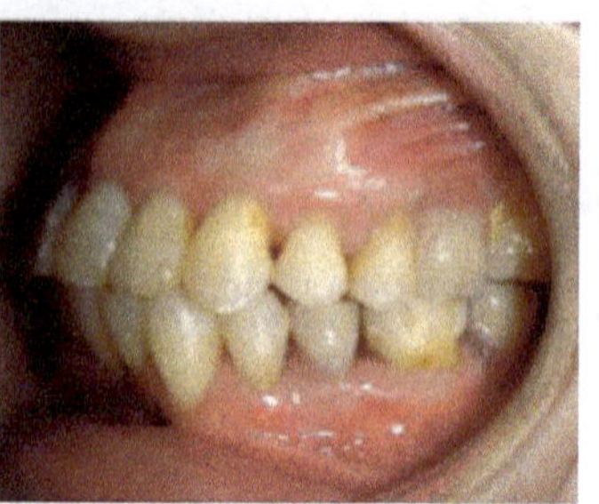

Figure 8. Orthodontic treatment was to correct malopositions and dental rotations and creates spaces for future prostheses. A provisional prosthesis was performed until achieve dental implants

5.3. Orthodontics-orthognathic surgery relationships

Skeletal malocclusion (dysgnathia) is defined as the congenital or acquired abnormal position or morphology of one or both jaws. There might be symmetry or asymmetry with disruption of the maxillomandibular relationship or the relationship of the jaws to the skull base combined with malocclusion or joint disruption [30]. The main treatment objectives for serious skeletal malocclusions are aesthetic, functional and psychological rehabilitation. For this kind of cases these goals may be achieved [31]. The orthodontist can move teeth and alveoli but this has no substantial impact on the adult basal jaw bone. The main orthodontist's task is teeth alignment. The oral & maxilofacial surgeon is responsible for the surgical correction of jaws and their associated structures. Generally speaking, the diagnosis and treatment plan of orthognathic cases require a systematic team approach [32].

Orthognathic surgery involves risks and this is why we need to proceed with it only after careful planning. It is particularly important to understand the patient's view; this establishes trust and communication and helps achieve high quality results [33].

Indications of orthognatic surgery [34, 35]

Given the relationship between facial skeletal deformities and masticatory dysfunction, as well as the limitations of non-surgical therapies to correct these discrepancies, orthognathic surgery should be considered medically appropriate in the following circumstances.

a. Anteroposterior discrepancies: established norm=2mm

   1. Maxillary/Mandibular incisor relationship:

      - Horizontal overjet of +5mm or more.
      - Horizontal overjet of zero to a negative value (fig. 9).

   2. Maxillary/Mandibular anteroposterior molar relationship discrepancy of 4mm or more (norm 0 to 1mm).

b. Vertical discrepancies

   1. Presence of a vertical facial skeletal deformity which is two or more standard deviations from published norms for accepted skeletal landmarks.

2. Open Bite
    - No vertical overlap of anterior teeth.
    - Unilateral or bilateral posterior open bite greater than 2mm
3. Deep overbite with impingement or irritation of buccal or lingual soft tissues of the opposing arch.
4. Supraeruption of a dentoalveolar segment due to lack of occlusion.

c. Transverse discrepancies

1. Presence of a transverse skeletal discrepancy which is two or more standard deviations from published norms.
2. Total bilateral maxillary palatal cusp to mandibular fossa discrepancy of 4mm or greater, or a unilateral discrepancy of 3mm or greater, given normal axial inclination of the posterior teeth.

d. Asymmetries

Anteroposterior, transverse or lateral asymmetries greater than 3mm with concomitant occlusal asymmetry.

Preoperative orthodontics (fig. 10)

The goals of preoperative orthodontic treatment are to allow for maximum surgical correction of the abnormality, to facilitate potential sectional surgical procedures and to provide the possibility for creating an ideal, stable occlusion (Tompach et al., 1995). The major part of orthodontic treatment takes place before surgery and might last one and a half to two years (Slavnic & Marcusson, 2010; Diaz et al., 2010) [36, 37, 38]

1. Arch alignment

The first goal of preoperative orthodontics is to align the dental arches or their parts so that they might be compatible with each other. Correcting crowding and rotations, management of impacted teeth and arch length discrepancies is mainly a concern of preoperative orthodontics, because it facilitates arch intercuspation; otherwise, the surgical result would be restricted. [37]

2. Arch flattening

The planning of dental arch flattening is particularly important. Dental flattening and alignment are usually a common one-step process in conventional orthodontics. This is not the case for all surgical cases. When the mandible is surgically moved forward or backward, the position of the lower incisor is what determines the lower facial height. [38]

3. Exacerbations

In serious skeletal discrepancies, the teeth try to maintain some contact, under the effect of external and internal forces, so as to compensate for the skeletal problem. Although this compensation improves occlusal relationships and the patient's appearance, it restricts the extent of surgical correction. In skeletal Class III cases, the upper incisors are often labially inclined, while the lower ones are lingually inclined. On the contrary, in cases of skeletal Class II the upper incisors are often upright and the lower labially inclined. A consequence of these compensatory changes is that the overjet is virtual in regard to the actual magnitude of the skeletal discrepancy. Preoperative orthodontics aims at exacerbating dental relationships, by removing the camouflage effect and placing the incisors in normal inclination for the skeletal bases, if this is feasible (Jacobs & Sinclair, 1983). [39]

4. Intercuspation of the two arches

One of the goals of preoperative orthodontics is to achieve harmonisation of dental arches at all levels during surgery. Before the end of the preoperative phase, upper and lower rigid rectangular wires need to be passively in position for eight weeks before surgery. Some type of hooks or brackets with thick attachments should be placed on the wires Kobayashi so as to facilitate immobilization during surgery. [40]

Surgical procedures. [41]

- Le Fort I Osteotomy (fig 11)

The vertical position of the maxilla is recorded by measuring the distance between the medial canthus and the orthodontic arch wire. These vertical measurements are absolutely critical. The cut should be made at least 5 mm above the apices of the teeth. If cuts are complete, the maxilla is downfractured with manual pressure. The amount the maxilla will be impacted or elongated was determined in the treatment plan.

- Surgically Assisted Rapid Palatal Expansion

Correction of transverse maxillary constriction can be corrected in adolescence with nonsurgical orthodontic appliances. As the sutures begin to close during late adolescence, relapse increases. A multipiece LeFort osteotomy can be performed to provide simultaneous maxillary expansion, but the degree of relapse is high. In the young adult, the preferred procedure is the surgically assisted rapid palatal expansion (SARPE). The orthodontist places a palatal expander prior to the procedure.

- Bilateral Sagittal Split Osteotomy

The cut is made with electrocautery about 1 cm from the lateral aspect of the molars and extends from midramus to the region of the second molar. If insufficient tissue is left on the dental side of the incision, closure is more difficult. A periosteal elevator is used to expose the lateral mandible and the anterior coronoid process in a subperiosteal plane.

- Two-Jaw Surgery

Moving the maxilla and the mandible in one procedure require osteotomizing both jaws and precisely securing them into the position determined by the treatment plan. If proper treatment planning, model surgery, and splint fabrication are performed, each jaw should be able to be placed into its desired position with precision. The mandibular bony cuts are made first but terminated prior to osteotomy completion. The maxillary osteotomy is made, and the maxilla is placed into its new position using the intermediate splint. The splint is used to wire the teeth into intermaxillary fixation. The intermediate splint indexes the new position of the maxilla to the preoperative (uncorrected) position of the mandible.

Postoperative orthodontics (fig 12)

The aim of postoperative orthodontics is to bring the teeth to their final positions and secure balanced occlusion; finally retention planning should be achieved. This phase of the treatment starts two to four weeks later, after a satisfactory range of mandibular movement has been achieved and there is good bone healing. [42] (fig 13)

Case n°5

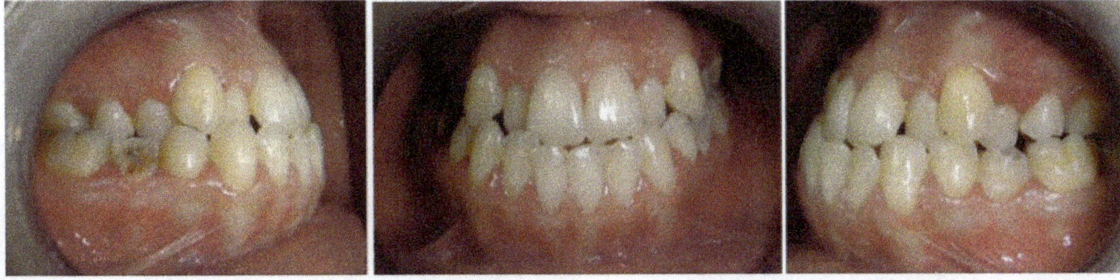

Figure 9. A patient aged 23 years presented to an aesthetic pattern with a skeletal Class III with facial asymmetry.

Clinical examination revealed anterior crossbite with a deviation of the median incisors on the right side

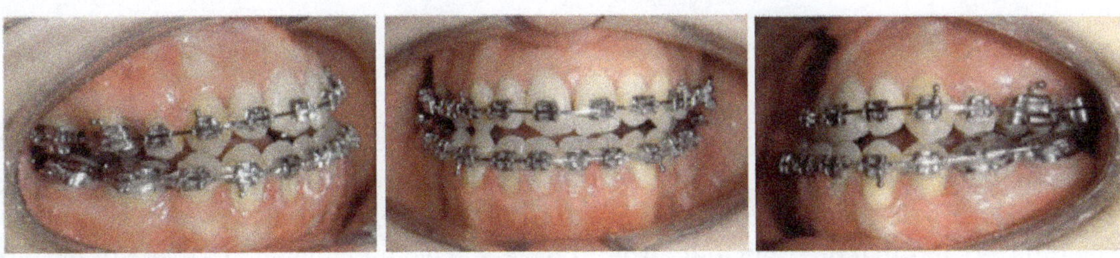

Figure 10. we opted for orthognathic surgery. Orthodontic treatment aimed to raise dental compensations with extraction: 14.24.34.44.

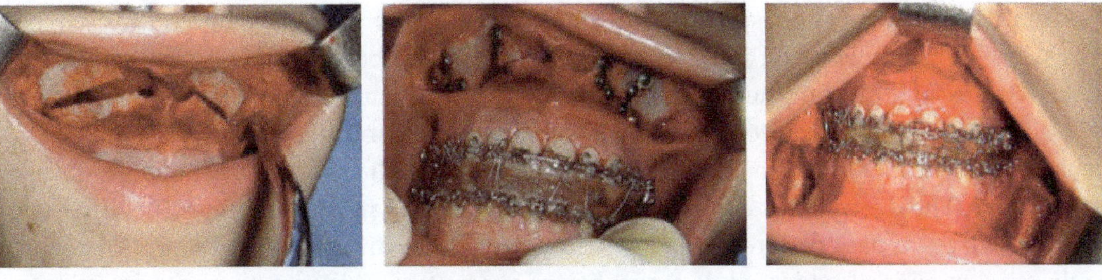

Figure 11. Orthognathic surgery consisted of an osteotomy Lefort 1 for maxillary advanced and sagittal mandibular osteotomy to go back and refocus the mandible

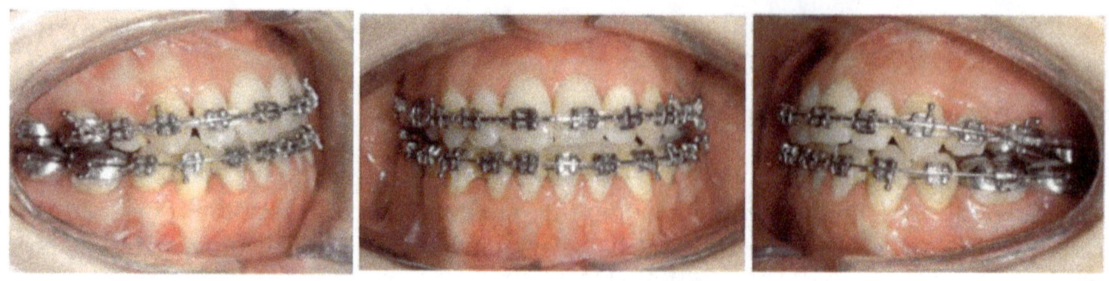

Figure 12. Some months after the surgery, orthodontic treatment is to install a good occlusion

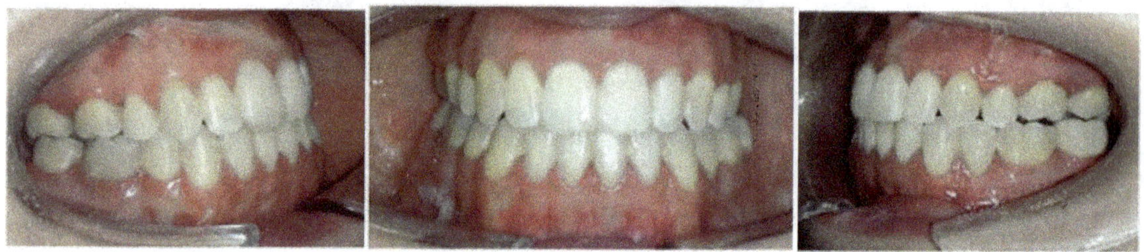

Figure 13. After 26 months, we were able to obtain a satisfactory aesthetic and functional result

6. Conclusion

Adult patients provide us the opportunity to render the greatest service possible in orthodontics. There is a great need for orthodontic treatment for the adult patient Treating adults is a very pleasant and gratifying experience both clinically and personally [43]. Adult patients are cleaner, more careful, more punctual, prompt payers, have much less pain than youngsters, and treatment time is either the same or less than that of younger patients. Continuing education of the general public will result in an increasing demand for this type of service. The orthodontist should update his knowledge and his thinking in this aspect of his responsibility, and should try as much as possible to co-ordinate his efforts with those of his confreres in other branches of dentistry in order to render to the population a better and more complete dental health service [46]. The problems that may arise are minimal in comparison with the great results that the clinician can obtain in consistently improving the function, aesthetics, and psychological outlook of the adult patient. With the adult, diagnosis is really simpler than it is for a child. The diagnosis more or less "leaps out at you" and, sometimes, the diagnosis is even made by the patient. Treatment is sometimes more difficult for the adult, because it requires the combined expertise of a number of specialties, and growth is not on your side. Without growth and with some of the symptomatology that occurs, requiring other specialists, orthodontic treatment of adults can be more complex than treatment of the child.

Author details

Mourad Sebbar[1*], Nassiba Fatene[2], Asmaa El Mabrak[2], Narjisse Laslami[2], Zouhair Abidine[1] and Zakaria Bentahar[2]

*Address all correspondence to: sebbar.mourad@gmail.com

1 Hospital Moulay Abdellah, Mohammedia, Morocco

2 Department of orthodontics; Faculty of dentistry, Casablanca, Morocco

References

[1] Fastlicht J. Adult orthodontics, Journal of clinical orthodontics 1982; 16 :606-618.

[2] Thomas M Graber, Rober t L Vanarsdall, Katherine W L Vig. Or thodontic: Current principles and technique, 4 th edition: 937-985.

[3] Seema G, Somesh G, Deepak A. psychological aspects of orthodontic treatment. J Ind Orthod Soc 2001;34:92-94.

[4] Pabari S, Mole DR. Cunninghamc SJ. Assessment of motivation and psychological characteristics of adult orthodontic patients. Am J Orthod Dentofacial Orthop. 2011;140(6):e263-72.

[5] Khan RS, Horrocks EN. A study of adult orthodontic patients and their treatment. Br J Orthod 1991;18:183-94.

[6] Nattrass C, Sandy JR. Adult orthodontics—a review. Br J Orthod 1995;22:331-7.

[7] ZachrissonBU.Global trends and paradigm shifts in clinical orthodontics. World J Orthod 2005;6(Suppl):3-7.

[8] Edgerton MT Jr, Knorr NJ. Motivational patterns of patients seek- ing cosmetic (esthetic) surgery. Plast Reconstr Surg 1971;48: 551-7.

[9] Hagg U, Corbet EF, Rabie AM. Adult orthodontics and its interface with other discipline. HKMJ 1996-2: 186-90.

[10] Shei O, Waerhaug J, Lovdal A, Arnulf A. Alveolar bone loss as related to oral hygiene and age. J Periodontol 1959; 26:7-16.

[11] Cohn SA. Disuse atrophy of the periodontium in mice. Arch Oral Biol 1965;10(6): 909-19.

[12] Melsen B. Tissue reaction following application of extrusive and intrusive forces to teeth in adult monkeys. Am J Orthod 1986;89(6):469-75.

[13] Melsen B. Limitations in adult orthodontics. Current controversies in orthodontics. Quintessence Publishing Co 1991;147-80.

[14] Meeran NA, Madhuri, Parveen J. The Scope and Limitations of Adult Orthodontics. Ind J Multidiscipl Dent 2011;2(1):383-387.

[15] Kharbanda O.P. Orthodontics: Diagnosis and Management of Malocclusion and Dentofacial Deformities 2nd edition, Elsevier; 2013.

[16] Kokich V.G, Spear F.M. Guidelines for managing the orthodontic-restorative patient. Semin Orthod 1997; 3: 3-20.

[17] Savana K, Ansari A, Hamsa R, Kumar M, Jain A, Singh A. Interdisciplinary Therapy in Orthodontics: An Overview. Int J Advanced Health Sci l 2014 ;1(5) :23-31.

[18] Hom BM, Turley PK. Effects of space closure of the mandibular first molar area in adults. Am J Orthod Dentofac Orthop 1984;105:25-34.

[19] Zachrisson BU, Buyukyilmaz T. Recent advances in bonding to gold, amalgam and porcelain. J Clin Orthod 1993;27:661-75.

[20] Forsberg CM, Brattstrom V, Malmberg E, Nord CE. Ligature wires and elastomeric rings: two methods of ligation and their association with microbial colonization of Streptococcus mutans and Lactobacilli. Eur J Orthod 1991;13:416-420.

[21] Ong MA, Wang HL, Smith FN. Interrelationships between periodontics and adult orthodontics. J Clin Periodontol 1998;25:271-277.

[22] Harris EF, Vaden JL, Dunn KL. Effects of patient age on post orthodontic stability in Class II, division 1 malocclusion. Am J Orthod Dentofac Orthop 1994;105:25-34.

[23] Kahl-Nieke B. Retention and stability considerations for adult patients. Dent Clin North Am 1996;40:961-994.

[24] Elliasson LA, Hugoson A, Kurol J, Siwe H. The effects of orthodontic treatment on periodontal tissues in patients with reduced periodontal support. Eur J Orthod 1982;4:1-9.

[25] Boyd RL, Leggot PJ, Quinn RS, Eakle WS, Chambers DW. Periodontal implications of orthodontic treatment in adults with reduced or normal periodontal tissues versus those of adolescents. Am J Orthod Dentofac Orthop 1989;96:191-8.

[26] Ong M A Wang HL. Periodontic and orthodontic treatment in adults. Am J Orthod Dentofac Orthop 2002;122:420-8.

[27] Del Santo M. Periodontium and Orthodontic Implications: Clinical Applications. Int J Stomatol Res 2012, 1(3): 17-23.

[28] Wennström JL, Stokland BL, Nyman S, Thilander B. Periodontal tissue response to orthodontic movement of teeth with infrabony pockets. Am J Orthod Dentofacial Orthop 1993;103(4):313-9.

[29] Bagga DK. Limitations in Adult Orthodontics: A Review. J Oral Health Comm Dent 2009;3(3):52-55.

[30] Slavnic S, Marcusson A. (2010). Duration of orthodontic treatment in conjunction with orthognathic surgery. *Swedish Dental Journal,* Vol. 34, No. 3, pp. 159-166, ISSN 0347-9994.

[31] Sabri R. (2006). Orthodontic Objectives in Orthognathic surgery: state of the art today. *World Journal of Orthodontics,* Vol. 7, No. 2, pp. 177-191, ISSN 1530-5678.

[32] Wolford LM, Stevao ELL, Alexander CM, Goncalves JR. (2004). Orthodontics for Orthognathic Surgery, In: Peterson's Principals of Oral and Maxillofacial Surgery, Miloro M, Ghali GE, Larsen PE, Waite P, pp. 1111-1134, BC Decker Inc, ISBN 1-55009-234-0, Canada.

[33] Wolford LM. (2007). Surgical Planning in Orthognathic Surgery, In: *Maxillofacial Surgery,* Booth PW, Schendel SA, Hausamen J-E, pp. 1155-1210, Churchill Livingstone Elsevier, ISBN-13 978-0-443-10053-6, St. Louis USA.

[34] Arnelt W, McLaughlin R. Overview, treatment goals re-stated. In: Facial and Dental Planning for Orthodontists and Oral Surgeons.St Louis, MO: Mosby/Elsevier; 2004:2-3

[35] Bousaba S, Siciliano S, Delatte M, Faes J, Reychler H, Indications for orthognathic surgery, the limitations of orthodontics and of surgery, Rev Belge Med Dent (1984). 2002;57(1):9-23.

[36] Tompach PC, Wheeler JJ, Fridrich KL. (1995).Orthodontic considerations in orthognathic surgery. The *International Journal of Adult Orthodontics and Orthognathic Surgery*.Vol.10, No2, pp.97-107, ISSN 0742-1931.

[37] Slavnic S, Marcusson A. (2010). Duration of orthodontic treatment in conjunction with orthognathic surgery. *Swedish Dental Journal,* Vol. 34, No. 3, pp. 159-166, ISSN 0347-9994.

[38] Diaz PM, Garcia RG, Gias LN, Aguirre-Jaime A, Pérez JS, de la Plata MM, Navarro EV, Gonzalez FJ.(2010). Journal of Oral and Maxillofacial Surgery. Vol. 68, No. 1, pp. 88-92, ISSN 0278-2391.

[39] Jacobs JD, Sinclair PM. (1983). Principles of orthodontic mechanics in orthognathic surgery cases. American journal of orthodontics. Vol. 84, No 5, pp. 399-407, ISSN 0002-9416

[40] Reyneke JP. (2003). *Essentials of Orthognathic Surgery,* Quintessence Publishing Co, ISBN 0- 86715-410-1, China

[41] Proffit WR, Sarver DM. Treatment planning: optimizing benefit to the patient. In: Proffit WR, White RP, Sarver DM, eds. Contemporary Treatment of Dentofacial Deformity. St. Louis: Mosby; 2003:213–223.

[42] Proffit WR, Sarver DM. (2003). Treatment planning: Optimizing benefit to the patient. In *Contemporary Treatment of Dentofacial Deformity*. Proffit WR, White RP, Jr, SarverDM, pp. 172-244, Mosby, ISBN 0-323-01697-9, St.Louis USA.

[43] Robert C. Chiappone. Special considerations for Adult Orthodontics. J clin orthod 1976; 10 :535- 545.

[44] Harvey L. Levitt. Adult Orthodontics. J clin orthod 1971; 5: 130-155.

8

Oral Health From Dental Paleopathology

Hisashi Fujita

1. Introduction

Since when have humans been afflicted with dental diseases? It is not easy to find an answer to this question. There are two main methods to examine what types of disease our ancestors suffered. One method involves the history of medicine or a study called "medical history," which mainly examines pathologies written in ancient documents and ancient writings and attempts to identify the diseases. Michinaga Fujiwara was a powerful individual in the Heian period of Japan (794-1192 AD) [1]. He was speculated to have died of complications of diabetes based on the records of his pathology in the literature. This type of finding is the result of research in the history of medicine (a study of medical history). The other method involves a field of study in physical anthropology called "paleopathology," in which the author of this paper specializes. In paleopathology, the research materials are hard tissues such as bones and teeth from humans of ancient times and obtained from archeological excavations (needless to say, the soft tissues have long decomposed and returned to soil). Thus, it is possible to learn about the frequency of certain diseases in the past in groups of people and about the true pathology at the time of death. In this paper, a few dental diseases were interpreted from the perspective of an anthropologist who handles ancient human skeletal remains. These diseases can be indicators of modern oral health.

2. Two major diseases in the oral cavity are caries and periodontal disease

This statement is believed to have been true since the ancient times. In a previous study, the author of this paper described that, before the introduction of modern dentistry, people were more affected by caries and periodontal disease, the main cause of tooth loss, because they were unable to receive scientific dental care. Modern humans can obtain nutrients parenterally and via gastrostomy with the advancement of modern medicine. For the majority of human history, the mouth was the only means through which people have taken in nutrients. Therefore, tooth loss was speculated to have caused malnutrition and even death in many pre-modern individuals with numerous missing teeth. In the pre-modern times, longevity was likely dependent on the preservation of one's own teeth to obtain sufficient nutrients.

2.1. Tooth loss in human skeletal remains of Japan

Trinkaus reported on the problem of tooth loss in the La Chapelle-aux-Saints Neanderthal from approximately 60,000 years ago, the most ancient material that has been examined for this purpose [2]. He reported that 51.7% of the teeth were missing antemortem in this Neanderthal. In another study, Trinkaus also reported that 25% of the teeth were missing in the Shanidar Neanderthals [3]. It is difficult to obtain a large sample size of ancient human fossils, and consequently adequate statistical analysis cannot be performed due to small sample size. Therefore, the information from these ancient human fossils is merely for reference.

There are some case reports worldwide on tooth loss in Homo sapiens [4-8], but the number of studies on ancient human skeletal remains is not large. These researchers, except the author of this paper, used all examined individuals as materials. Thus, a bias likely occurred regarding the types of teeth, which were sometimes located in areas of defects in ancient human skeletal remains. The author of this paper examined remaining teeth in ancient human skeletal remains excavated from archeological sites of the pre-modern periods in Japan: the Kofun period (3rd–early7th century), Kamakura period (1192–1333 AD), Muromachi period (1335–1573 AD), and Edo period (1603–1868 AD). A total of 329 individuals were examined, of whom 145 individuals were selected as materials because their sex was determinable and their maxillary and mandibular alveolar bones were fully examinable (Table 1). This material selection method enabled data collection without bias for all tooth types. The estimation of age and determination of sex were performed by morphological observations of anthropological bones. Since the number of materials was not large, the individuals of different sexes were pooled together. The individuals were divided into three groups: early middle age group (approximately 20-39 years), late middle age group (approximately 40-49 years), and old age group (50 years or older).

In this study, the ancient human skeletal remains used as materials were grouped by time period and by age group. Table 1 shows the number of individuals and the number of examinable teeth. In all time periods as shown in Table 2, there was a tendency for the number of missing teeth to increase with age, progressing from early middle age to late middle age to old age. In the Kofun period, the mean number of missing teeth was 2.67 (SD: 1.63) in early middle age, 6.00 (SD: 2.00) in late middle age, and 16.00 in old age. In the Kamakura period, the mean number was 1.17 (SD: 1.47), 2.22 (SD: 2.10), and 4.50 (SD: 2.12), respectively. In the Muromachi period, the mean number was 1.80 (SD: 0.84), 5.80 (SD: 4.55), and 21.00, respectively. In the Edo period, the mean number was 2.31 (SD: 2.58), 5.18 (SD: 4.57), and 29.67 (SD: 4.04), respectively. Table 3 shows whether there is a difference in the number of missing teeth by age group after combining all the materials of different time periods. The results revealed that the number of missing teeth differed significantly ($p<0.01$) between the early middle age and late middle age groups and between the late middle age and old age groups, statistically indicating increasing tooth loss with age in pre-modern Japanese people. Table 4 shows the number of missing teeth in the maxilla and mandible. The number of missing teeth is shown by time period and by age group, but there were many time periods without a sufficient number of materials. Therefore, the lower portion of the table shows the number of maxillary missing teeth and the number of mandibular missing teeth of all time periods. A significance test was used to determine the difference in the number of missing teeth between the maxilla and mandible, and there was no significant difference between the jaws in any age group. Figures 1 and 2 show the percentages of missing teeth of all tooth types in the maxilla and mandible, respectively. In general, the percentage of missing teeth tended to be lower in the anterior teeth and the percentage tended to be higher in the posterior teeth.

Period	Group	Number of individuals	Number of Observed teeth[a]
Kofun	Early middle age	6	192
	Late middle age	7	224
	Old age	1	32
Kamakura	Early middle age	18	576
	Late middle age	18	576
	Old age	2	64
Muromchi	Early middle age	5	160
	Late middle age	5	160
	Old age	1	32
Edo	Early middle age	45	1440
	Larly middle age	34	1088
	Old age	3	96
Total		145	4640

[a]The number of observed teeth includes ante-mortem tooth loss and post-mortem tooth loss.

Table 1. The archaeological materials used from Kofun, Kamakura, Muromachi and Edo periods in Japan.

Period	Group	Lost teeth	Observed teeth	Average of number of ante-mortem teeth per person	SD
Kofun	Early middle age	16	192	2.67	1.63
	Late middle age	42	224	6.00	2.00
	Old age	16	32	16.00	-
Kamakura	Early middle age	21	576	1.17	1.47
	Late middle age	40	576	2.22	2.10
	Old age	9	64	4.50	2.12

Period	Group	Lost teeth	Observed teeth	Average of number of ante-mortem teeth per person	SD
Muromachi	Early middle age	9	160	1.80	0.84
	Late middle age	29	160	5.80	4.55
	Old age	21	32	21.00	-
Edo[a]	Early middle age	104	1440	2.31	2.58
	Late middle age	176	1088	5.18	4.57
	Old age	89	96	29.67	4.04

[a]Data were cited from Fujita[18].

Table 2. The number of ante-mortem tooth loss by age distribution.

	Significant
Early middle age-Late middle age	***
Late middleage-Old age	***

***: *P* <0.001

Table 3. Comparison of number of missing teeth by age distribution.

	Tooth type						
	Upper			Lower			
Early middle age	URM1	ULM1	Total	LRM1	LLM1	Total	Grand total
Observed	36	34	70	31	31	61	131
Average	3.13	3.24	3.19	2.16	2.27	2.23	2.74
SD	0.99	1.05	1.01	0.9	0.87	0.86	1.06
Early middle age vs Late middle age	P=0.165 ns	P=0.104 ns	P<0.05 L>E	P<0.05 L>E	P=0.218 ns	P<0.01 L>E	P<0.05 L>E
Late middle age	URM1	ULM1	Total	LRM1	LLM1	Total	Grand total
Observed	11	9	20	8	7	15	35
Average	3.91	3.89	3.9	3.13	2.71	2.93	3.49
SD	1.64	1.05	1.37	1.25	0.76	1.03	1.31

ns: not significance

E: Early middle age; L: Late middle age

Table 4. Alveoler resession of Somali people in Early middle age and Late middle age.

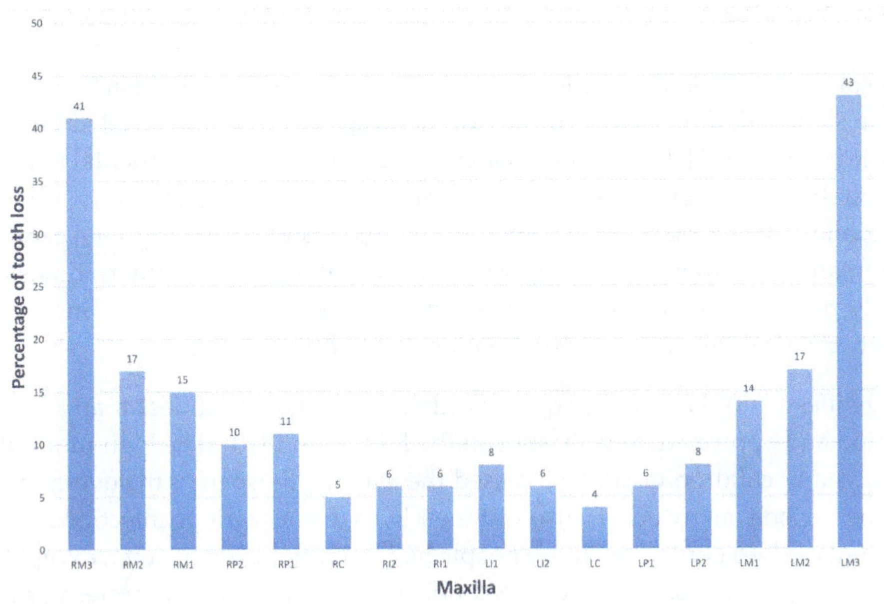

Figure 1. The rate of loss by tooth type in Maxilla in pre-modern periods in Japan.

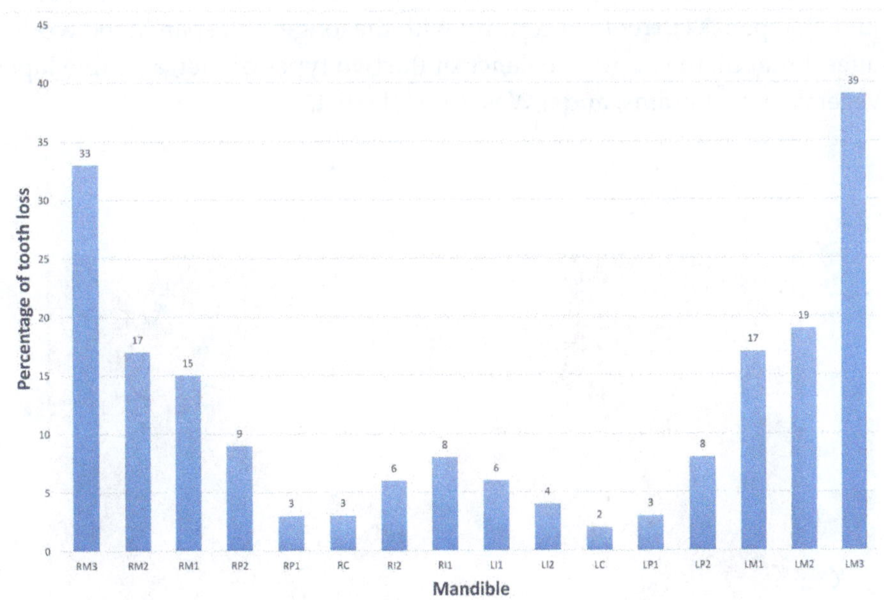

Figure 2. The rate of loss by tooth type in mandible in pre-modern periods in Japan.

In the early and late middle age individuals, the low number of missing teeth had been maintained at 1.11 to 6.00 teeth from the Kofun period to Edo period, spanning 1500 years. This result might be very surprising for health care providers as well as for the general public. The assumption is that people in olden times lost many teeth at an early age, but it is not consistent with the results of this study. At least to late middle age, the number of missing teeth was lower in pre-modern times than in modern time. Lopez *et al.* made a similar finding in a study comparing people of the Mediaeval Ages and modern people in Spain [5]. Sikanjic also made a similar finding in the number of missing teeth in human skeletal remains from the Iron Age in Croatia [6]. Diet and ingredients used in meals (i.e., nutrients) are expected to differ by country. Although it is difficult to generalize, modern people can receive scientific dental care, and tooth extraction can be performed easily and frequently. One cannot say that the dental treatment of tooth extraction was non-existent in the pre-modern times. However, it was likely not performed frequently, and the general public in those times were not as familiar with medical care as the general public of modern time [9].

The average lifespan of Japanese people is estimated to have been less than 15 years in the Jomon period and approximately 20 years in the Edo period [10]. The high mortality rates of infants and young children greatly decreased the average lifespan of the overall population. In these time periods, many adults also lost their lives due to various infections and parasitic diseases. Until the Edo period, Japanese people had a simple and plain diet, except for a small segment of the upper class. Such a diet did not contain much animal protein or fat. Diet in Japanese people began to change due to the introduction of more "American" foods, mainly with the post-war American occupation. Japanese people gradually began to consume more animal protein and fat. It is clearly consistent with the high correlation between increased average lifespan in Japanese people and increased consumption of animal protein and fat (Figures 3 and 4). Japan is currently a country with the longest lifespan in the world. This fact seems to suggest that there is a good balance of the two types of diet, a simple Japanese diet, mainly of vegetables and grains, and a Western-style diet.

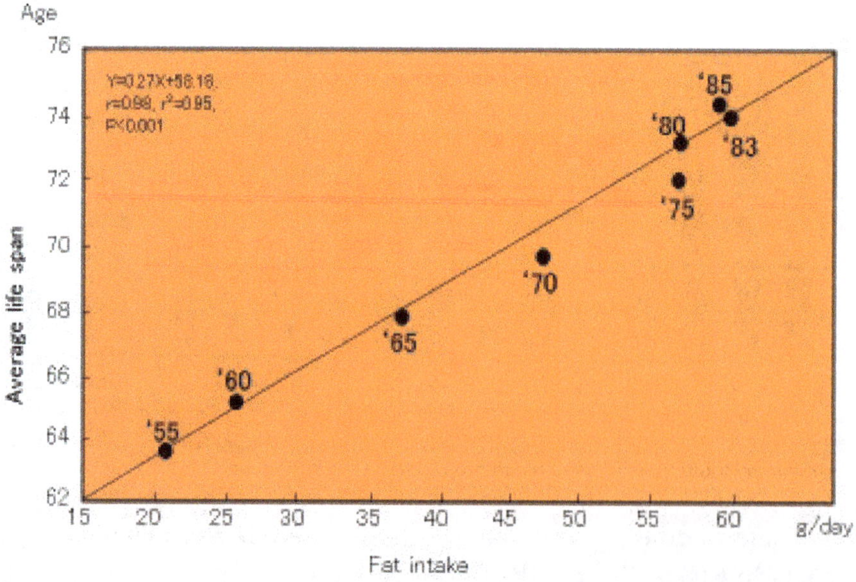

Figure 3. Relation between fat intake and Japanese life span

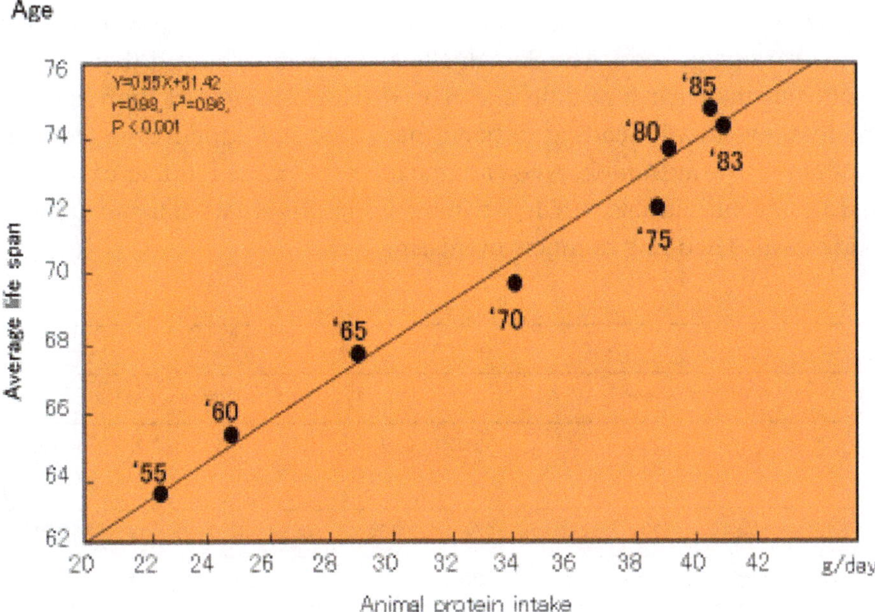

Figure 4. Relation between the animal protein intake and Japanese life span

Intravenous infusion was first introduced to Japan around 1960, and non-parenteral nutrition via gastrostomy was introduced much more recently. There are many restrictions and limitations when using these methods. In the time periods with only pre-modern medical care, the preservation of one's teeth was the only available way for people to get nutrients effectively. Thus, when people lost many of their teeth, they likely faced early death.

2.2. Tooth loss in ancient human skeletal remains from countries other than Japan

How was tooth loss in ancient human skeletal remains from other countries? The status of missing teeth was examined in human skeletal remains of the 3rd-7th centuries from the Yean-ri site in South Korea [11]. There were 2.7 missing teeth in the early middle age individuals and 8 missing teeth in the late middle age individuals, which are not large numbers. The status of missing teeth was also examined in modern Nigerian individuals who lived in the early 20th century and whose skeletal remains are stored at the University of Cambridge [12]. There were 1.3 missing teeth in the early middle age individuals and 3.3 missing teeth in the late middle age individuals, indicating very low numbers. No caries was observed in the examination of a total of 15 Nigerian individuals and 272 teeth. Similarly, when tooth loss was examined in Somali individuals living in the late 19th century to the early 20th century, AMTL was 2.60% in individuals in early middle age [13]. This percentage is a very low value, indicating the loss of at the most 1 tooth out of 32 teeth. In individuals in late middle age, AMTL was 17.02%, which is an approximate loss of 5.4 teeth. Thus, the number of missing teeth clearly increased with aging. There was a significant increase in alveolar bone loss with aging as shown in Table 4, while there was no change in caries rate with aging as shown in Table 5. It is speculated from these results that tooth loss in Somalis was due to periodontal disease and not caries. Although it is difficult to speculate on the details of their diet, they were believed to have had a low intake of simple sugars and carbohydrates. Thus, the diet of Somalis likely consisted of low cariogenic food. The Somali skeletal remains showed that they had periodontal disease from their early middle age. The disease progressed with age and caused alveolar bone loss, eventually leading to bone that could not support the teeth and consequently to tooth loss. The author observed an unexpectedly large number of remaining teeth in the late middle age individuals, much like in the Edo individuals in Japan. It indicated that Somali individuals also had low numbers of missing teeth.

					Tooth type						
			Upper					**Lower**			
Early middle age	I	C	P	M	Total	I	C	P	M	Total	Grand total
Observed	168	84	170	252	674	130	65	130	195	520	1194
Loss	9	3	1	8	21	0	0	3	7	10	31
SD	0.23	0.19	0.08	0.18	0.17	—	—	0.15	0.19	0.14	0.16
% AMTL	5.36	3.57	0.59	3.17	3.12	0	0	2.31	3.59	1.92	2.60
Early middle age vs Late middle age	P=0.135 ns	P=0.333 ns	P<0.01 L>E	P<0.001 L>E	P<0.001 L>E	P<0.001 L>E	P<0.05 L>E	P=0.051 ns	P<0.001 L>E	P<0.001 L>E	P<0.001 L>E
Late middle age	I	C	P	M	Total	I	C	P	M	Total	Grand total
Observed	52	26	52	78	208	44	22	43	65	174	382
Loss	7	3	5	18	33	6	3	5	18	32	65
SD	0.32	0.33	0.3	0.42	0.37	0.35	0.35	0.32	0.45	0.39	0.38
% AMTL	13.46	11.54	9.62	23.08	15.87	13.64	13.64	11.63	27.69	18.39	17.02

I: Incisors; C: Canines; P: Premolars; M: Molars in tooth type distribution.

ns: not significant

E: Early middle age; L: Late middle age

Table 5. Antemortem tooth loos (AMTL) of Somali people in Early middle age and Late middle age.

The lifespan remains short in developing countries of the 21st century. Similar types and proportions of disease are thought to have been maintained in modern populations (likely even in present-day populations) as in the populations of 1000-2000 years ago. It is speculated that missing teeth of populations of 1000-2000 years ago were maintained at very low numbers until late middle age despite the presence of periodontal disease, much like ancient human skeletal remains from Japan.

Early middle age				Late middle age				P-value
Tooth type	Observed	Caries	% Caries	Tooth type	Observed	Caries	% Caries	
UI	168	0	0	UI	52	0	0	-
UC	84	0	0	UC	26	0	0	-
UP	170	0	0	UP	52	1	1.92	P=0.537
UM	252	6	2.38	UM	78	0	0	P=0.384
U-total	674	6	0.89	U-total	208	1	0.48	P=0.896
LI	130	0	0	LI	44	0	0	-
LC	65	0	0	LC	22	0	0	-
LP	130	0	0	LP	43	0	0	-
LM	195	4	2.05	LM	65	2	3.08	P=0.991
L-total	520	4	0.77	L-total	174	2	1.15	P=0.994
Grand Total	1194	10	0.84	Grand Total	382	3	0.79	P=0.820

Table 6. Prevalence of dental caries of Somali people in Early middle age and Late middle age.

3. Stress markers and enamel hypoplasia

Stress in modern-day people signifies mainly "psychological stress" in the majority of cases. In ancient skeletal human remains, the focus is on the examination of signs of "physical stress" remaining in bones and teeth as a result of surviving in a very harsh environment. It is desirable to examine the level of such stress not in one or a few individuals but in a group, if possible in at least a few dozen to a few hundred individuals. Otherwise, the stress level in a certain group and differences in stress level among groups cannot be known.

Stress marker might not be a commonly used term. It is a lesion that is used to compare the level of health particularly among groups such as mentioned above. Stress markers on teeth are not very common. Enamel hypoplasia is one such marker and will be discussed below pertaining to ancient human skeletal remains.

Teeth are formed relatively early and enamel matrix is formed at approximately the sixth week of gestation for primary teeth. Enamel matrix formation begins early even for permanent teeth. For example, it begins to form at birth for permanent first molars. Enamel hypoplasia occurs when there is poor enamel formation at such stages. The cause is hypocalcemia due to conditions such as starvation and impaired food intake due to serious disease [14].

Enamel hypoplasia is a useful stress marker because: (1) it is a lesion which is found relatively frequently in ancient human skeletal remains, and (2) it is a lesion that occurs due to environmental factors such as those affecting the nutritional status. Briefly explained, the ancient human skeletal remains that we encounter represent one individual in a few thousands or a few tens of thousands of individuals who lived in the past from a certain time period. They represent a very fortunate discovery and are very important representatives. Therefore, if a disease occurred only in one in a few tens or hundreds of thousands, finding this disease in the excavated remains is greatly affected by chance. Therefore, such disease is not suitable for examining the stress level in a group or comparing the stress level with other groups.

As shown in Figure 5, enamel hypoplasia often appears linearly on the enamel surface. The crowns of healthy teeth should be smooth, but aplasia occurs in depressions of the crowns of teeth with enamel hypoplasia.

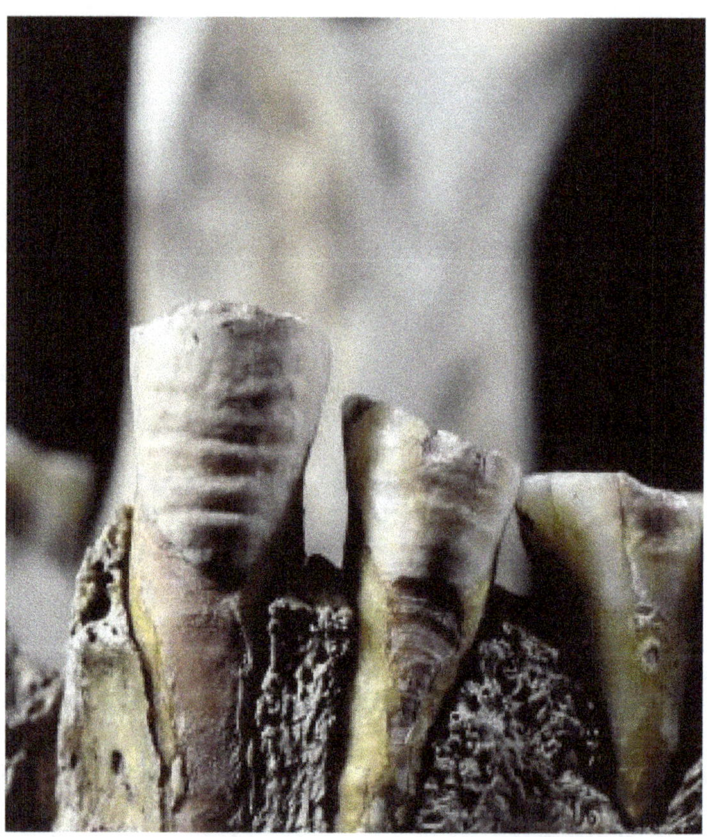

Figure 5. Linear enamel hypoplasia found in Jomon people of Japan

Although there are individual differences, the timing of crown formation by tooth type is roughly the same among individuals. Therefore, when enamel hypoplasia is seen in a certain site of a certain tooth, one can estimate the age at which the enamel hypoplasia occurred. If several lines can be seen in an individual (Figure 5), it can be speculated that this individual experienced multiple bouts of starvation or malnutrition due to serious disease. Some individuals have linear enamel hypoplasia of the entire dentition as in Figure 6. It shows that the individual was exposed to stress causing enamel hypoplasia during crown formation of different tooth types [14]. Therefore, this case is very important as such evidence.

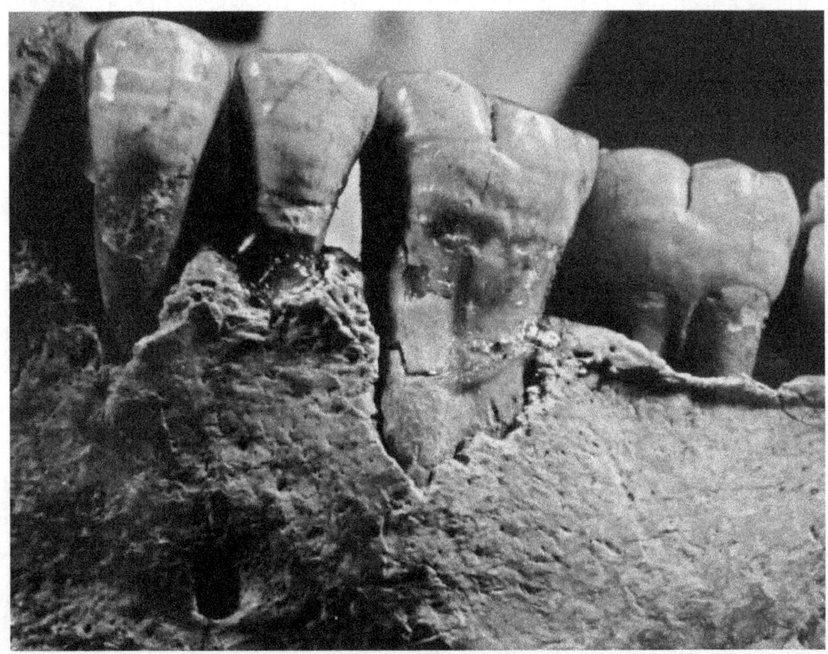

Figure 6. Linear enamel hypoplasia found some tooth type in Jomon people of Japan

When does enamel hypoplasia occur? There have been several studies on this topic, including one by Yamamoto, who examined ancient human skeletal remains of Japanese individuals [15]. According to the study of Yamamoto, enamel hypoplasia occurs repeatedly between 3.5-5.5 years of age in the majority of the cases and very rarely occurs at ages younger than 3 years. Yamamoto gave as reasons for the onset: such stress was likely fatal in individuals at ages younger than 3 years in a pre-modern environment, and even if individuals survived the stress, they could not have tolerated subsequent stress and would have died before the eruption of permanent teeth. In contrast, enamel hypoplasia in modern-day individuals occurs repeatedly at 0-12 months after birth but rarely beyond 34 months [15]. That is, it occurs repeatedly early after birth but rapidly decreases thereafter. Thus, the ancient skeletal remains indicate that timing of hypoplasia differed between ancient people and modern-day people. It is speculated that improved health status, including due to medical advancement, helps modern-day individuals face conditions recorded in crowns as enamel hypoplasia without causing death.

The above findings show that it was very difficult for very young children, particularly infants, to survive in pre-modern times during which bouts of starvation were common and medical care was not advanced. This tendency was likely stronger in more ancient times, and countless young lives must have been lost before these individuals were able to leave any signs of enamel hypoplasia.

Stress markers develop on bones and teeth when individuals continue to survive under a poor environment. If individuals die in a short period of time due to disease or malnutrition, then there will be no stress marker on bones or teeth. For example, when individuals die of acute infections, including dysentery and influenza, it is very difficult to find signs of such infections in excavated bones and teeth. If individuals had chronic diseases such as advanced tuberculosis, leprosy, and syphilis of the bone for a few years to decades, then signs of such diseases will remain in their bones.

The frequency of enamel hypoplasia was 48.1% in the Jomon population, 36.4% in the Kofun population, approximately 60% in the Edo population, and 39.5% in the present-day population of Japan [15]. These numbers seem to indicate that the environment in the Jomon period was better than that in the Edo period. However, these numbers can be explained in another way. When Jomon people suffered various diseases or malnutrition, they likely did not recover and died a short time later. Therefore, they probably did not live long enough to develop enamel hypoplasia, resulting in a lower frequency of enamel hypoplasia in the Jomon period. Edo people also likely lived in a much harsher environment than present-day people. However, medical care and nutritional conditions were improved in the Edo period compared with those in the Jomon period. Therefore, Edo people with various diseases and malnutrition likely had higher chances of survival than Jomon people with such conditions. As a result, signs of enamel hypoplasia remain in individuals from the Edo period. Present-day people can have high-quality medical care and nutrition readily and sufficiently, and the infant mortality rate has consequently decreased. Thus, only a modest frequency of enamel hypoplasia is seen. Therefore, in this type of a situation, one should conclude that a group with a low frequency of stress markers had a worse environment and that a group with a high frequency had a better environment. This phenomenon is called a "paleopathological paradox." One needs to be mindful of this paradox when examining nutritional conditions, health status, and the difference in frequency of disease among groups or time periods.

What are the frequencies of enamel hypoplasia in various countries? When the frequency of enamel hypoplasia was examined in former inhabitants of what is now the State of Illinois in the U.S., it was 45% in the excavated individuals from the hunting and gathering period, 60% in the excavated individuals from the transition to the agricultural period, and a high frequency of 80% in the excavated individuals from the agricultural period [16]. Similarly, when the frequency was examined in former inhabitants of what is now Ohio, it was higher in the excavated individuals from the agricultural period than those from the hunting and gathering period [17, 18]. These findings indicate that poor harvests more greatly affected people in an agricultural society than frequent food shortages affected people in a hunting and gathering society. In addition, the agricultural people who lived in these areas had a diet which depended heavily on corn. Such a diet resulted in increased caloric intake and nutritional quantity but decreased animal protein intake and nutritional quality. Weaning diets were deficient in protein, and nutritional stress occurred such as diarrhea due to bacterial infection. Some researchers interpret the high frequency of enamel hypoplasia as a result of increased population density in the agricultural period, leading to a higher risk for infection and increased environmental stress such as outbreaks of endemic diseases [19, 20].

The author of this paper is not in agreement with the above explanations. There is no evidence that a hunter-gatherer economy enabled people to maintain necessary and sufficient proteins. There is also no evidence that people in an agricultural economy had repeated poor harvests and had lower animal protein intake than people in a hunter-gatherer economy. The term "hunters and gatherers" gives the image of hunting. However, it is speculated that people in a hunter-gatherer economy did not necessary have sufficient animal-derived foods, and the majority of their diet consisted of plant-derived foods. Even natural-born hunters like lions have very low hunting success rates. Therefore, it is valid opinion that hunters and gatherers must have had great difficulties maintaining a constant intake of animal protein even with human intelligence and use of tools. The diet of an agricultural economy could not have consisted entirely of plant-derived foods. Instead, it is speculated that hunting must have continued, and its techniques must have evolved from previous time periods to the agricultural period. Therefore, people must have continued to consume animal-derived foods in the agricultural period.

Even when societies transitioned from a hunting-gathering type to an agricultural type, it is very unlikely that the consumption of animal protein decreased sharply. Instead, the aforementioned enamel hypoplasia frequencies should be interpreted in the following ways: the types of people who were unable to survive in a hunter-gatherer society were more likely to survive in an agricultural society, and the average lifespan, an index of cumulative stress, increased.

4. TMD in human skeletal remains from the Edo period in Japan

Prolonged retention of primary teeth rarely poses clinical problems in modern people if these teeth are extracted and the eruptive paths of permanent teeth are normalized. A report in a Japanese journal has shown that when primary teeth were retained beyond the normal period, their extraction resulted in gradual improvement of TMD and in normal occlusion. In the field of physical anthropology, very few report has been published that simultaneously discussed prolonged retention of primary teeth, temporomandibular joint (TMJ) arthritis, and TMD [21]. The material discussed in this section was skeletal human remains from the Edo period (17-19th centuries) in Japan. The mandible showed signs of TMJ arthritis and TMD likely due to bilateral primary second molars. The skeletal remains were excavated from the Suhgen temple site in Shinjuku-ku in Tokyo and were of a woman in the early part of early middle age. Retention of primary molars was observed in the left and right mandible (Figure 7). Since first premolars were present anterior to them, the over-retained primary teeth were both believed to be primary second molars. Radiographs showed no formation of left or right second premolars, confirming that they were missing congenitally (Figures 8a and 8b). It was speculated that bilateral primary second molars remained in adulthood because second premolars were missing congenitally. Other permanent mandibular teeth, including the third molars, were erupted bilaterally, and it is consistent with the individual being in the early part of early middle age. Bilateral primary molars had more severe occlusal attrition of the distal area than on the mesial area, and dentin was markedly exposed. The occlusal attrition of the mesial area was confined to near the proximal aspect adjacent to the first premolar.

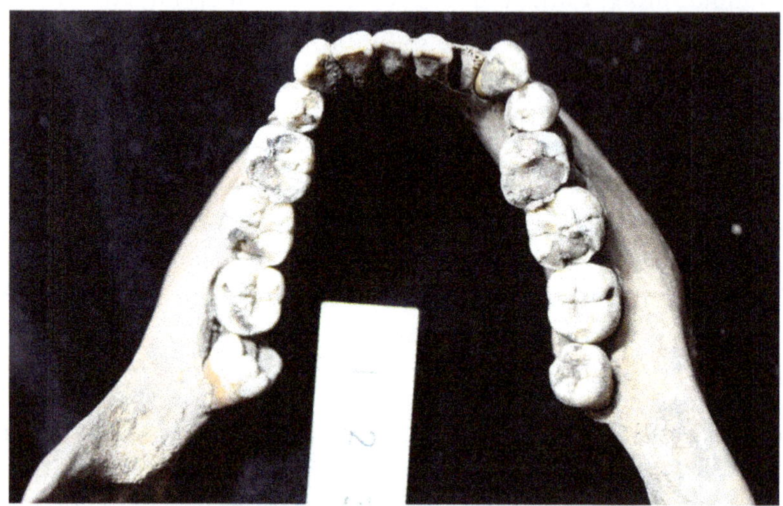

Figure 7. Persistence of both sides of second deciduous molars.

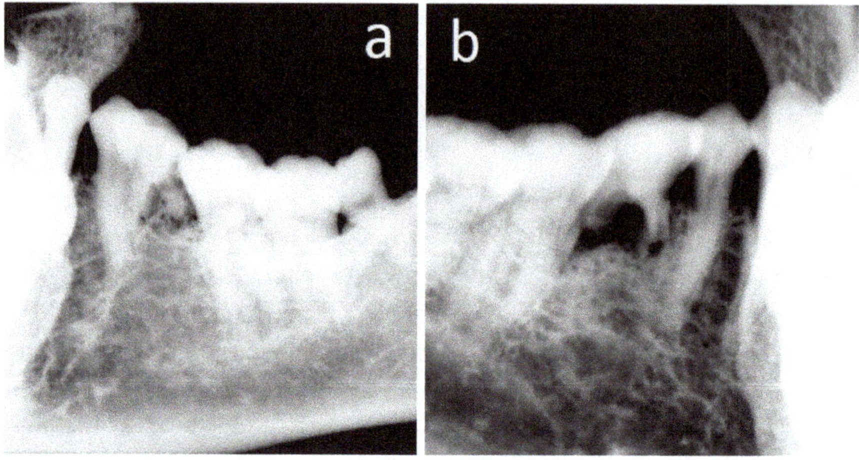

Figure 8. The lack of permanent second premolars are admitted in the roentgenograms. a: right side, b: left side, respectively. a: right mandibular condyle is normal. b: left mandibular condyle has caused the deformity by TMJ arthritis.

The right mandibular condyle was normal, but TMJ arthritis had developed in the left mandibular condyle with overall deformation (Figures 9a and 9b). It was of minimum expression under the Rando and Waldron classification [22]. The right mandibular fossa was normal. In the left mandibular fossa, a new articular facet had formed accompanying inflammation and deformation of the mandibular condyle, and it was evident that TMJ arthritis and accompanying TMD had developed (Figures 10a and 10b).

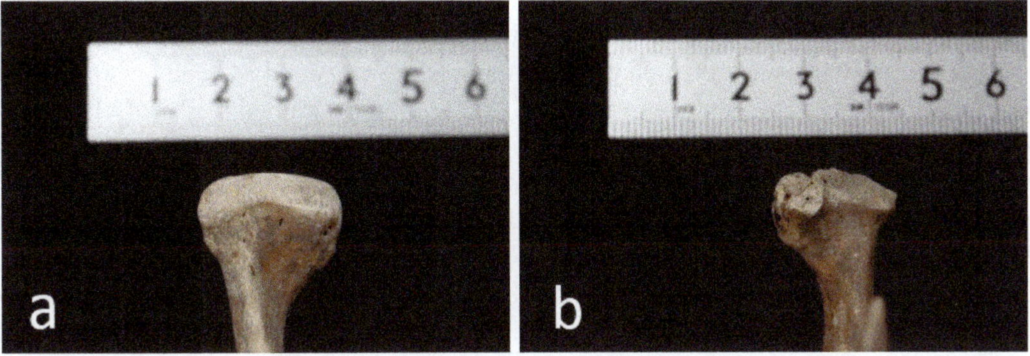

Figure 9. a: mandibular fossa of both sides. b: left mandibular fossa forms the false joint (arrow) and porosity is recognized in frame area.

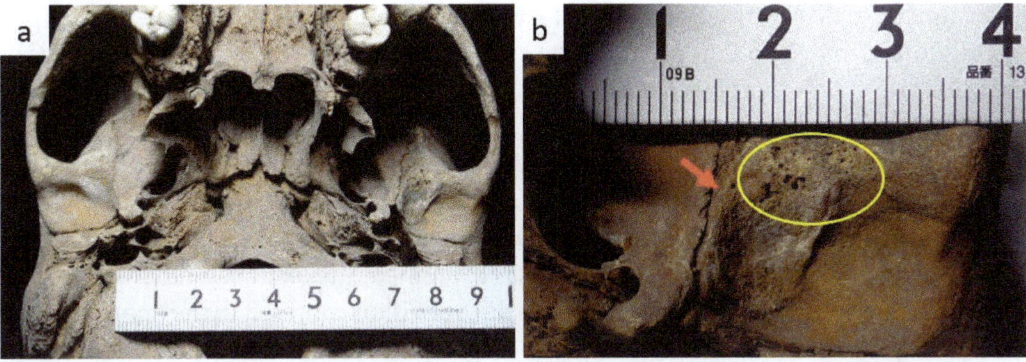

Figure 10. Periostitis found in the alveolar bone at right second deciduous molar (a) and left second deciduous molar (b).

There was bilateral periostitis of the alveolar bone supporting the primary teeth (Figures 11a and 11b). Periostitis was severe in the areas with over-retained primary second molars, and there was mild periostitis in all other areas, which was almost the entire maxilla and mandible.

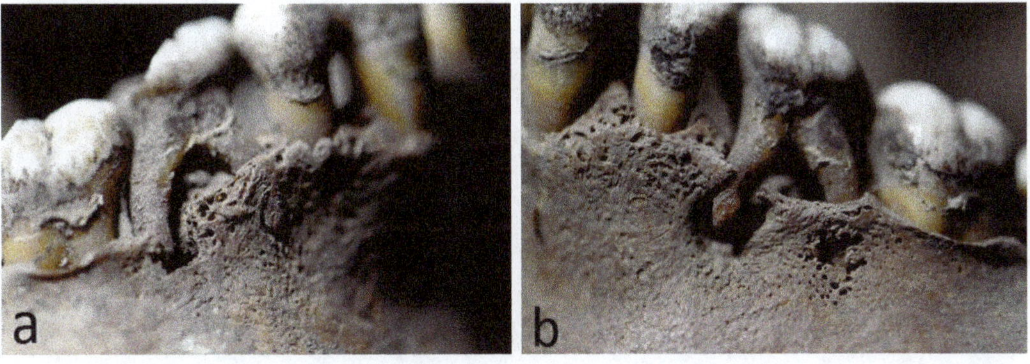

Figure 11. Slight periostitis is admitted in the widespread area of the alveolar bone.

Sumiya reported that the prevalence of prolonged retention was 0.58% for primary second molars in both Japanese men and women aged 21-25 years [23]. Onizuka examined 151 teeth in 106 individuals with over-retained primary teeth who were aged 14-47 years and reported that 63% had one over-retained tooth and 32% had two over-retained teeth [24]. It should be noted that over-retained teeth occurred symmetrically in the left and right sides of the maxilla or mandible in 33 of 34 patients with two over-retained teeth, indicating a very high proportion of patients [24]. The most commonly over-retained tooth was the primary second molar at 52.3% [24]. In the individual from the Suhgen temple site, there was prolonged retention of two mandibular primary second molars with bilaterally symmetry. The occurrence rate was 0.19% based on simple calculation, suggesting that such prolonged retention occurred in approximately 2 in 1000 adults. When one takes into account that the excavated skeletal remains were of the Edo period, this individual can be said to represent a valuable case of over-retained primary teeth in ancient human skeletal remains.

Although some reports have discussed that over-retained primary teeth can frequently cause TMD, treatment such as extraction of such teeth has been reported to improve the symptoms. In the individual from the Suhgen temple site, occlusal attrition was observed in the distal area of the left and right first molars. In the right first molar, the occlusal surface gently sloped upward from the distal to the mesial direction until there was no attrition. One area of the left first molar showed severe attrition where its distal area contacted the left second molar. It is nearly impossible to reproduce an accurate antemortem occlusion using a mandible and maxilla without soft tissue. However, there was likely abnormal occlusal force on the areas with attrition. When the maxillary dentition was examined, the teeth had normal positions in the left and right molar regions and there was slight attrition confined to the enamel. Attrition was confined to the lingual aspect for the left and right maxillary first molars. In this individual, the findings were strongly suggestive of malocclusion such as cusp-to-cusp occlusion. It is not known whether TMD occurred at a transition period from primary teeth to permanent teeth or after eruption of all permanent teeth. In any case, prolonged retention of primary second molars was thought to have somehow contributed to the development of TMD.

There are limitations in discussing TMD based on archeological materials, but there can be reports of new valuable cases of archeological materials. Modern-day individuals can have prolonged retention of primary teeth causing TMD and can have concurrent periodontal disease. Therefore, it is desirable to appropriately treat individuals with such conditions in modern clinical dental medicine. The material from the Suhgen temple site was an excavated archeological sample, but the implication of its findings can be important in modern dental medicine.

5. Conclusions

This paper discussed three topics from the perspective of physical anthropology which handles ancient human skeletal remains: antemortem tooth loss and problems of periodontal disease and caries, enamel hypoplasia as a stress marker, and occurrence of TMD due to prolonged retention of primary teeth. There are many other oral diseases in ancient skeletal remains that the author of this paper would like to discuss but was unable to, due to limitation of space. The diseases discussed in this paper are all in the oral region and have afflicted people from a few thousand years ago until the present day, i.e., diseases which have also afflicted our ancestors. The author hopes that the readers were able to appreciate that many new findings can be obtained from examination of diseases in the past. It is important to focus on the present to save patients who suffer from modern-day diseases. However, when one examines only the present, one will likely be unable to properly envision dental health of the future. The author is of the opinion that "knowing the past" or "learning from the past" is a very important point. Modern humans have existed for a long time, the ancestors of whom emerged about 7 million years ago. Thus, humans have a long past and modern humans should be thought of as being on the leading edge of this long human history.

Cooperation of physical anthropologists will be important in the creation of guidelines in modern medicine and future oral health. Such an effort can organically link the past, present, and future for the first time and can contribute to a better future. Another hope of this author is that the information and findings of this paper will be useful to many readers.

Author details

Hisashi Fujita*

Address all correspondence to: rxh05535@nifty.com

Department of Bioanthropology, Niigata College of Nursing, Japan

References

[1] Sakai S. Japanese History from the diseases. Tokyo: Kodansha; 2014. (in Japanese)

[2] Trinkaus E.; Pathology and Posture of the La Chapelle-aux-Saints Neandertal. Am. J. Phys. Anthropol. 1985, 67, 19-41.

[3] Trinkaus E. The Shanidar Neandertals. Academic Press, New York, USA, 1983.

[4] Nelson GC, Lukacs JR, Yule P. Dates, Caries, and Early Tooth Loss During the Iron Age of Oman. Am J. Phys. Anthropol. 1999, 108, 333-343.

[5] Lopez B, Pardinas AF, Gacia-Vazquez E. Dopico E. Socio-cultural fractures in dental diseases in the Medieval and early Modern Age of northern Spain. Homo. 2012, 63, 21-42.

[6] Sikanjic PR. Bioarchaeology research in Croatia—a historical review. Coll Anthropol. 2005, 29(2): 763-768.

[7] Fujita H. The number of missing teeth in people of the Edo period in Japan in the 17th to 19th centuries. Gerodontol. 2012, 29, e520-e524.

[8] Oyamada J, Igawa K, Manabe Y, Kato K, Matsushita T, Rokutanda A, Kitagawa Y. Preliminary analysis of regional differences in dental pathology of early modern commoners in Japan. Anthropol. Sci. 2010, 118, 1-8.

[9] Takehara T, Sakashita R, Fujita H, Matsushita T, Simoyama A. History of dental caries. : Tokyo; Sunashobo, 2001. (in Japanese)

[10] Fujita H. Were the Jomon People healthy or not? Speculation of total health condition of ancient people. J. Lipid Nutrition, 2007 16(2), 205-210.

[11] Fujita H., Suzuki, T., Shoda, S., Kawakubo, Y., Ohno, K., Giannakopoulou, P. and Harihara, S.: Contribution on antemortem tooth loss (AMTL) and dental attrition to oral palaeopathology in the human skeletal series from the Yean-ri site, South Korea. International Journal of Archaeology, 2013 1:1-5.

[12] Fujita H. Dental Diseases and Stress Markers on Crania in the Early Modern People of Nigeria. Japanese Journal of Gerodontology, 2013 28(1): 10-19.

[13] Fujita H. Health status in early modern Somali people from their skeletal remains. Int J Archaeol 2014, 2(3), 1-5.

[14] Jalevik B, Noren JG. Enamel hypomineralization of permanent first molars: a morphological study and survey of possible aetiological factors. Int. J. Paediatr. Dent., 2000 10: 278-289.

[15] Yamamoto M. Enamel Hypoplasia of the Permanent Teeth in Japanese from the Jomon to the Modern Periods. J. Anthrop. Soc. Nippon 1988 96(4) 417-433.

[16] Goodman AH, Armelagos GJ, Rose JC. Enamel hypoplasia as as indicators of stress in three prehistoric populations from Illinois. Human Biol. 1980 52: 515-528.

[17] Sciulli PW, Developmental abnormalities of the permanent dentition in prehistoric Ohio Valley Amerindians. Am. J. Phys. Anthropol., 1978 48: 193-198.

[18] Cook DC. Subsistence and health in the Lower Illinois Valley: Osteological evidence. In: Cohen M and Aemelagos GJ (ed.) Paleopathology at the Origins of Agriculture. Academic Press, 1984 235-269.

[19] Lallo JW, Rose JC. Patterns of stress, diseases and mortality in two prehistoric populations from North America. J. Human Evolution, 1979 8: 323-335.

[20] Cassidy CM. Nutrition and health in agriculturalist and hunter-gatherers. In: Jerome NW, Kandel RF, Pelto GH (ed.) Nutritional Anthropology, Redgrave Press, 1980 117-145.

[21] Fujita H, Suzuki T, Harihara S. Simultaneous Dental Anomalies (Polyanomalodontia) in Mediaeval Japanese Skeletal Remains. Jpn. J. Oral. Biol. 1997 39: 257-262.

[22] Rando C, Waldron T. TMJ Osteoarthritis: A New Approach to Diagnosis. Am. J. Phys. Anthropol. 2012 148: 45-53

[23] Sumiya Y. Statistic Study on Dental Anomalies in the Japanese. J. Anthropol. Soc. Nippon. 1959 64: 215-233. (in Japanese)

[24] Onizuka Y. Statistical Observation on the Multiple Cases (106 Cases) of the Retained Deciduous Teeth. Kyushu Shika Gakkai Zasshi 1979 33: 52-67. (in Japanese)

9

A New Protocol of Tweed-Merrifield Directional Force Technology Using Micro-Implant Anchorage (M.I.A.)

Jong-Moon Chae

1. Introduction

Edward H. Angle [1] introduced the edgewise appliance and presented numerous case reports that supported its efficacy. Charles H. Tweed [2] identified his orthodontic treatment objectives, and presented modifications in both the edgewise appliance and its use. Anchorage preparation was the cornerstone of Tweed's treatment. He prepared anchorage with coordinated bends in the mandibular arch wire, Class III elastics, and maxillary headgear.

L. Levern Merrifield [3, 4] enhanced, expanded and simplified Tweed's concepts and treatment mechanics. He developed force systems that simplify the use of the edgewise appliance. Directional forces can be defined as controlled forces that place the teeth in the most harmonious relationships with their environment.

A hallmark of Tweed-Merrifield edgewise treatment is the use of directional force systems to control the mandibular anterior and posterior teeth and the maxillary anterior teeth. The resultant vector of all orthodontic forces should be counterclockwise so that the opportunity for a favorable skeletal change is enhanced particularly for dentoalveolar protrusion and Class II malocclusion corrections. Such an upward and forward force system requires that the mandibular incisors be upright over basal bone so that the maxillary incisors can be moved distally and superiorly. For the upward and forward force system to be a reality, vertical control is critical. To control the vertical dimension, the clinician must control the mandibular plane, the occlusal plane, and the palatal plane. If Point B drops down and back, the face becomes lengthened, the mandibular incisor is pushed forward off the basal bone, and the maxillary incisor drops down and back instead of being moved up and back [5, 6].

Vertical control is the key to successful orthodontic treatment. The control of the horizontal movement of the dentition depends on how the vertical dimension of the maxillomandibular complex is controlled. Vertical control can make horizontal correction possible [7]. This might be the single most important mechanical consideration that has to be accomplished during the treatment of the patient with a high angle Class II malocclusion. Successful correction of various orthodontic problems depends on the control of the horizontal planes, particularly the occlusal plane. The occlusal plane is the key to counterclockwise rotation of the horizontal planes. The clinician should control extrusion of the maxillary and mandibular posterior teeth, and control anterior vertical dimension, particularly the maxillary anterior segment [8] during mechanotherapy to maintain or close the occlusal plane. A large increase in horizontal mandibular response for Class II correction, chin enhancement, and Z-angle improvement can be achieved by vertical control [9].

Tweed-Merrifield directional force technology is a very useful concept, particularly for the treatment Class I and Class II dentoalveolar protrusion malocclusions. It has contributed to creating a favorable counter-clockwise skeletal change and balanced face, while the headgear force, using high pull J-hook (HPJH) in an appropriate direction is also essential to influence such results. Although the headgear force using HPJH in an appropriate direction can be used to provide directional forces and stable anchorage, a high degree of patient compliance is required. Clinicians have encountered some problems concerning patient compliance; however, skeletal anchorage has been used widely because it does not necessitate patient compliance, yet produces absolute anchorage.

To obtain an absolute anchorage without patient cooperation, endosseous implants [10], miniplates [11], and screws [12-22] have been used as orthodontic anchorage. Of those, screws have many advantages such as ease of implantation and removal, low cost, possible immediate loading, and possible placement in most areas of the alveolar bone. Micro-implants are very effective in maintaining or closing the occlusal plane and mandibular plane with counter-clockwise movement of the chin by vertical control of maxillomandibular complex.

The present new protocol demonstrates the usefulness of micro-implants as anchorage aid in Tweed-Merrifield directional force technology.

2. New protocol of directional force treatment using MIA – 4 steps

4 steps can achieve tweed-Merrifield Sequential Edgewise Directional Force Treatment: denture preparation, denture correction, denture completion, and denture recovery. During each step of the treatment, there are certain objectives that must be attained prior to initiating the next step.

1. Denture preparation

The first step of treatment is denture preparation. Each case is sequentially banded or bonded with a. 22 non-tipped, non-torqued appliance. Sequential banding allows the operator to use edgewise archwire at the outset of treatment. The use of the edgewise archwire enhances control of tooth movement as well as the leveling and the distal tipping of the terminal molar.

During canine retraction, anchorage has always been a major concern for the orthodontist, especially in those cases in which maximum anchorage is needed. Maxillary and mandibular posterior micro-implants (MIs) are installed and elastomers are applied for maximum retraction of canines and anchorage preparation of the terminal molars (Figure 1.A). At the end of the denture preparation step of treatment, the mandibular arch should be leveled, the maxillary and mandibular canines should be retracted, all rotations should be corrected, and the mandibular terminal molars should be tipped distally into an anchorage prepared position of approximately 15° (Figure 1.B).

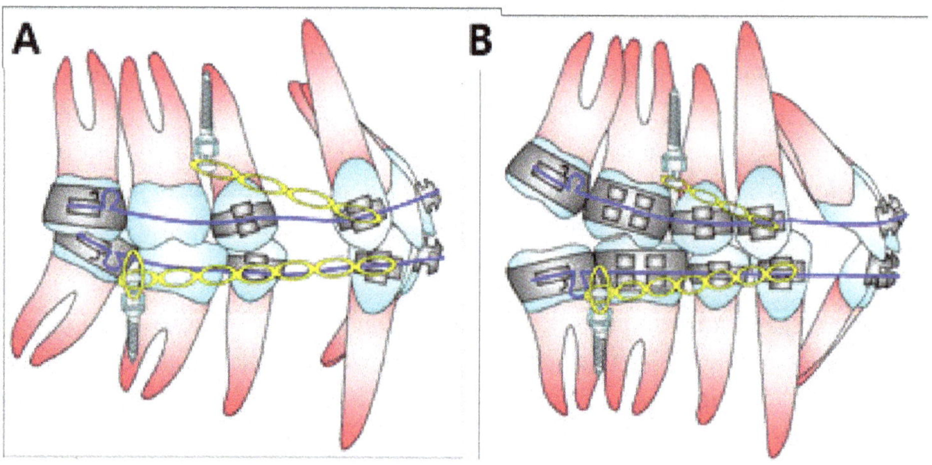

Figure 1. A. Denture preparation : An .022 × .028″ edgewise appliance is sequentially placed. .017 × .022″ maxillary and .018 × .025″ mandibular archwires are inserted. Maxillary and mandibular posterior micro-implants, and elastomers are applied to the canine brackets and mandibular archwire just mesial to omega stop loop. **B. End of denture preparation** : The arches are leveled, the rotations are corrected, the canines have been retracted, and the mandibular terminal molar has been tipped to an anchorage prepared position.

2. Denture correction

The second step of treatment is denture correction. During denture correction, spaces are closed with maxillary and mandibular closing loops which are supported by maxillary anterior micro-implants and elastomers attached to the soldered hooks or main archwire between the maxillary centrals and laterals for control of vertical dimension and torque of the maxillary anterior segment. During en masse retraction of anterior teeth, vertical and horizontal anchorage loss of posterior teeth can be prevented by maxillary and mandibular posterior micro-implants (Figure 2.A).

During en masse retraction of anterior teeth, both arch should be leveled with maintenance of compensating curve in maxillary arch and 15° distal tip of the mandibular second molar (Figure 2.B).

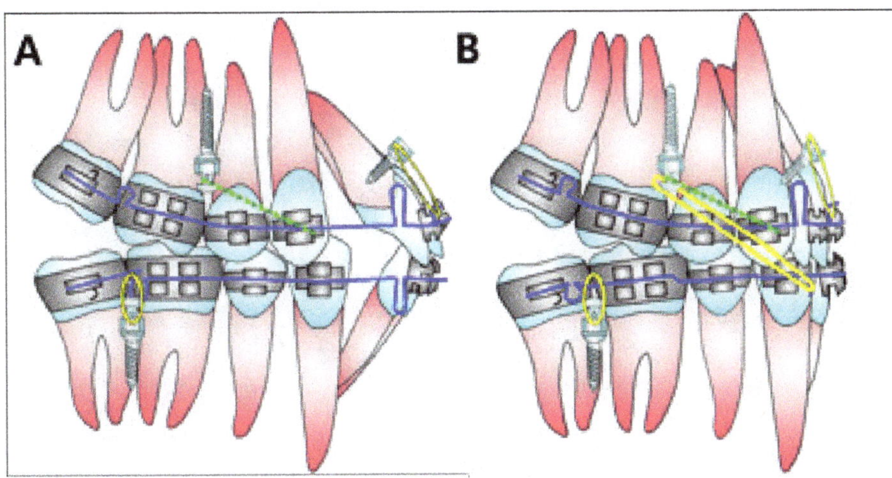

Figure 2. A.Denture correction : A mandibular .019 × .025″ closing loop archwire and a maxillary .020 × .025″ closing loop archwire are fabricated. Maxillary and mandibular posterior micro-implants and elastomers are attached to hooks, brackets and archwires. **B. Mandibular anchorage preparation:** First molar Anchorage preparation : The .019 × . 025″ mandibular archwire biases the first molar bracket at a 10° angle. Second premolar anchorage preparation : A compensation bend is placed mesial to the mandibular first molar and an anchorage bend of 5° is placed 1mm mesial to the second premolar bracket. Mandibular anchorage preparation is supported by Class III elastics between maxillary posterior micros-implants and anterior hooks in mandibular archwire and/or elastomers between mandibular posterior micro-implants and mandibular archwire just mesial to omega stop loop.

After space closure, mandibular anchorage is sequentially prepared. This sequential anchorage preparation was initiated by tipping the terminal molar during denture preparation and is continued after space closure by tipping the first molar and second bicuspid.

Each tooth is moved individually into its anchorage prepared position with Class III elastics between maxillary posterior micro-implants and mandibular anterior hooks between mandibular lateral incisors and canines. During anchorage preparation, elastomers are applied on the mandibular posterior dental segment to prevent extrusion of mandibular posterior teeth and to encourage counterclockwise mandibular rotation.

At the end of denture correction, space closure in both arches, sequential anchorage preparation in the mandibular arch, enhanced curve of occlusion in the maxillary arch and Class I relationship should be accomplished.

3. Denture completion

The third step of treatment is denture completion. During this step of treatment, the idealization and finishing of the case is done with elastics attached to cusp seating spurs soldered to archwires with the proper first, second and third order bends (Figure 3.A and 3.B).

At the end of denture completion, well alignment, tight closure of all space, overcorrection to a Class I relationship, Tweed occlusion (slight out of occlusion on the distal cusps of the first molars and second molars) should be accomplished.

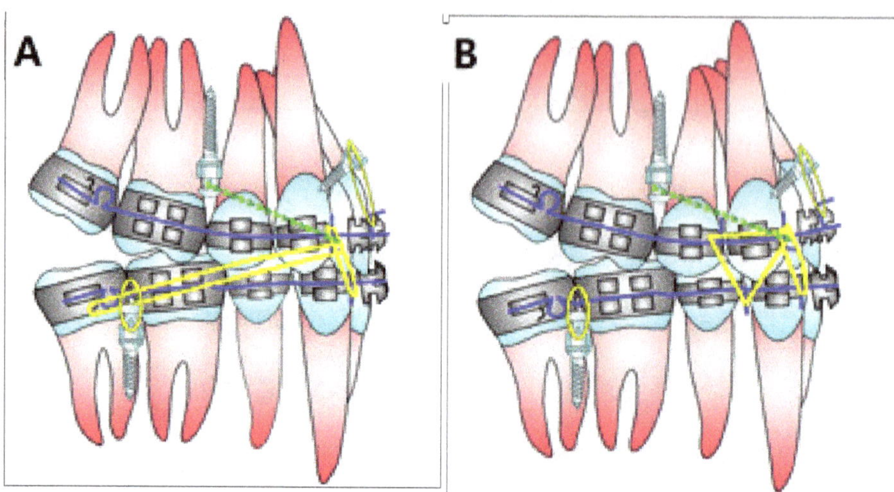

Figure 3. Denture completion: **A.** Class II elastics, anterior vertical elastics, and microscrew implants and elastomeric threads or chains are used for directional force control. **B.** Maxillary and mandibular.0215 ×.028″ archwires are fabricated. Hooks are soldered for the use of micro-implants and elastomeric threads or chains, cusp seating and anterior vertical elastics. The force system used depends on final tooth positions that need to be achieved.

4. Denture recovery

At the end of the denture completion stage of treatment, the appliances are removed, and Tweed occlusion, anchorage prepared positions of the mandibular posterior teeth, and a gentle curve of Spee in the maxillary arch exists (Figure 4.A). As time goes by, functional forces place the teeth into a beautiful inter-digitation (Figure 4.B).

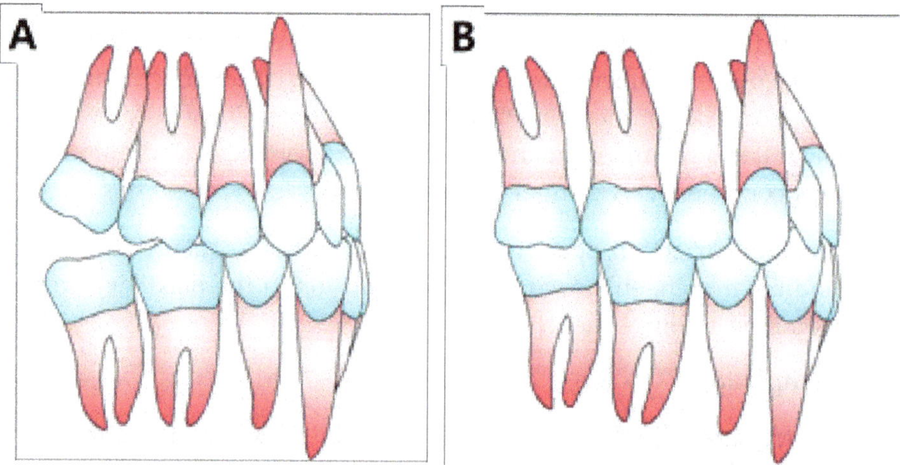

Figure 4. Denture recovery: A. Tweed post-treatment occlusion. Note the distal inclination of the maxillary and mandibular second molars. The maxillary first molar occludes with its mesial buccal cusp in the mesial buccal groove of the mandibular first molar. The canines are in an ideal Angle Class I relationship. The overjet and overbite have been overcorrected. **B.** Functional occlusion. Settling places both the maxillary and mandibular posterior and anterior teeth into their ideal occlusal relationships.

3. Case report

3.1. Case 1. skeletal class II with lip protrusion, gummy smile and asymmetry [18]

3.1.1. *Diagnosis*

A 23-year old woman presented with the chief complaints of lip protrusion and gummy smile. She showed a convex profile with marked protrusion of the lips and retrognathic mandible, mentalis strain, excessive lower anterior facial height, facial asymmetry and gummy smile. Intraorally, she had a Class I relationship with minor crowding and anterior edge-to-edge bite; all third molars were present (Figure 5 and Figure 6).

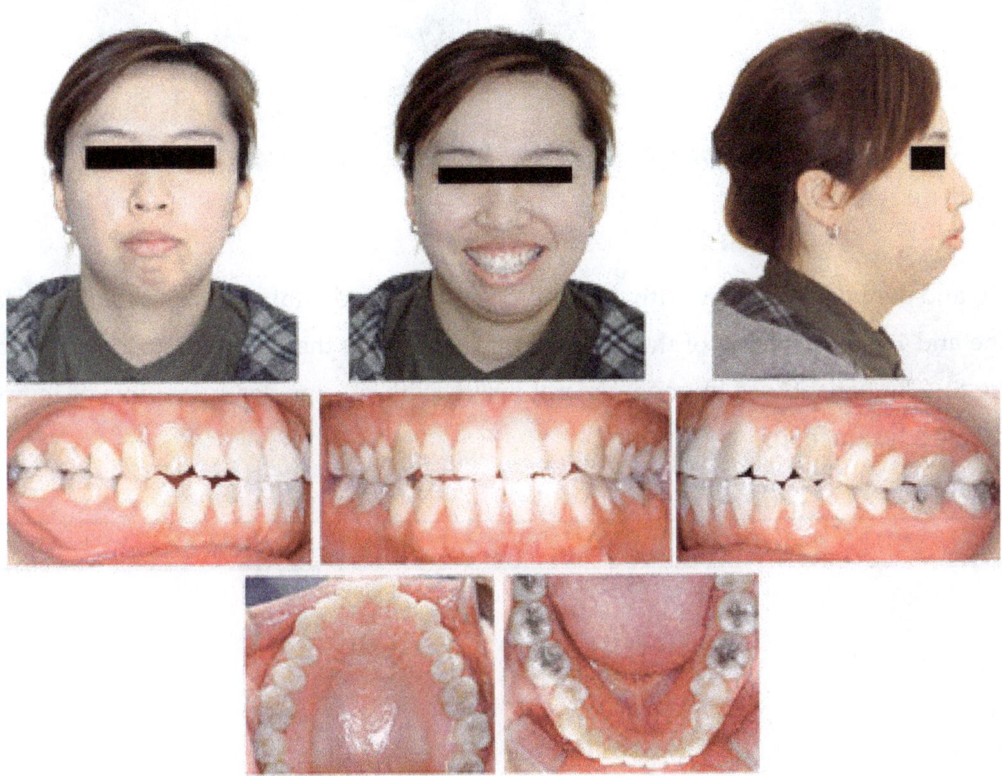

Figure 5. Pretreatment facial and intraoral photographs. (Case 1)

The lateral cephalometric radiograph showed severe facial and skeletal problems (Figure 7). The skeletal pattern was hyperdivergent as indicated by the Frankfort mandibular plane angle (FMA) of 32.0° and the facial height index (FHI) of 65.0%. The ANB angle of 5.5° reflected the class II skeletal problem and the occlusal plane angle of 13.5° showed vertical dental problem. The FH/U1 of 115.5° indicated the normal inclination of upper incisors, and the incisor–mandibular plane angle (IMPA) of 100.5° reflected the proclination of the lower incisors. The Z-angle of 53.0° was a measure of the facial imbalance (Table 1). The posteroanterior cephalogram showed skeletal asymmetry with canting of the maxilla and a deviation of the chin to

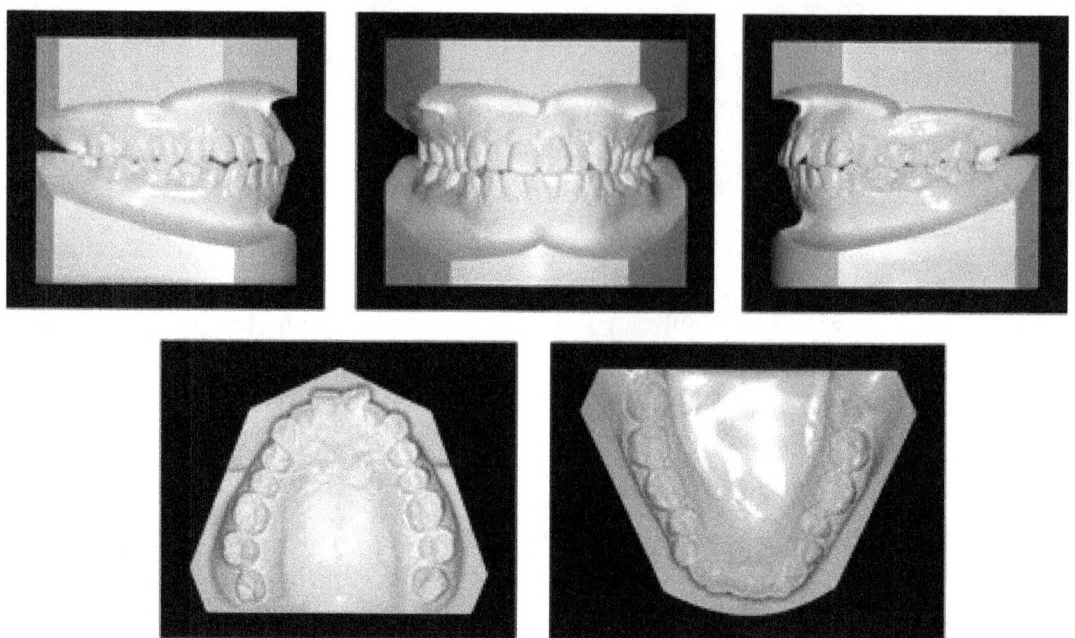

Figure 6. Pretreatment dental casts. (Case 1)

the left, and dental asymmetry with deviation of the upper dental midline to the left of facial midline and 1-mm deviation of the lower dental midline to the left of upper dental midline (Figure 8). The patient was in good general health with no signs or symptoms of temporomandibular dysfunction.

	Pretreatment	Post-treatment
FMIA (°)	47.5	60.0
FMA (°)	32.0	29.5
IMPA (°)	100.5	90.5
SNA (°)	83.0	82.0
SNB (°)	77.5	78.0
ANB (°)	5.5	4.0
AO-BO (mm)	-1.5	1.0
Occlusal plane angle (°)	13.5	7.0
FH to U1(°)	115.5	112.0
Z angle (°)	53.0	67.5
PFH	48.0	48.0
AFH	73.5	71.5
FHI (PFH/AFH) (%)	0.65(48.0/73.5)	0.67(48.0/71.5)

Table 1. Cephalometric measurements (Case 1)

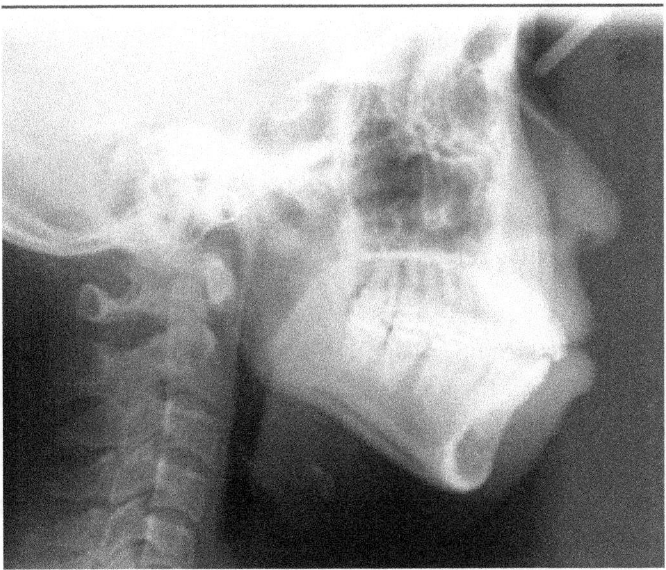

Figure 7. Pretreatment lateral cephalometric radiograph. (Case 1)

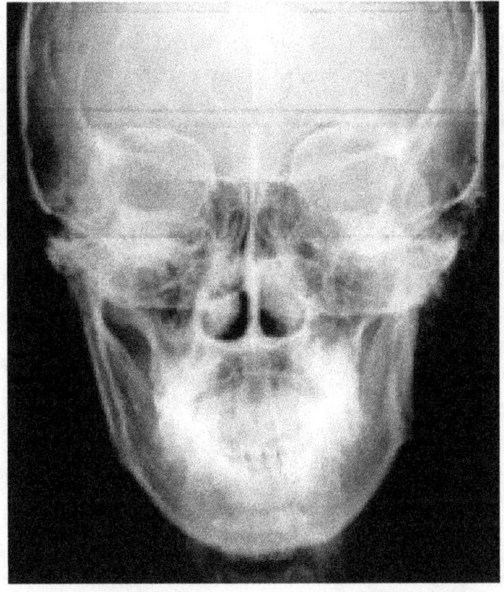

Figure 8. Pretreatment posteroanterior cephalometric radiograph. (Case 1)

3.1.2. Treatment alternatives

The first treatment plan was orthognathic surgery. Extraction of the maxillary second premolars and the mandibular first premolars would be done to resolve the arch-length discrepancy and upright the mandibular anterior teeth. Following this, two jaw surgeries with genioplasty would be necessary for mandibular advancement, reduction of lower anterior facial height and correction of asymmetry. However, the patient not want to undergo orthognathic surgery, therefore another treatment plan was needed.

The second treatment plan was orthodontic camouflage treatment with removal of the four first premolars and four 3rd molars using MIA to achieve a balanced facial profile.

3.1.3. Treatment progress

Before treatment, the mandibular second premolars were inadvertently extracted instead of the mandibular first premolars by an oral surgeon. However, that did not prove to be problematic since our plan was to use micro-implant anchorage (MIA).

.022 ×.028-in nontipped, nontorqued standard edgewise appliances were placed in both arches after extraction. Maxillary posterior MIs (1.2 mm in diameter, 8 mm in length; Absoanchor AX12-108, Dentos, Taegu, South Korea) were installed into the buccal alveolar bone between the maxillary second premolars and the first molars, and mandibular posterior MIs (1.2 mm in diameter, 7 mm in length; Absoanchor ATX 1311-107, Dentos) were installed into the buccal alveolar bone between the mandibular first and second molars. Then, elastomers were placed immediately after installation of the MIs, from the maxillary and mandibular posterior MIs to the canine brackets for retraction of the maxillary canines and simultaneously retraction of the mandibular canines and first premolars (Figure 9.A).

Following the retraction of canines and first premolars, closing loop archwires were placed on both arches. Maxillary anterior MIs (1.2 mm in diameter, 6.0 mm in length; Absoanchor ATX1311-106, Dentos) were installed into the labial alveolar bone between the maxillary central and lateral incisors and elastomers were placed for torque control, bodily movement, and intrusion of the maxillary anterior teeth. Elastomers were also placed to the omega stop areas of the mandibular archwire for intruding mandibular posterior teeth (Figure 9.B).

After en-masse retraction of anterior teeth, directional force was applied to achieve mandibular response (Figure 9.C). Ideal archwires were inserted and elastomers were placed for finishing the treatment (Figure 9.D). Fixed lingual retainers were placed on the six anterior teeth and circumferential clear retainers were placed on both arches for retention. Total treatment period was 24 months.

3.1.4. Treatment results

After treatment, she showed a nicely balanced and harmonious face by retracting lips, reducing the mentalis strain, and reducing lower anterior facial height. Excessive gingival display when smiling was successfully reduced by intruding the maxillary anterior segment (Figure 10). Dentally, a good interdigitation of the teeth and acceptable overjet-overbite relationship were achieved (Figure 11). The postero-anterior cephalometric radiograph showed improvement in skeletal and dental asymmetry (Figure 12).

Cephalometric superimposition showed the bodily retraction with intrusion of the maxillary anterior teeth, intrusion and distal movement of the maxillary posterior teeth, retraction with uprighting of the mandibular anterior teeth, and uprighting with intrusion of the mandibular posterior teeth. A good mandibular response with chin advancement was achieved by the counterclockwise autorotation of the mandible caused by vertical control of dentition (Figure

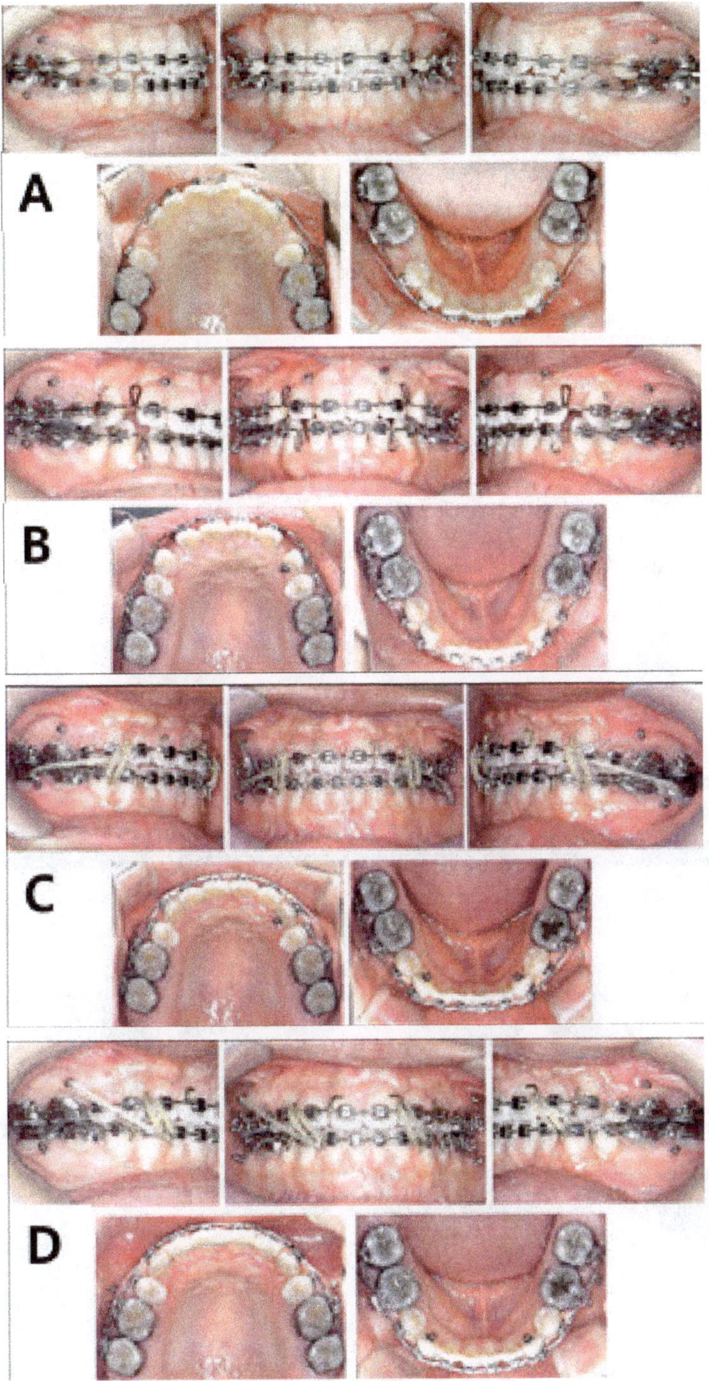

Figure 9. A. Denture preparation: retraction of maxillary and mandibular canines and first premolars with elastomeric chain, and maxillary and mandibular posterior MIs. **B.** Denture correction: en-masse retraction with closing loop arch-wires supported by maxillary posterior and anterior MIs and mandibular posterior MIs. **C.** Denture completion: directional force. **D.** Denture completion: finishing with cusp-seating elastics for good interdigitation and additional unilateral Class III elastics for correction of asymmetry. (Case 1)

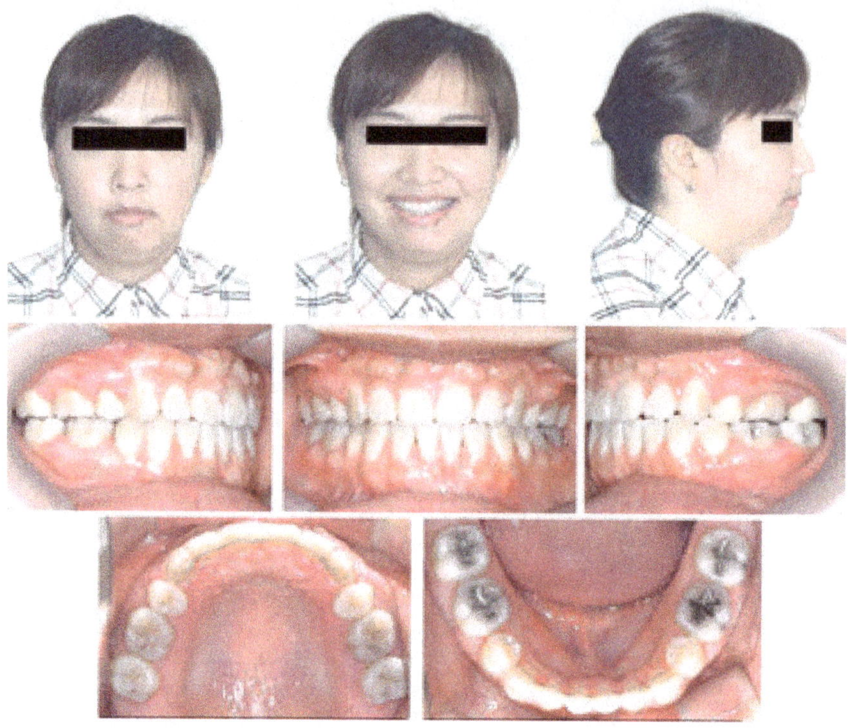

Figure 10. Post-treatment facial and intraoral photographs. (Case 1)

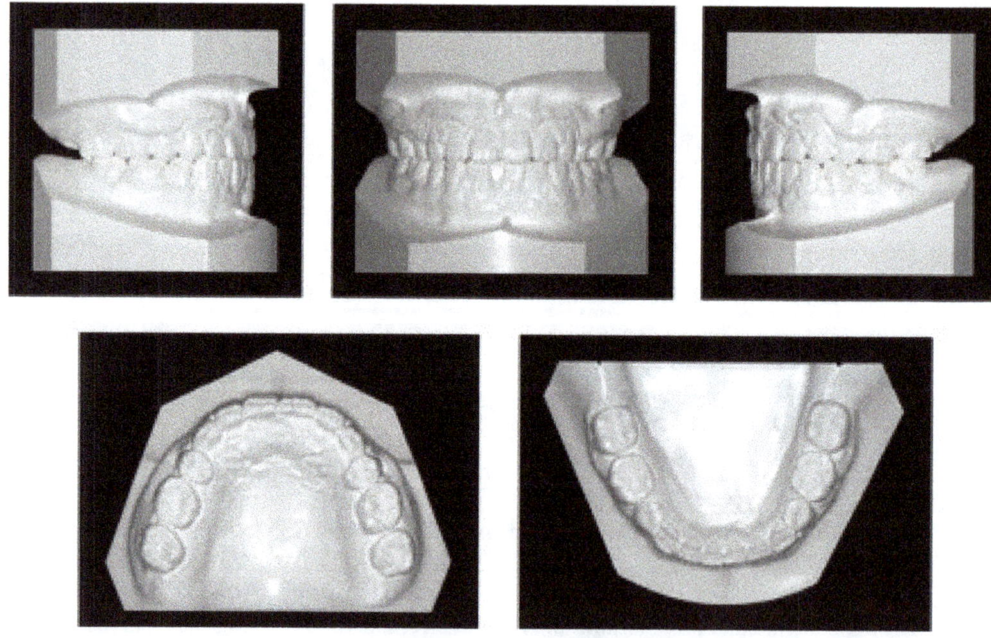

Figure 11. Post-treatment dental casts. (Case 1)

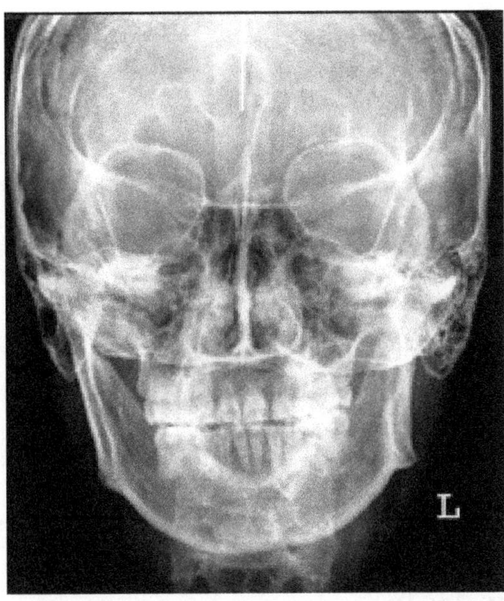

Figure 12. Post-treatment lateral cephalometric radiograph. (Case 1)

13). As a result of vertical control, the FMA, ANB angle, occlusal plane angle, and anterior facial height were reduced by 2.5°, 1.5°, 6.5°, and 2mm, respectively. The IMPA and was reduced by 10° and the Z-angle was increased by 14.5° (Table 1). All of the above changes resulted in significant improvement of the facial profile.

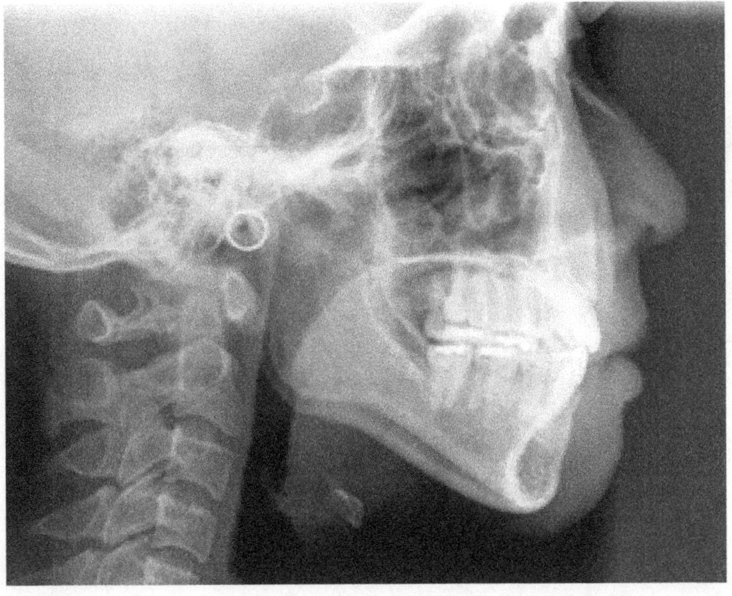

Figure 13. Post-treatment posteroanterior cephalometric radiograph. (Case 1)

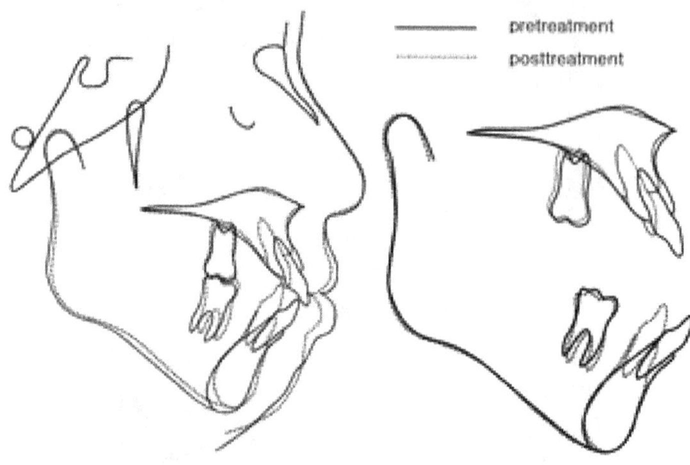

Figure 14. Cephalometric superimposition. (Case 1)

3.2. Case 2. skeletal class II with lip protrusion and nasal airway obstruction [21]

3.2.1. Diagnosis

A 22-year-old male presented with the chief complaints of lip protrusion and difficulty in nasal breathing. Facially, he showed a convex profile with marked protrusion of the lips and retrognathic mandible, mentalis strain, excessive lower anterior facial height and a typical "adenoid face". He had a Class I relationship with moderate crowding, severe constricted "V" shaped arch forms of both jaws, an anterior open bite, several restorations on the posterior teeth; upper left and lower right third molars were present (Figure 15 and Figure 16).

	Pretreatment	Post-treatment	13-month retention
FMIA (°)	53.5	73.0	71.5
FMA (°)	33.5	30.5	32.0
IMPA (°)	93.0	76.5	76.5
SNA (°)	84.0	83.0	83.0
SNB (°)	79.5	80.0	79.5
ANB (°)	4.5	3.0	3.5
AO-BO (mm)	-2.0	-1.0	-1.5
Occlusal plane angle (°)	10.0	8.0	10.0
FH to U1(°)	112.0	103.0	98.0
Z angle (°)	51.5	61.5	60.5
PFH	54.5	57.5	57.0
AFH	91.0	88.0	89.0
FHI (PFH/AFH) (%)	0.61(54.5/91.0)	0.65(57.5/88.0)	0.64(57.0/89.0)

Table 2. Cephalometric measurements (Case 2)

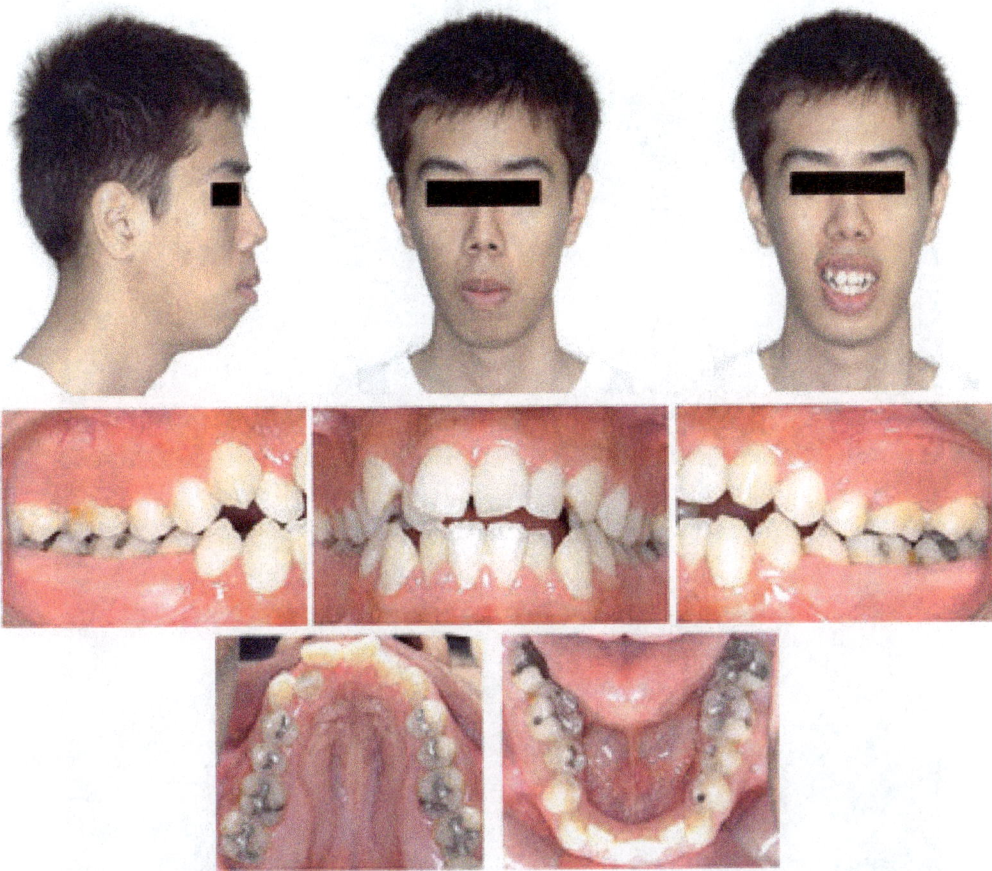

Figure 15. Pretreatment facial and intraoral photographs. (Case 2)

The lateral cephalometric radiograph showed severe facial and skeletal problems (Figure 16). The skeletal pattern was hyperdivergent and Class II as indicated by the FMA of 33.5°, the FHI of 61% and the ANB angle of 4.5°. The FH/U1 of 112.0° and the IMPA of 93.0° indicated the normal inclination of upper and lower incisors. The Z-angle of 51.5° was a measure of the facial imbalance (Table 2). The posteroanterior cephalogram showed a dental midline deviation of 2 mm to the left to the maxillary dental midline which was coincident to the facial midline and slight canting of the maxilla and transverse constriction of both arches (Figure 16). The patient was in good general health with no signs or symptoms of any temporomandibular disorders.

3.2.2. *Treatment alternatives*

The first treatment plan was orthognathic surgery. Expanding maxillary arch by surgical assisted rapid maxillary expansion (SARME) and mandibular arch by Schwarz appliance would be done to resolve the arch-length discrepancy and achieve normal arch form. Then, two jaw surgeries with genioplasty would be necessary for mandibular advancement and reduction of lower anterior facial height. However, the patient did not want to undergo orthognathic surgery o another treatment plan was chosen.

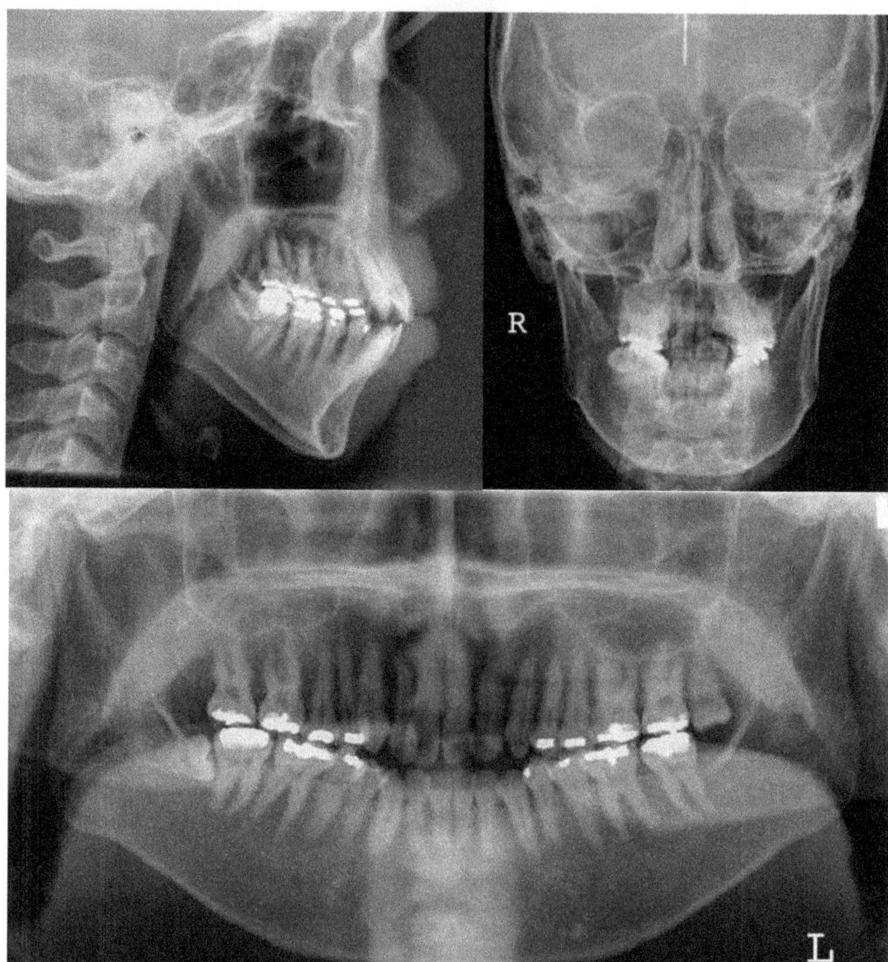

Figure 16. Pretreatment radiographs. (Case 2)

The second treatment plan was orthodontic camouflage treatment with expansion of the constricted upper and lower arches with SARME and Schwarz appliance, respectively, followed by orthodontic treatment with extraction of the four first premolars and all third molars using MIA. As mentioned previously [15], MIA can provide absolute anchorage for vertical control, which would induce a horizontal mandibular response resulting in a balanced facial profile.

3.2.3. Treatment progress

The treatment was divided into 2 phases. Phase I treatment was consisted of SARME in the maxilla and Schwarz appliance in the mandible (Figure 17). Schwarz appliance was activated once a week for about 5 months. SARME with Hyrax palatal expansion appliance cemented to the maxillary first molars and first premolars was activated two turns per day (0.5 mm) for 20 days and then 1 turn per week for a further 28 days until the desired level of expansion was achieved (Figure 18). After the desired expansion, a Hyrax palatal expander in the maxilla remained in place for an additional 3.5 months during the completion of mandibular expansion (Figure 19).

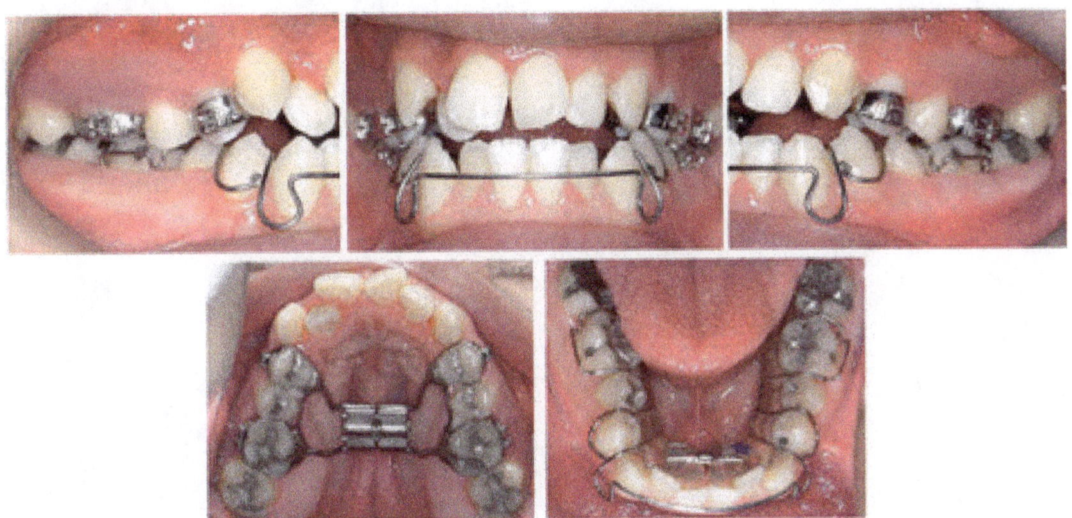

Figure 17. Surgical assisted rapid maxillary expansion on the maxilla and Schwarz appliance on the mandible. (Case 2)

The phase II treatment plan was consisted of Tweed- Merrifield directional force technology with MIA with extraction of four first premolars and two third molars. 0.022 × 0.028-in nontipped, nontorqued edgewise appliances were placed in both arches after the extractions. Maxillary posterior MIs (1.3 - 1.2 mm in diameter, 8 mm in length; Absoanchor SH1312-08, Dentos, Taegu, South Korea) were installed into the buccal alveolar bone between the maxillary second premolars and first molars, and the mandibular posterior MIs (1.3 - 1.2 mm in diameter, 7 mm in length; Absoanchor SH1312-08, Dentos) were installed into the buccal alveolar bone between the mandibular first and second molars. Elastomers were placed immediately after installation of the MIs, from the maxillary and mandibular posterior MIs to the canine brackets for retraction of the canines to level the six anterior teeth (Figure 20.A).

Two months into the treatment, 0.019 × 0.025-in stainless steel closing loop archwire was placed in the lower arch for en masse retraction of the six anterior teeth. Elastomers were applied from the mandibular posterior MIs to the omega loop areas of the mandibular archwire for intruding mandibular posterior teeth. Three months into the treatment, a 0.017 × 0.022-in stainless steel archwire was inserted and elastomers were placed from the maxillary MIs to the maxillary archwire for intrusion of the maxillary posterior teeth. Unilateral Class III elastomer was added from the maxillary posterior MIs to the right-side loop of the mandibular archwire for reduction of the dental asymmetry (Figure 20.B).

Four months into the treatment, 0.020 × 0.025-in stainless steel closing loop archwire was placed in the upper arch for en masse retraction of the six anterior teeth. At this time, maxillary anterior MIs (microimplants, 1.3 - 1.2 mm in diameter, 8 mm in length; Absoanchor SH1312-08, Dentos)

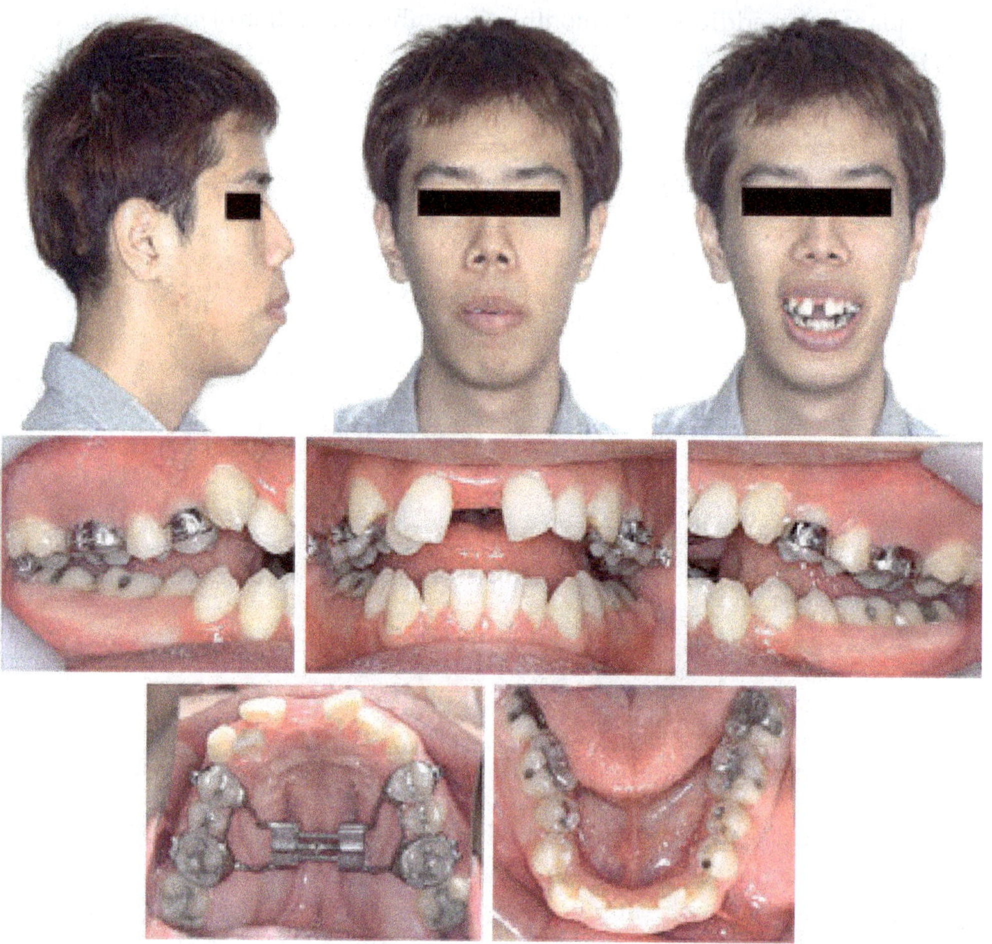

Figure 18. Photographs after 28-day expansion of the maxilla and mandible. (Case 2)

were installed into the labial alveolar bone between the maxillary central incisors for torque control, bodily movement and intrusion of the maxillary anterior teeth (Figure 20.C).

After en masse retraction, directional force was applied to achieve a mandibular response. Ideal archwires (0.020 × 0.025-in stainless steel archwire in the upper arch and 0.019 × 0.025-in stainless steel archwire in the lower arch) were inserted and elastomers were placed for finishing the treatment (Figure 20.D). Fixed lingual retainers were placed on the six anterior teeth and circumferential clear retainers were placed on both arches for retention. Total treatment period of phase II was 24 months.

3.2.4. Treatment results

After phase I treatment, considerable expansion on both arches was achieved in the anterior and posterior segments, which provided the space for dental alignment. The postero-anterior cephalometric radiograph showed a remarkable increase in transverse intermolar width (between the buccal surfaces of the first molar) by 10.0 mm after 1 month of expansion with

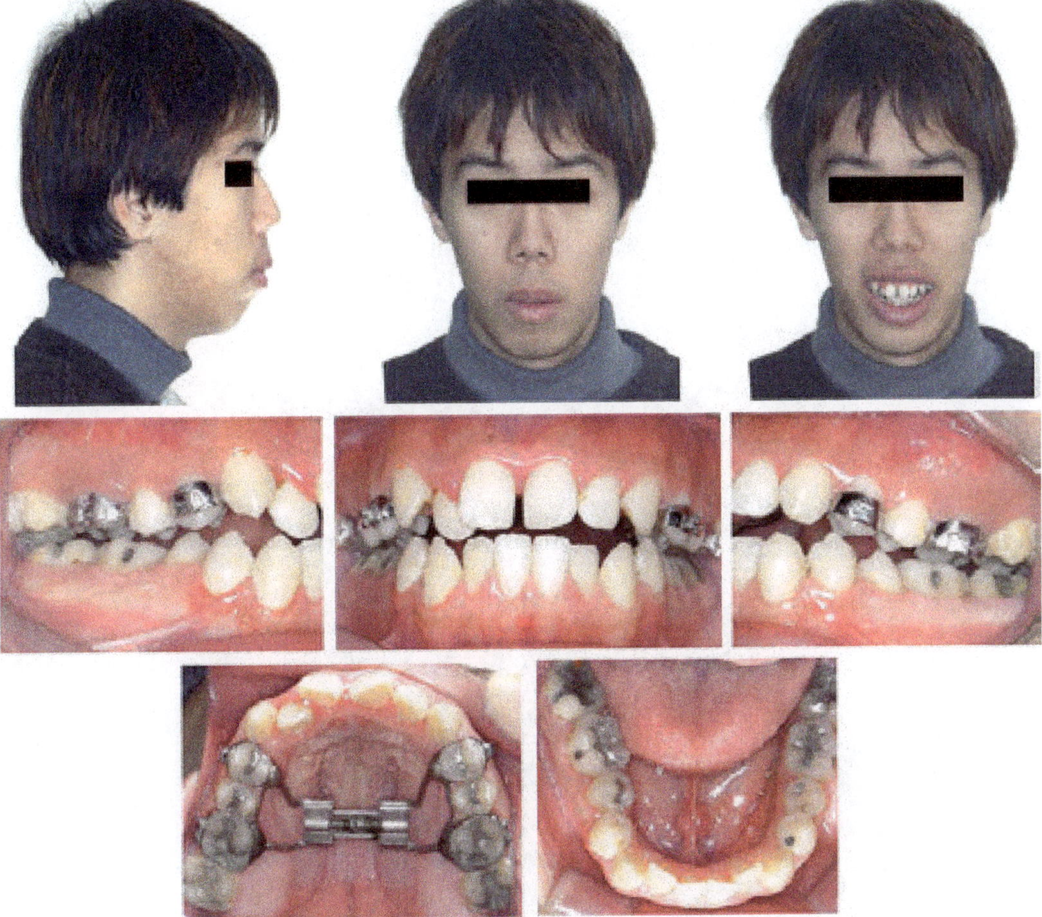

Figure 19. Photographs after 3.5 months of retention of the maxilla and 5 months of expansion of the mandible. (Case 2)

SARME in the maxillary arch and by 5.5 mm after 5 months of expansion with Schwarz appliance in the mandibular arch. Facially, he showed a slightly worsened appearance by the clockwise rotation of the mandible due to molar extrusion as a result of expansion of both arches. However, it was recovered during the retention period of phase I and he was pleased with the slightly peaceful looking facial appearance with easier nasal breathing.

After phase II treatment, he showed a well-balanced and harmonious face by retracting both upper and lower lips, reducing the mentalis muscle strain, and decreasing lower anterior facial height. Excessive gingival display during smiling was successfully reduced by intruding the maxillary anterior segment. Dentally, a good interdigitation of the teeth, acceptable arch form and a normal overjet-overbite relationship, and good overall root parallelism with no significant root resorption was achieved. The postero-anterior cephalometric radiograph showed relapse of transverse dimension of the maxillary intermolar width by 5.5 mm and an additional increase of the mandibular width by 3.5 mm (Figure 21 and Figure 22). After retention of thirteen months, he showed good retention without any obvious relapse (Figure 23).

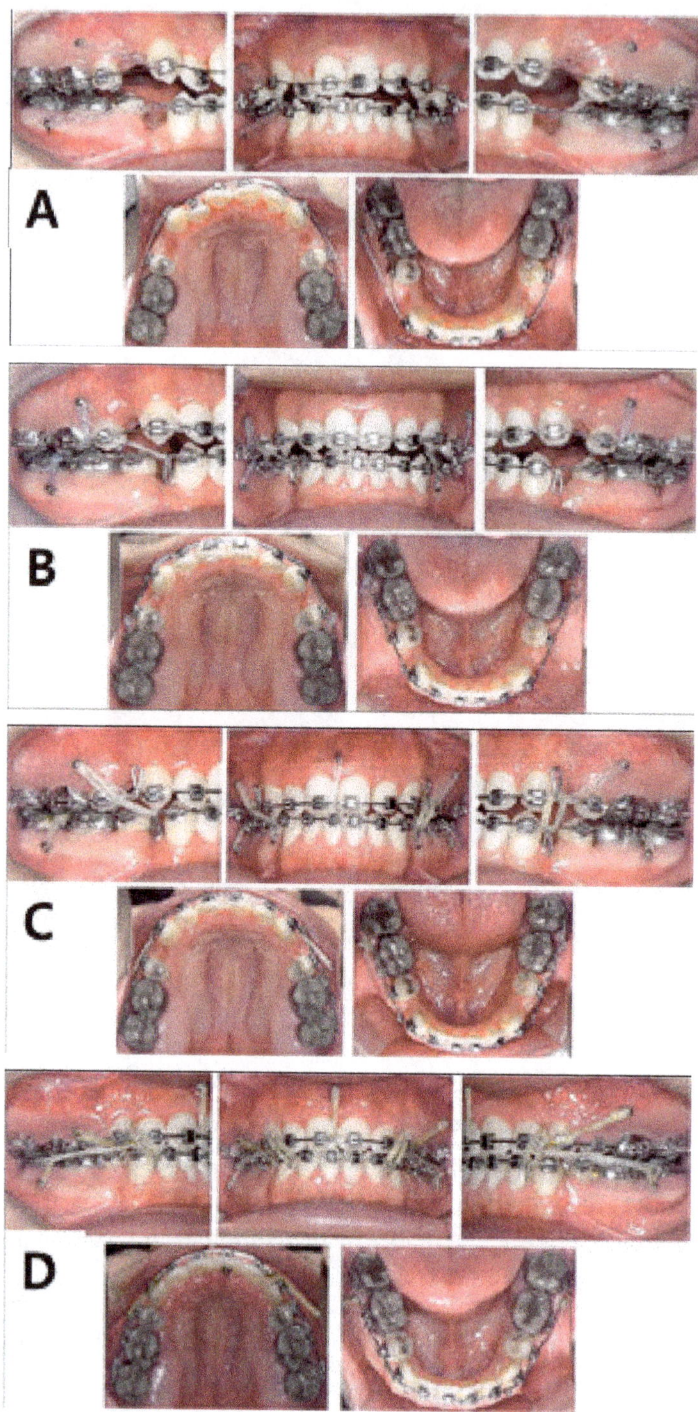

Figure 20. A. Denture preparation: retraction of the maxillary and mandibular canines to level six anterior teeth. (Case 2) **B.** Denture correction: en masse retraction with a closing loop archwire supported by mandibular posterior MIs, intruding forces with elastomeric chain between the main archwires and maxillary and mandibular posterior MIs, and unilateral Class III elastics to correct asymmetry. (Case 2) **C.** Denture correction: en masse retraction with closing loop archwire supported by maxillary posterior and anterior MIs. (Case 2) **D.** Denture completion: directional force and finishing with Class II and cusp seating elastics, and elastomeric chain and MIs. (Case 2)

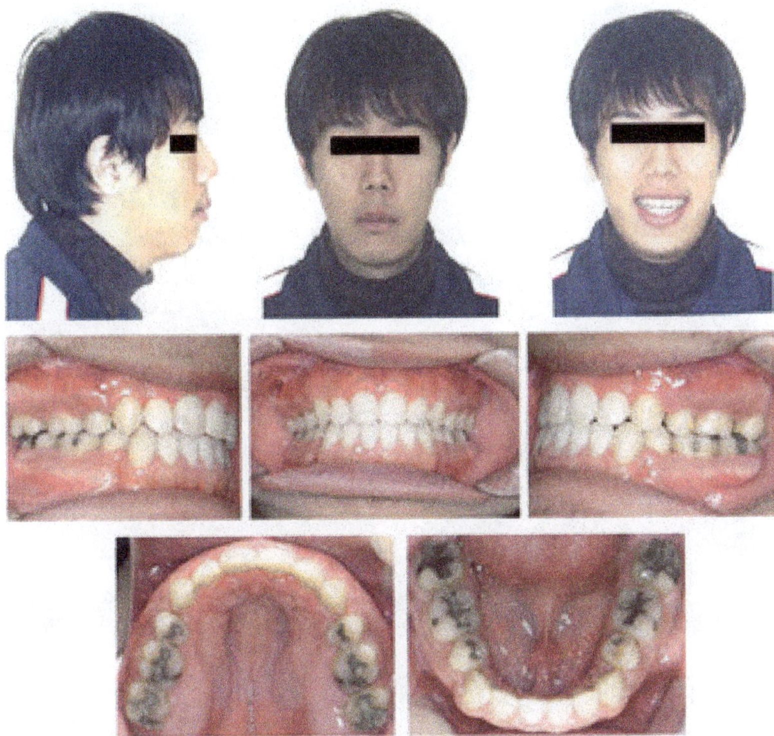

Figure 21. Post-treatment facial and intraoral photographs. (Case 2)

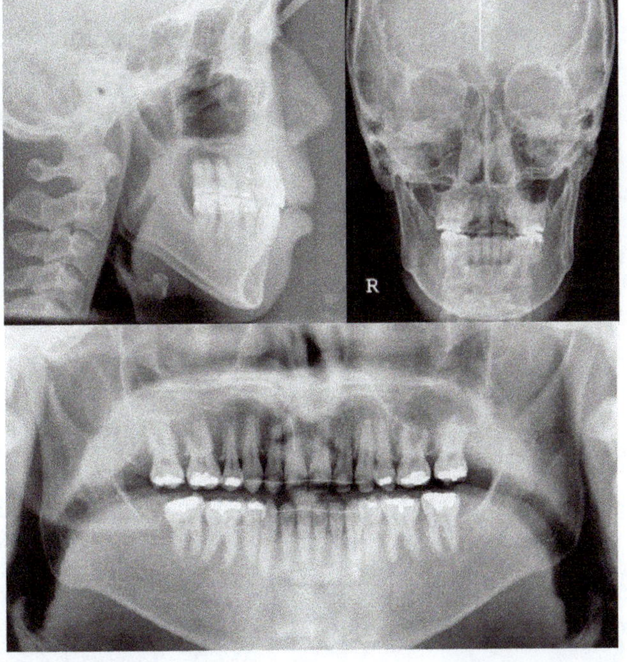

Figure 22. Post-treatment radiographs. (Case 2)

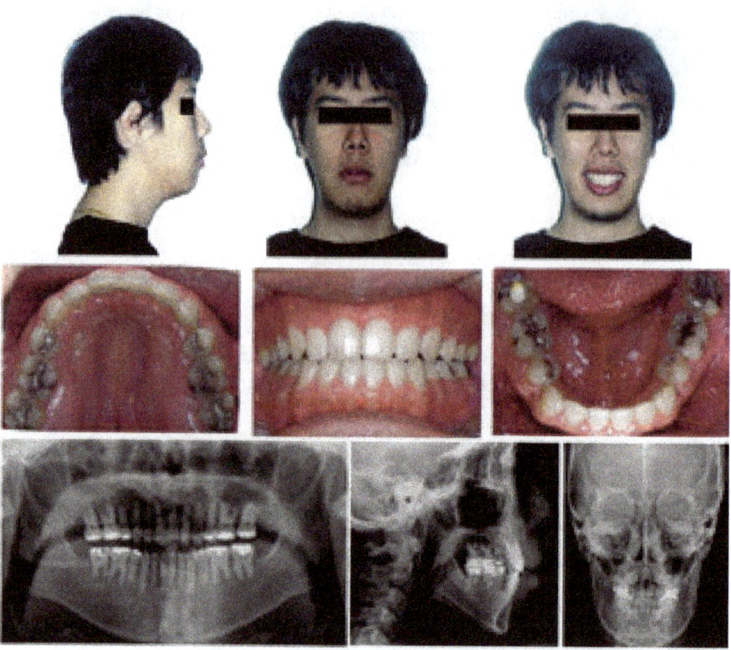

Figure 23. month retention photographs and radiographs. (Case 2)

Cephalometric superimposition showed the bodily retraction with intrusion of the maxillary anterior teeth, intrusion of maxillary posterior teeth, retraction with uprighting of mandibular anterior teeth and uprighting of mandibular posterior teeth. A good mandibular response with chin advancement was obtained by the counterclockwise autorotation of the mandible facilitated by vertical control of dentition (Figure 24.A). As a result of vertical control, the FMA, ANB angle, and anterior facial height were decreased by 3.0°, 1.5° and 3 mm, respectively. The IMPA was decreased by 16.5 ° and Z-angle was increased by 10 ° (Table 2). Facial profile was improved by all these changes.

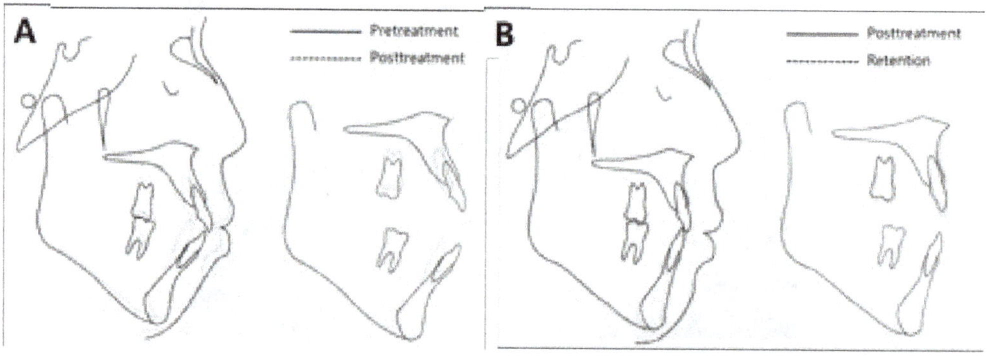

Figure 24. A. Pretreatment and post-treatment cephalometric superimposition; **B.** post-treatment and 13-month retention cephalometric superimposition. (Case 2)

After 13 months of retention, as a result of relapse due to extrusion of the maxillary anterior and posterior teeth, the FMA, ANB angle, and anterior facial height were increased by 1.5°, 0.5°, and 1 mm, respectively (Figure 24.B and Table 2).

3.3. Case 3. skeletal class II div.1 with lip protrusion, gummy smile and deep bite [16]

3.3.1. *Diagnosis*

A 13-year-old male presented with the chief complaints of lip protrusion and gummy smile. Facially, he exhibited a convex profile due to a retrognathic mandible. The facial photographs showed a convex facial profile with marked protrusion of the lips, mentalis strain and a gummy smile. Intraorally, he had Class II canine and molar relationships with slight crowding, "V" shaped arch forms of both jaws, an anterior deep bite, deep curve of Spee, caries and restoration on the posterior teeth; all third molars were present (Figure 25).

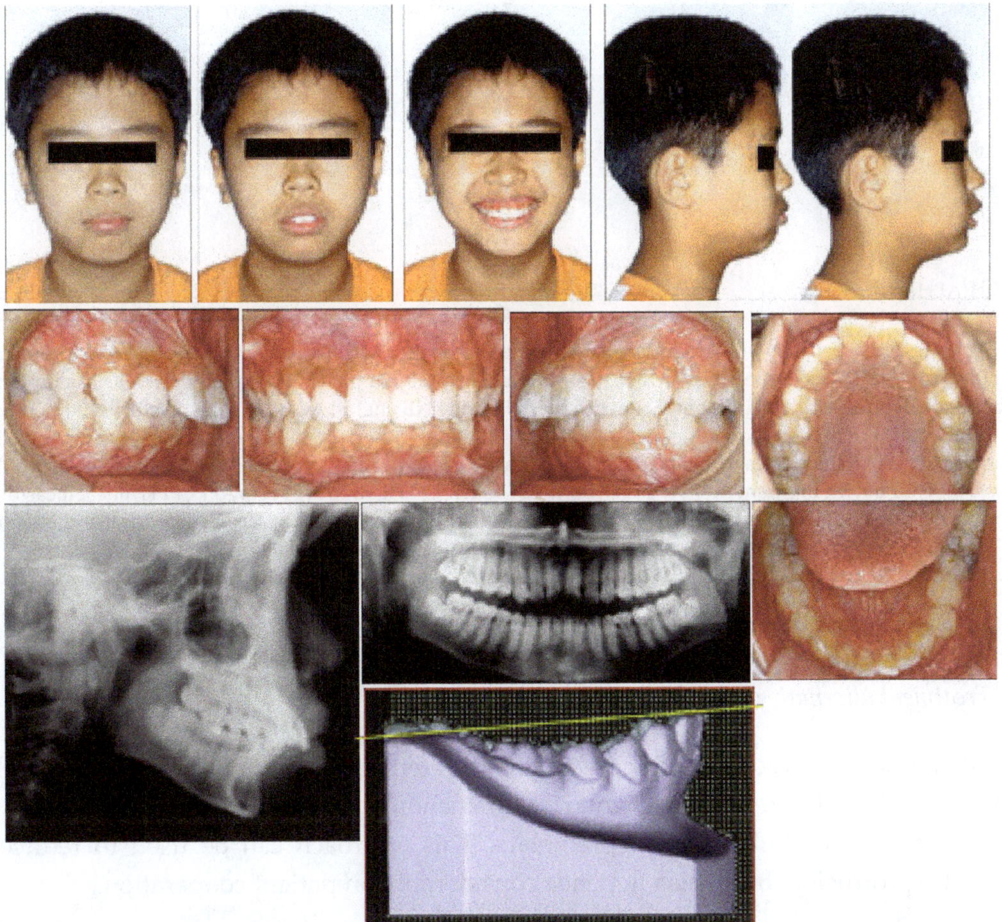

Figure 25. Pretreatment facial and intraoral photographs, mandibular cast, and cephalometric and panoramic radiographs. (Case 3)

The lateral cephalometric radiograph showed severe facial and skeletal problems (Figure 25). The skeletal pattern was hypodivergent and Class II as indicated by the FMA of 22.0° and the FHI of 71.0%, and the ANB angle of 6.5°. The Z-angle of 58.5° was a measure of the facial imbalance. The IMPA of 106.0° indicated severe protrusion of mandibular incisors (Table 3). There were no significant signs or symptoms of any temporomandibular disorders.

	Pretreatment	Post-treatment	30-month retention
FMIA (°)	52.0	60.0	57.5
FMA (°)	22.0	20.0	17.0
IMPA (°)	106.0	100.0	105.5
SNA (°)	83.5	81.5	82.0
SNB (°)	77.0	78.5	80.0
ANB (°)	6.5	3.0	2.0
AO-BO (mm)	5.0	2.0	1.0
Occlusal plane angle (°)	6.0	3.5	2.5
FH to U1(°)	124.5	121.5	122.5
Z angle (°)	58.5	78.0	79.0
PFH	44.0	48.5	53.5
AFH	62.0	65.5	68.0
FHI (PFH/AFH) (%)	0.71(44.0/62.0)	0.72(48.5/65.5)	0.79(53.5/68.0)

[a] FMIA indicates angle between Frankfort plane and mandibular incisor axis; FMA, angle between Frankfort plane and mandibular plane; IMPA, angle between lower incisor axis and mandibular plane; SNA, angle between SN and NA; SNB, angle between SN and NB; ANB, difference between the SNA and SNB angles; AOBO, distance between perpendiculars drawn from point A and point B onto the occlusal plane; FH, Frankfort horizontal plane; UI, maxillary incisor axis; FH to UI, angle between Frankfort plane and maxillary incisor axis; Z angle, angle between FH and Z line; Z line, profile line tangent to the chin and the more anterior vermilion border of both lips; FHI, ratio of PFH to AFH; PFH, linear measurement from articulare, along a line tangent to the posterior border of the mandible, to the intersection with the mandibular plane; and AFH, linear measurement from palatal plane to mention, measured perpendicular to palatal plane.

Table 3. Cephalometric measurements (Case 3)

3.3.2. *Treatment alternatives*

The first alternative was orthodontic treatment with retraction and intrusion of the maxillary anterior teeth by using headgear for maximum anchorage after extraction of maxillary first premolars and mandibular second premolars. This approach can be used to reduce the patient's lip protrusion, but it also depends considerably on patient cooperation.

The second alternative was orthodontic treatment with retraction and intrusion of the maxillary anterior teeth by using MIA and headgear for absolute and maximum anchorage after extraction of maxillary first premolars and mandibular second premolars, respectively.

The second option would provide good results with minimum patient compliance. Therefore, this treatment plan was chosen.

3.3.3. *Treatment progress*

The treatment plan involved Tweed-Merrifield directional force technology with MIA and HPJH, after the extraction of the maxillary first premolars and mandibular second premolars.

After the extractions,.022 ×.028-in pre-adjusted appliances and.022 ×.028-in nontipped, nontorqued edgewise appliances were placed in upper and lower arches, respectively. And leveling began with a.014-in nickel-titanium archwire and.018 stainless steel archwires. Maxillary posterior MIs (2.0 mm in diameter, 7 mm in length; Martin, Tuttlingen, Germany) were implanted into the buccal alveolar bone between the maxillary second premolars and the first molars (Figure 26).

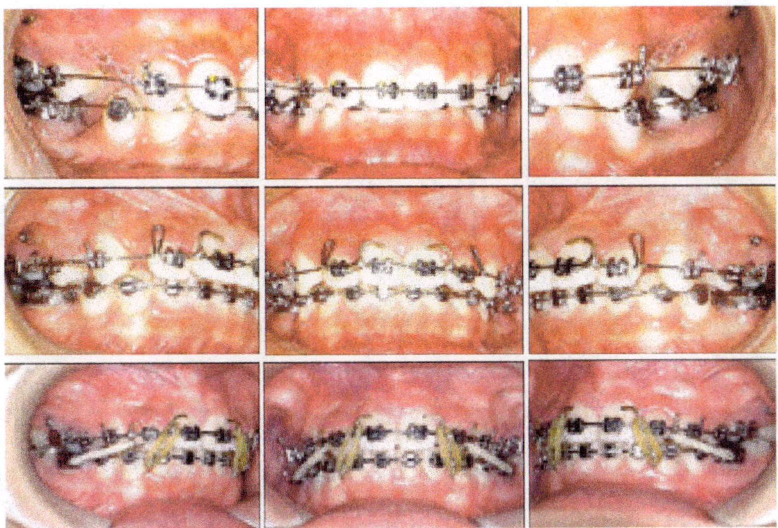

Figure 26. Intraoral photographs during treatment showing micro-implants implanted in the maxilla, elastomeric chains, class II and up and down elastics, soldered hooks for elastics and J-hook. (Case 3)

Elastic chain force was loaded one month after placement of the MIs, from the maxillary MIs to the maxillary canine brackets, to retract the maxillary canines. Two months into treatment,. 018 ×.025-in stainless steel archwire with running loops and elastomers were placed in the lower arch, for retracting to level mandibular anterior teeth, uprighting and mesial movement of mandibular first molars, and closing the spaces (Figure 26). During the retraction of maxillary canines and en masse retraction of maxillary anterior teeth, maxillary posterior MIs were loosened twice, so they were re-implanted into the buccal alveolar bone between the maxillary second premolars and the first molars (1.2mm in diameter, 8mm in length; Osteomed Co, Addison, Texas, U.S.A.) and between the maxillary first molars and the second molars (1.2mm in diameter, 7mm in length; Dentos Co, Taegu, Korea). During the period of bone healing, HPJH was substituted for MIs.

After the retraction of the maxillary canines into half of the extraction space, closing loop archwire was placed and was supported by the HPJH for torque control, bodily movement, and intrusion of the maxillary anterior teeth. After en-masse movement, directional force control was performed to promote mandibular response (Figure 26). The treatment was completed with ideal archwires and cusp-seating elastics. Total treatment time was 31 months.

3.3.4. Treatment results

The post-treatment facial photographs and lateral cephalometric radiograph showed a well-balanced and harmonious face through retraction of the upper and lower lips, reduction of the mentalis muscle strain, and favorable nasal and mandibular growth. The intrusive forces used on the maxillary anterior segment successfully reduced the excessive gingival display during smiling. The post-treatment intraoral photographs and dental casts showed a good interdigitation of the teeth, an acceptable arch form, a normal overjet-overbite relationship and a flat curve of Spee. The post-treatment panoramic radiograph showed good overall root parallelism with no significant resorption of root and alveolar bone (Figure 27). After retention of thirty-month retention, the patient showed good retention without any obvious relapse (Figure 28).

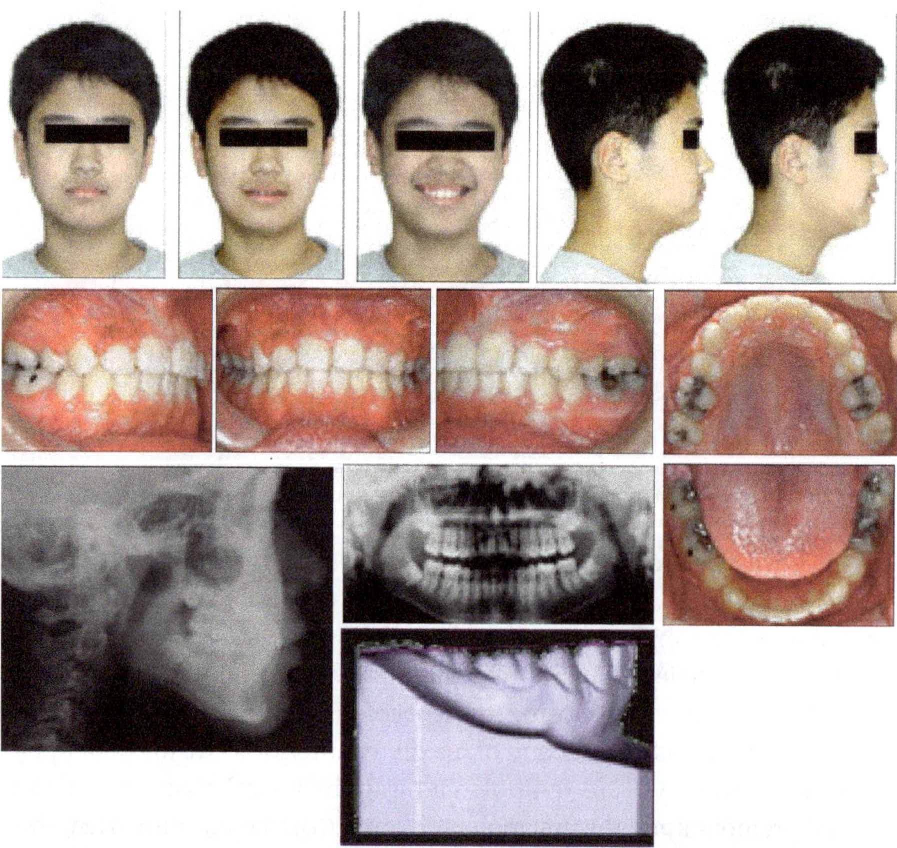

Figure 27. Post-treatment facial and intraoral photographs, mandibular cast, and cephalometric and panoramic radiographs. (Case 3)

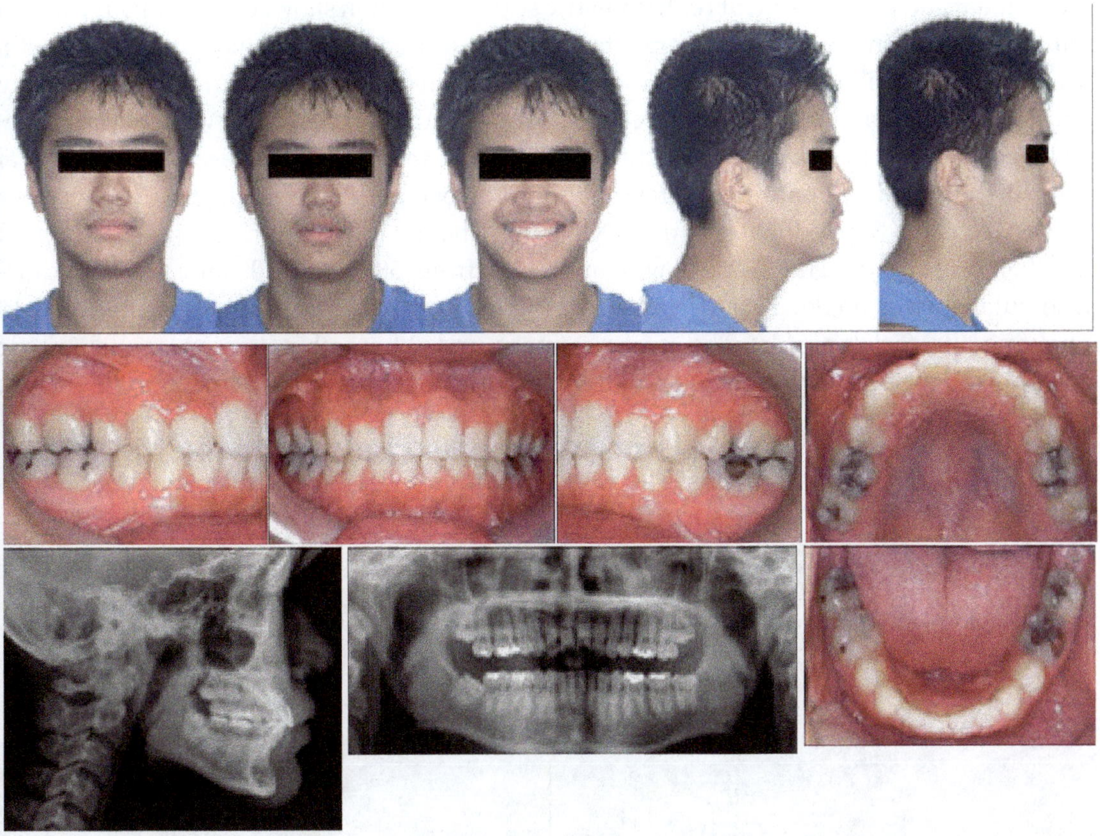

Figure 28. 30-month retention facial and intraoral photographs and cephalometric and panoramic radiographs. (Case 3)

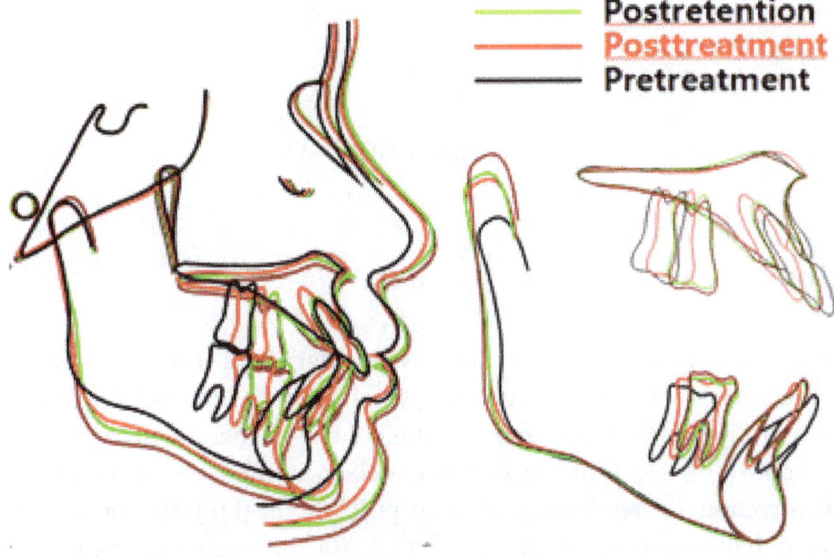

Figure 29. Pretreatment, post-treatment 30-month retention cephalometric superimposition. (Case 3)

Pretreatment and post-treatment cephalometric superimposition showed the bodily retraction with intrusion of the maxillary anterior teeth, slight intrusion of maxillary posterior teeth, retraction with uprighting of the mandibular anterior teeth, and uprighting with mesially extrusion of the mandibular posterior teeth. A good mandibular response with chin advancement was achieved by the counterclockwise rotation of the mandible caused by the vertical control of the maxillary dentition and favorable growth of mandible, resulting in a 2.0° decrease in the FMA, and a 3.5° reduction of the ANB angle. The mandibular incisors were uprighted from 106.0° to 100.0°. The Z-angle was improved from 58.5° to 78.0° and the Frankfort-mandibular incisor angle (FMIA) was increased by 8.0°. All these changes contributed to improving the facial profile. The post-treatment and 30-month retention cephalometric superimposition showed favorable growth such as maintenance of ANB and Z-angle (Figure 29 and Table 3).

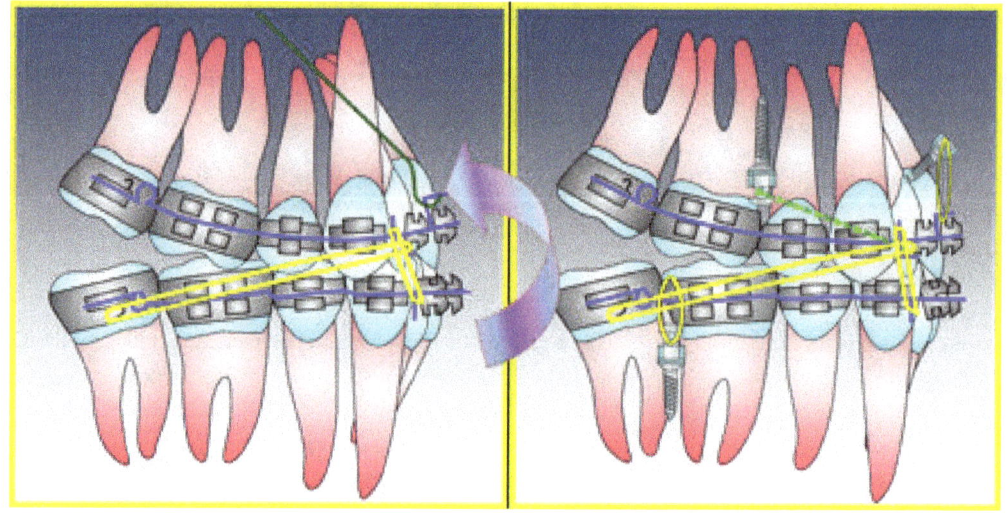

Figure 30. Counterclockwise directional force technology with HPJH and MIA.

4. Conclusion

A good facial balance could be obtained by Tweed-Merrifield directional force technology using HPJH together with skeletal anchorage, which provide anchorage control in the maxillary and mandibular posterior area, torque control in the maxillary anterior area, and mandibular response. These indicate that skeletal anchorage could be used to reinforce anchorage for directional force instead of high pull J-hook (HPJH). Consequently, Tweed-Merrifield directional force technology using M.I.A. for the treatment of Class I and Class II bialveolar protrusion not only maximizes the result of treatment but can also minimize patient compliance (Figure 30).

Author details

Jong-Moon Chae[1,2,3]

Address all correspondence to: jongmoon@wonkwang.ac.kr

1 Department of Orthodontics, School of Dentistry, University of Wonkwang, Daejeon Dental Hospital, Wonkwang Dental Research Institute, Iksan, South Korea

2 The Korean Orthodontic Research Institute Inc, Daejeon and Seoul, South Korea

3 The Charles H. Tweed International Foundation, Tucson, Arizona, USA

References

[1] Angle EH. The latest and best in orthodontic mechanism. Dent Cosmos; 1928. p1154.

[2] Tweed CH. Clinical Orthodontics, vol 1 and 2. St. Louis: C.V. Mosby; 1966.

[3] Merrifield LL, Cross JJ. Directional forces. Am J Orthod 1970;57:435-64.

[4] Merrifield L. The systems of directional force. J Charles H. Tweed Int Found 1982;10:15-29.

[5] Gebeck TR, Merrifield LL. Orthodontic diagnosis and treatment analysis— concepts and values: part I. Am J Orthod Dentofacial Orthop 1995;107:434-43.

[6] Gebeck TR, Merrifield LL. Orthodontic diagnosis and treatment analysis— concepts and values: part II. Am J Orthod Dentofacial Orthop 1995;107:541-7.

[7] Ward DM. Angle Class II, Division 1 malocclusion. Am J Orthod Dentofacial Orthop 1994;106:428-33.

[8] Lamarque S. The importance of occlusal plane control during orthodontic mechanotherapy. Am J Orthod Dentofacial Orthop 1995;107:548-58.

[9] Vaden JL, Harris EF, Behrents RG. Adult versus adolescent Class II correction: a comparison. Am J Orthod Dentofacial Orthop 1995;107:651-61.

[10] Roberts WE, Nelson CL, Goodacre CJ. Ridgid Implant Anchorage to Close a Mandibular First Molar Extraction site. J Clin Orthod 1994;28:693-704.

[11] Umemori M, Sugawara J. Mitani H, Nagasaka H, Kawamura H. Skeletal anchorage system for open-bite correction. Am J Orthod Dentofacial Orthop 1999;115:166-74.

[12] Creekmore TD, Eklund MK. The possibility of skeletal anchorage. J Clin Orthod 1983;17:266-69.

[13] Kanomi R. Mini-implant for Orthodontic Anchorage. J Clin Orhod 1997;31:763-7.

[14] Park HS, Bae SM, Kyung HM, Sung JH. Micro-implant anchorage for treatment of skeletal Class I bialveolar protrusion. J Clin Orthod 2001;35:417-22.

[15] Park HS, Kwon TG, Kwon OW. Treatment of open bite with microscrew implants anchorage. Am J Orthod Dentofacial Orthop 2004;126:627-36.

[16] Chae JM. Directional forces using skeletal anchorage for treatment of skeletal Class II div.1 malocclusion. Korean J Orthod 2004;34(2):197-203.

[17] Chae JM. Indirect palatal skeletal anchorage (PSA) for treatment of skeletal Class I bialveolar protrusion. Korean J Orthod 2004;34(5):458-64.

[18] Chae JM. A new protocol of Tweed-Merrifield directional force technology with microimplant anchorage. Am J Orthod Dentofacial Orthop 2006;130(1):100-9.

[19] Chae JM. Unusual extraction treatment of Class I bialveolar protrusion using microimplant anchorage. Angle Orthod 2007;77(2):367-76.

[20] Chae J, Kim S. Running loop in unusual molar extraction treatment. Am J Orthod Dentofacial Orthop 2007;132(4):528-39.

[21] Chae JM, Chang NY, Cho JH, Kang KH, Kim SC. Treatment of skeletal Class II adult patient with vertical and transverse problems caused by nasal airway obstruction using microimplant anchorage. Korean J Orthod 2009;39(4):257-72.

[22] Chae JM, Paeng JY. Orthodontic treatment of an ankylosed maxillary central incisor through single-tooth osteotomy by using interdental space regained from microimplant anchorage. Am J Orthod Dentofacial Orthop 2012;141(2):e39-51.

10

Caries Risk and Prevention in Orthodontic Patients

Anas H. Al-Mulla

1. Introduction

The human oral cavity is a complex ecosystem, inhabited by more than 300 bacterial species, mycoplasmas, protozoa, and yeasts [1]. Any external interference could disturb the balance between components of the microflora in this environment. Fixed orthodontic appliances are an example of such an interference. Bonding of brackets usually includes acid etching of enamel, which results in changes in the morphology and chemical nature of the tooth surface. It has been found that decalcified enamel constitutes good support for adhesion and proliferation of mutans streptococci [2]. It is also known that living cells easily adhere and colonize polymeric surfaces [3-5]. Thus, composite resins, containing polymers used for attaching brackets to etched enamel, provide surfaces especially prone to adhesion and growth of microorganisms [6-8]. In effect, fixed dental appliances induce development and retention of bacterial plaque [9-14]. Development of dental plaque usually leads to an increased level of caries-inducing bacteria in the oral cavity (e.g. mutans streptococci and lactobacilli) [2, 15, 16]. These observations indicate that fixed orthodontic appliances induce a certain risk for development of caries.

2. Caries risk in orthodontic patients

The risk of developing a caries lesion around a bracket, placed on the buccal tooth surfaces during orthodontic treatment with fixed appliances, is high [10, 17, 18]. This risk is attributed to the presence of brackets, arch wires, ligatures, and other orthodontic auxiliaries that complicate conventional oral hygiene measures, which in turn, leads to increased plaque accumulation at the base of the brackets [12, 19]. In the presence of fermentable carbohydrates, demineralization of the enamel around the bracket occurs rapidly [10, 12, 20]. Despite improvements in materials and preventive efforts, demineralization may occur around orthodontic appliances after only one month [11]. Children between 11 and 14 years, the age group in which orthodontic treatment is usually carried out, are considered to be at high risk of developing caries [21]. Fixed orthodontic appliances create extra retention sites, leading to more mutans streptococci soon after the start of treatment [22, 23]. A study concluded that measures including intensive brushing and careful cleaning with dental floss of the spaces around brackets under arch wires and between teeth were insufficient to decrease mutans streptococcus and lactobacillus levels. Thus, patients with fixed appliances carry a high caries risk.

2.1. Caries prevalence in orthodontic patients

The prevalence of new enamel lesions among orthodontic patients treated with fixed appliances and using fluoride toothpaste is reported to range from 13 to 75% [10, 14, 24, 25].

Although demineralized enamel can remineralize after de-bonding, the lesions are often irreversible [11-13, 17]. Inactive demineralized enamel was found to be present five years after the completion of orthodontic treatment [18]. The lesions have been reported to develop on all teeth, but are most frequently observed on the cervical and middle third of the buccal surface of the lateral maxillary incisors, the mandibular canines and the first premolars [10, 17]. The long-term presence of enamel lesions, which appear as white spots, is a concern for both the patient and the orthodontic profession.

2.2. Fluoride toothpaste

Fluoride toothpaste has been widely used for more than four decades and remains a benchmark for the prevention of dental caries [26-28]. It reduces caries in both primary and permanent teeth [28]. For this reason, fluoride toothpaste plays an important role as an effective caries prevention measure worldwide [28]. Topical fluoride (mouth rinses, gels, and varnishes), used in addition to fluoride toothpaste, achieves a modest reduction in caries compared with toothpaste used alone [29]. Numerous studies have shown that even low levels of fluoride, resulting from the regular use of toothpaste, have a profound effect on enamel demineralization and remineralization [30, 31]. Considering the widespread use of fluoride toothpaste during orthodontic treatment, there is little evidence as to which method to deliver the fluoride paste is the most effective.

At least four factors influence the anti-caries efficacy of fluoride toothpaste: (1) frequency of brushing, (2) duration of brushing, (3) fluoride concentration in the toothpaste, and (4) post-brushing rinsing behavior. Brushing should be recommended minimum twice daily [32] and patients should be persuaded to brush for longer periods of time [33]. A recent study by Zero et al. [34] concluded that both brushing time and dentifrice quantity might be important determinants both of fluoride retention in the oral cavity and of consequent enamel remineralization.

There seems to be a correlation between the fluoride concentration of dentifrices and caries prevention [35]. Treatment of demineralized dentin with a toothpaste containing 5, 000 ppm fluoride reduces mineral loss and lesion depth on exposed dentin [36]. In a randomized clinical trial comparing 5, 000 and 1, 450 ppm fluoride, the high fluoride toothpaste reversed non-cavitated fissure caries lesions [37]. Moreover, the group using 5, 000 ppm fluoride showed a significantly higher decrease in laser fluorescence of enamel than the 1, 450 ppm fluoride group. Furthermore, dentifrice containing 5, 000 ppm fluoride was significantly better at remineralizing root caries lesions than a dentifrice with 1, 100 ppm fluoride [38]. In addition, caries active adolescents using the 5, 000 ppm toothpaste had significantly lower progression of caries compared to subjects using the 1, 450 ppm toothpaste, after two years [39].

Rinsing method after brushing teeth has been found to correlate with caries experience and caries increment [40]. Salivary fluoride concentration measured after dentifrice application decreases significantly with increasing water volume, rinse duration, and frequency of rinsing [41, 42]. A toothpaste technique where a slurry rinse with the toothpaste is carried out after brushing increases the efficacy of fluoride toothpaste and reduces approximal caries in preschool children by an average of 26% [43]. A recent study by Sonbul et al. [43] reported 66% preventive fraction effect on approximal caries between the group that used a modified fluoride toothpaste technique compared to the group who continued with their regular oral hygiene habits. Furthermore, eating immediately after brushing reduces the salivary fluoride level about 12-15 times compared with brushing alone [44]. There is an increase of fluoride in both proximal saliva and plaque, using a dentifrice with 5, 000 ppm fluoride without post-brushing water rinsing compared to with rinsing [39]. Post-brushing rinsing habits may play an important role in the oral retention of fluoride from dentifrices that may, in turn, affect their clinical efficacy [41].

The specific aim of the chapter is to test the hypothesis that toothpaste slurry rinsing, combined with some other simple post-brushing advice (in this thesis called modified fluoride toothpaste technique [MFTT]), would reduce the number of decayed and filled tooth surfaces (DFS) in a two-year randomized clinical trial in orthodontic patients.

3. Material and methods

3.1. Subjects

The study population consisted of 150 orthodontic patients at baseline, recruited consecutively during a period of six months at a well-established orthodontic clinic in Riyadh, KSA. They were randomly divided into two groups (test group and control group) with 75 individuals in each group. After six months, we had dropout recession around 33% to achieve a final sample size of 100 orthodontic patients (Figure 1).

A power analysis with an assumption significance level of 5%, standard deviations of 3.0 DFS, least detectable difference of 2.0 ΔDFS, and a power for that detection of 90% was performed and produced a minimum sample size of 45 observations per group.

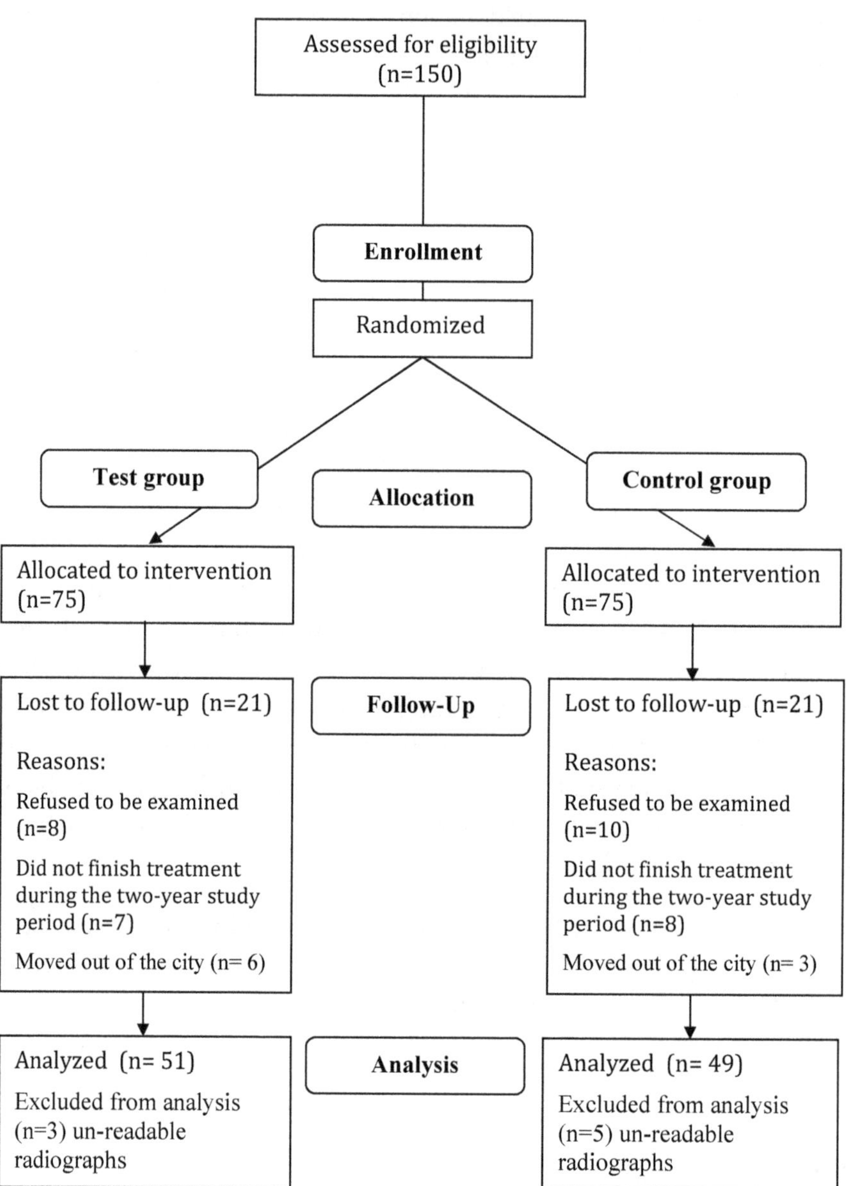

Figure 1. Study IV CONSORT flow chart.

3.2. Examination

The examination consisted of recording the plaque index according to Silness and Löe [45] Registration of caries was done according to WHO [46] after prophylaxis, flossing, and radiographic exam according to Mejàre et al. [47], which consisted four bitewings. A total of 24 surfaces were included in the radiographic DFS index, from the distal of the first pre-molars to the mesial surface of the second molars. Filled surfaces underlined with caries were scored as recurring caries.

Upon completion of the examination, the patients in both test and control groups received a Colgate Max Cavity fluoride toothpaste containing 1450 ppm (Colgate, Riyadh, KSA).

3.3. Oral hygiene instructions including MFTT

The test groups received verbal and written instructions of the MFTT. They were as follows: (1) use 2 cm (1 gram) of dentifrice on a wet toothbrush, (2) spread the toothpaste evenly in the lower and upper arches, (3) brush all surfaces for 2 min, (4) use a small amount of water, equivalent to a handful, together with the dentifrice remaining in the mouth and filter the dentifrice slurry between the teeth by active cheek movements for 30 s before expectorating, (5) avoid further rinsing with water, (6) avoid drinking or eating for 2 h, (7) brush at least twice a day, after breakfast and at night before going to bed, and (8) abstain from all other types of dentifrice during the treatment and until its completion (Figure 2). To ensure that all patients in both groups had a supply of the toothpaste used in the study, they were supplied with the toothpaste at each visit or on request.

The control group was given the routine clinic oral hygiene instructions, which consisted of brushing at least twice a day after breakfast and after dinner before going to bed. At each patient visit to the clinic for the treatment follow-up, the instructions were repeated by the assigned nurse/assistant.

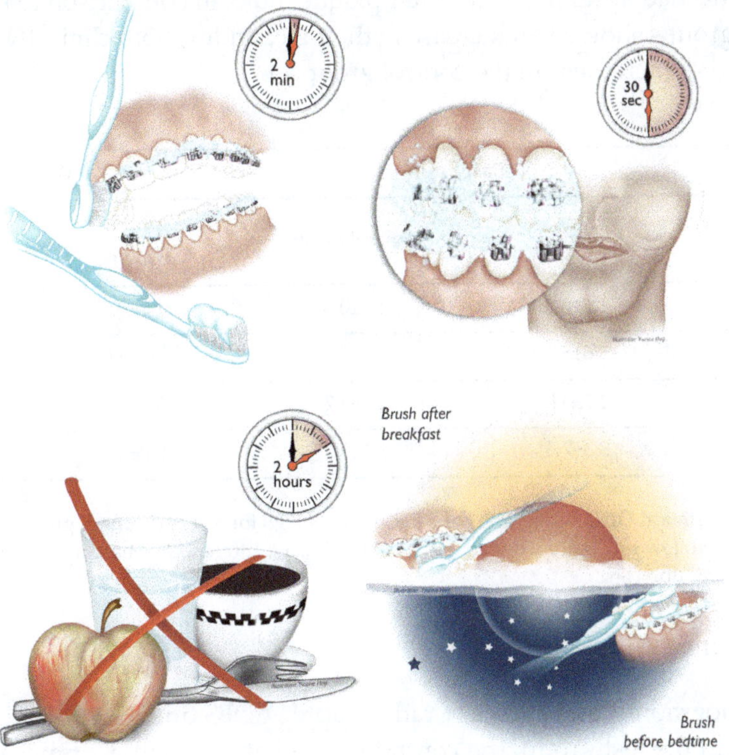

Figure 2. The Modified Fluoride Toothpaste Technique (MFTT).

3.4. Statistical analysis

The Statistical Package for Social Sciences (SPSS Inc., Chicago, IL, USA, version 18.0, Mac OSX) was used for the statistical analysis of the determined measurements in all four studies. ΔDFS and prevented fractions (PF) were calculated according to these two formulas (ΔDFS = follow-up DFS - baseline DFS), (PF = [control group ΔDFS - test group ΔDFS]/control group ΔDFS × 100). For the descriptive statistics, the mean values with standard deviations were calculated. To determine statistically significant differences between the groups, the independent sample t-test was applied between the groups. The paired t-test was utilized to check intra-examiner reliability for the radiographic analysis. The 25 randomly selected radiographs were checked within one-week interval. In all the analyses, $P < 0.05$ was considered statistically significant.

4. Results

4.1. Plaque index, clinical and radiographic DFS

The test and control groups' baseline and follow-up plaque index, clinical DFS, radiographic DFS, and clinical + radiographic DFS values are shown in Table 1. At baseline, there were no significant differences between the groups. At follow-up, the total number of teeth available was almost the same in both groups (26.9±1.7 test vs. 26.8±1.7 control). At the end of the study, test group patients had a significantly better plaque index in comparison to the control group ($P < 0.05$). Both groups showed an increase in their DFS index, both clinically and radiographically, with a higher increment in the control group.

	Baseline		Follow-up	
	Test (n=51)	Control (n=49)	Test (n=51)	Control (n=49)
Plaque Index	1.4±0.5	1.5±0.6	1.1±0.8	1.6±0.7
Clinical DFS	5.6±5.7	5.7±5.4	5.8±6.0	7.4±7.7
Radiographical DFS	2.7±3.0	2.3±3.2	3.1±3.0	4.1±4.0
Total DFS	8.3±7.5	8.1±8.4	9.0±8.0	11.6±10

Table 1. Plaque index, clinical DFS, radiographical DFS, and total DFS for test and control groups. Mean±SD are given both at baseline and at follow up. There were no statistical significant differences at baseline and only plaque index was significant at follow-up.

4.2. Caries incidence

The clinical, radiographic, and clinical + radiographic ΔDFS (incidences) are shown in Figure 3. Compared with the test group, the control group patients had > 7 times clinical DFS ($P < 0.001$), > 4 times radiographic DFS ($P < 0.001$), and > 5 times clinical + radiographic DFS ($P < 0.001$), with preventive fraction of 87%, 78%, and 83%, respectively.

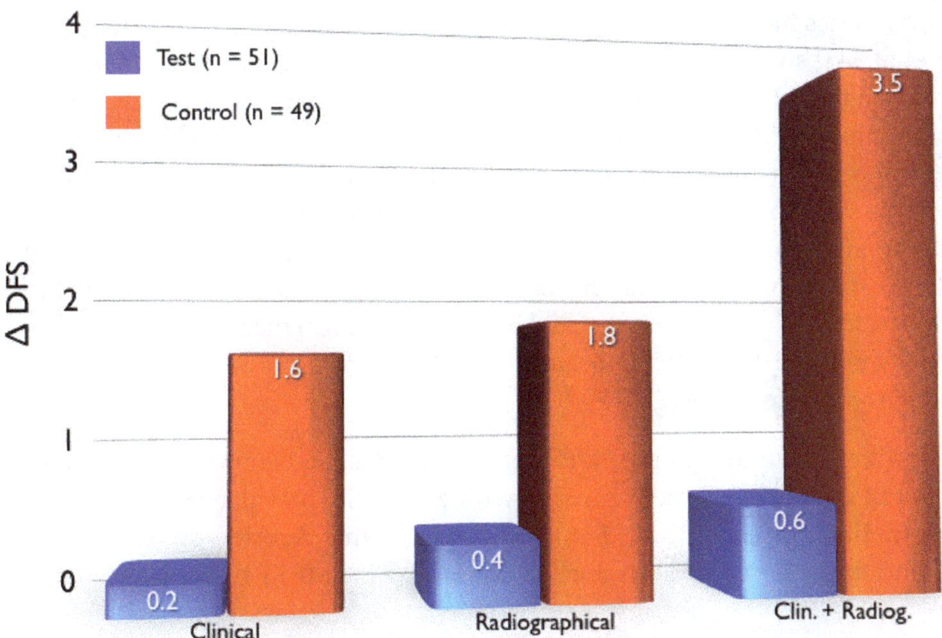

Figure 3. Caries incidence (ΔDFS) in the test and control groups after two years. The mean ± SD values are given on top of each column. There were statistically significant differences ($P < 0.001$) between the groups in the clinical, radiographic and total DFS.

5. Discussion

This chapter focuses on caries risk and prevention in orthodontic patients. High concentrated fluoride toothpaste combined with no post-brushing water rinsing and the MFTT could be a suitable regime for patients with high caries risk.

The MFTT aimed to both increase the fluoride concentration and prolong the time during which the fluoride level is elevated in the oral cavity. Spreading dentifrice on the teeth prior to brushing and rinsing with toothpaste slurry immediately after brushing can be expected to produce a more even distribution of the dentifrice and an enhanced fluoride concentration compared with a more conventional technique. Brushing twice daily has been shown to be a very important factor for caries prevention [48], while not eating or drinking for two hours secures a longer time period of elevated fluoride concentration. It must be remembered that the MFTT contains a package of advice. It is possible to speculate about the factor that is most important, but it is not possible to identify a specific one that made our test group patients develop significantly less caries.

Duckworth et al. [49] found that the fluoride concentration in saliva after brushing vanished rapidly as a result of thorough rinsing. Chesters et al. [50] showed that the water-rinsing pattern among children after brushing influences the cariostatic effect of fluoride toothpaste. They concluded that children who did not use water beakers for rinsing had a significantly lower (16%) caries incidence, during a three-year period than those who used water beakers. Sjögren et al. [43] studied different types of post-brushing behavior; they also evaluated the caries reducing effect of a technique very similar to the one used in Study IV. They concluded that mouth rinsing with the toothpaste foam-water slurry after brushing elevates the concentration of fluoride in saliva for a prolonged period of time as compared to tooth brushing followed by a single or double water rinse; children who used the MFTT developed fewer DFS. These observations are in agreement with Study IV, i.e. the test group patients had a significantly lower mean caries incidence in comparison to the control group. The MFTT technique is easy to teach. Patients can be instructed on how to perform the technique; they can perform it personally in the orthodontic clinic and a pamphlet can be handed to the patients with clear illustrations and instructions.

The large difference found in the ΔDFS between the test and control group patients in KSA should not be expected in other countries with a low DFS prevalence. For example, Sweden has long tradition of using fluoride toothpaste and other fluoride products in orthodontic patients and the expected caries reduction after using the MFTT is therefore lower.

5.1. How to treat orthodontic patients in the sagacity of caries risk and prevention - personal reflections

Orthodontic patients are special kind of patients. They usually come to our clinic complaining about mal-alignment, and few come asking us to solve a functional or prophylactic problem. Most of them underestimate the importance of having excellent oral hygiene practices before and throughout their active prolonged orthodontic treatment. For patients with active caries or having a high risk to develop caries, delaying orthodontic treatment would be my preferred choice. For patients with DMFT index above the mean of their corresponding population, orthodontic treatment should be initiated only when they have been followed over a period of time sustaining excellent oral health habits.

There is a huge responsibility on an orthodontist before bonding brackets and ligating wires. It is simplified in something I call PDE (patient diet education). PDE is highly recommended, particularly for patients with a high DMFT index. The cariogenic potential of foods should be explained, the significant effect of fermentable carbohydrates (sugar containing food as an example) on the number of Lactobacilli should be mentioned and the frequency of meals per day and its effect on the pH should be explained.

Patients should be taught the MFTT and should then be asked to demonstrate their ability to perform the technique. They should understand the importance of each step of the technique, brushing after meals while timing themselves when they brush (2 min brushing), rinsing with the toothpaste for 30 seconds and avoiding eating, drinking or further rinsing for 2 h after. The beauty of the MFTT that it can be applied to any regular toothpaste and have significant effect on caries incidence, it can be prescribed in any situation (low, medium or high risk to develop caries) and in any dental clinic (ortho, perio, endo, etc.).

Compared with other dental specialties, orthodontists have a great opportunity to place the emphasis on MFTT in their clinics, as they usually visit the clinic every 6 -12 weeks. During active orthodontic treatment, orthodontist and the hygienist should work as a team, continuously reminding the patient of MFTT, encouraging proper diet, and evaluating caries risk on every appointment. Any signs of decalcification or poor oral health status should be documented (taking photos as an example) and potential risks re-explained to the patient and their guardians, in case the patient is a child. If repeated episodes of bad oral hygiene are occurring, wires can be removed and patients are asked to improve their oral hygiene. They should be followed up and evaluated for 3 months. If active caries developed at anytime during treatment, wires and brackets should be removed, preventive caries measures should be explained and applied, and later after 6 months of evaluation, treatment can be re-initiated.

It is not difficult to reduce orthodontic patients' caries risk and prevent the incidence of new caries lesions, but it is only challenging to an orthodontist to establish a routine regime and spare few more minutes evaluating, educating, and advising his or her patients. Hopefully this chapter will aid orthodontists around the world to achieve these goals.

6. Conclusions

The use of the MFTT significantly reduces the incidence of new caries lesions in orthodontic patients.

Author details

Anas H. Al-Mulla

Address all correspondence to: a.almulla@mac.com

Department of Orthodontics, European University College, Dubai Health Care City, Dubai, United Arab Emirates

No part of this chapter may be reproduced or transmitted, in any form or by any means, without written permission. Dr. Anas Hasan Al-Mulla.

References

[1] Marcotte H, Lavoie MC: Oral microbial ecology and the role of salivary immunoglobulin A. Microb and Molec Bio Rev 1998:63:71-109.

[2] Boyar R M, Thylstrup A, Holmen L, Bowden GH: The microflora associated with the development of initial enamel decalcification below orthodontic bands *in vivo* in children living in fluorinated-water area. J Dent Res 1989:68:1734-1738.

[3] Zühlke A, Röder B, Widdecke H, Klein J: Synthesis and application of new microcarriers for animal cell culture. Part I: design of polystyrene based microcarriers. J Biom Sci Polymer Edition 1993:5:65-78.

[4] Langer R: Polymers for drug delivery and tissue engineering. Ann Biomed Eng 1995:23:101-111.

[5] West JL, Hubbell JA: Polymeric biomaterials with degradation sites for proteases involved in cell migration. Macromolecules 1999:32:241-244.

[6] Weitman RT, Eames WB: Plaque accumulation on composite surfaces after various finishing procedures. J Am Den Assoc 1975:91:101-106.

[7] Gwinnett AJ, Ceen RF: Plaque distribution on bonded brackets: a scanning microscope study. Am J Orthod 1979:84:667-677.

[8] Sukontapatipark W, El-Agroudi MA, Selliseth NJ, Thunold K, Selvig KA: Bacterial colonization associated with fixed orthodontic appliances. A scanning electron microscopy study. Eur J Orthod 2001:23:475-484.

[9] Zachrisson BU: Cause and prevention of injuries to teeth and supporting structures during orthodontic treatment. Am J of Orthod 1976:69:285-300.

[10] Gorelick L, Geiger AM, Gwinnett AJ: Incidence of white spot formation after bonding and banding. Am J Orthod Dentofacial Orthop 1982;81:93-98.

[11] O'Reilly MM, Featherstone JDB: Demineralization and remineralization around orthodontic appliances: an in vivo study. Am J Orthod 1987:92:33-40.

[12] Øgaard B, Rølla G, Arends J: Orthodontic appliances and enamel demineralization. Part 1: Lesion development. Am J Orthod Dentofacial Orthop 1988a;94:68-73.

[13] Øgaard B, Rølla G, Arends J, ten Cate JM: Orthodontic appliances and enamel demineralization. Part 2: Prevention and treatment of lesions. Am J Orthod Dentofacial Orthop 1988b; 94:123-128.

[14] Mitchell L: Decalcification during orthodontic treatment with fixed appliances: An overview. Br J Orthod 1992;19:199-205.

[15] Balenseifien J W, Madonia J V: Study of dental plaque in orthodontic patients. J Dent Res 1970:49:320-324.

[16] Diamandi-Kiopioti A, Gusberti F A, Lang N P: Clinical and microbiological effects of fixed orthodontic appliances. J Clin Periodontol 1987:14:326-333.

[17] Årtun J, Brobakken BO: Prevalence of carious white spots after orthodontic treatment with multibonded appliances. Eur J Orthod 1986;8:229-234.

[18] Øgaard B: Prevalence of white spot lesions in 19-year-olds: A study on untreated and orthodontically treated persons 5 years after treatment. Am J Orthod Dentofacial Orthop 1989;96:423-427.

[19] Chang HS, Walsh LJ, Freer TJ: Enamel demineralization during orthodontic treatment: Aetiology and prevention. Austr Dent J 1997;42:322-327.

[20] Mizrahi E: Surface distribution of enamel opacities following orthodontic treatment. Am J Orthod Dentofacial Orthop 1983;84:323-331.

[21] Axelsson P: An introduction to risk prediction and preventive dentistry. Carol Stream, Quintessence Publishing, 1999, pp 107-111.

[22] Scheie AA, Arneberg P, Krogstad O: Effect of orthodontic treatment on prevalence of *Streptococcus mutans* in plaque and saliva. Scand J Dent Res 1984;92:211-217.

[23] Jordan C, LeBlanc DJ: Influences of orthodontic appliances on oral populations of mutans streptococci. Oral Microbiol Immunol 2002;17:65-71.

[24] Wenderoth CJ, Weinstein M, Borislow AJ: Effectiveness of a fluoride-releasing sealant in reducing decalcification during orthodontic treatment. Am J Orthod Dentofacial Orthop 1999;116:629-634.

[25] Fornell AC, Sköld-Larsson K, Hallgren A, Berg- strand F, Twetman S: Effect of a hydrophobic tooth coating on gingival health, mutans streptococci, and enamel demineralization in adolescents with fixed orthodontic appliances. Acta Odontol Scand 2002;60:37-41.

[26] Marinho VC, Higgins JP, Sheiham A, Logan S: Fluoride toothpastes for preventing dental caries in children and adolescents. Cochrane Database Syst Rev 2003:CD002278.

[27] Twetman S, Axelsson S, Dahlgren H, Holm AK, Källestål C, Lagerlöf F, Lingström P, Mejàre I, Nordenram G, Norlund A, Petersson LG, Söder B: Caries-preventive effect of fluoride toothpaste: A systematic review. Acta Odontol Scand 2003;61:347-355.

[28] Twetman S: Caries prevention with fluoride toothpaste in children: An update. Eur Arch Paediatr Dent 2009;10:162-167.

[29] Marinho VC: Cochrane reviews of randomized trials of fluoride therapies for preventing dental caries. Eur Arch Paediatr Dent 2009;10:183-191.

[30] Bowen WH: The role of fluoride toothpastes in the prevention of dental caries. J R Soc Med 1995;88:505-507.

[31] Lynch RJ, Navada R, Walia R: Low-levels of fluoride in plaque and saliva and their effects on the demineralisation and remineralisation of enamel; role of fluoride toothpastes. Int Dent J 2004;54:304-309.

[32] Davies RM, Ellwood RP, Davies GM: The rational use of fluoride toothpaste. Int J Dent Hyg 2003;1:3-8.

[33] Creeth JE, Gallagher A, Sowinski J, Bowman J, Barrett K, Lowe S, Patel K, Bosma ML: The effect of brushing time and dentifrice on dental plaque removal in vivo. J Dent Hyg 2009;83:111-116.

[34] Zero DT, Creeth JE, Bosma ML, Butler A, Guibert RG, Karwal R, Lynch RJ, Martinez-Mier EA, Gonzalez-Cabezas C, Kelly SA: The effect of brushing time and dentifrice quantity on fluoride delivery in vivo and enamel surface microhardness in situ. Caries Res 2010;44:90-100.

[35] Travess H, Roberts-Harry D, Sandy J: Orthodontics. Part 6: Risks in orthodontic treatment. Br Dent J 2004;196:71-77.

[36] Bizhang M, Chun YH, Winterfeld MT, Altenburger MJ, Raab WH, Zimmer S: Effect of a 5000 ppm fluoride toothpaste and a 250 ppm fluoride mouth rinse on the demineralisation of dentin surfaces. BMC Res Notes 2009;2:147-151.

[37] Schirrmeister JF, Gebrande JP, Altenburger MJ, Monting JS, Hellwig E: Effect of dentifrice containing 5000 ppm fluoride on non-cavitated fissure carious lesions in vivo after 2 weeks. Am J Dent 2007;20:212-216.

[38] Baysan A, Lynch E, Ellwood R, Davies R, Petersson L, Borsboom P: Reversal of primary root caries using dentifrices containing 5, 000 and 1, 100 ppm fluoride. Caries Res 2001;35:41-46.

[39] Nordström A, Birkhed D: Fluoride retention in proximal plaque and saliva using two NaF dentifrices containing 5, 000 and 1, 450 ppm F with and without water rinsing. Caries Res 2009;43:64-69.

[40] Chestnutt IG, Schafer F, Jacobson AP, Stephen KW: The influence of toothbrushing frequency and post-brushing rinsing on caries experience in a caries clinical trial. Community Dent Oral Epidemiol 1998;26:406-411.

[41] Duckworth RM, Knoop DT, Stephen KW: Effect of mouthrinsing after toothbrushing with a fluoride dentifrice on human salivary fluoride levels. Caries Res 1991;25:287-291.

[42] Attin T, Hellwig E: Salivary fluoride content after toothbrushing with a sodium fluoride and an amine fluoride dentifrice followed by different mouthrinsing procedures. J Clin Dent 1996;7:6-8.

[43] Sjögren K, Birkhed D, Rangmar B: Effect of a modified toothpaste technique on approximal caries in preschool children. Caries Res 1995;29:435-441.

[44] Sjögren K, Birkhed D: Effect of various post-brushing activities on salivary fluoride concentration after toothbrushing with a sodium fluoride dentifrice. Caries Res 1994;28:127-131.

[45] Silness J, Löe H: Periodontal disease in pregnancy. II. Correlation between oral hygiene and periodontal condition. Acta Odontol Scand 1964;22:121-135.

[46] World Health Organization. Oral health surveys: Basic methods, 4th ed. Geneva: World Health Organization, 1997.

[47] Mejàre I, Källestål C, Stenlund H, Johansson H: Caries development from 11 to 22 years of age: A prospective radiographic study. Prevalence and distribution. Caries Res 1998;32:10-16.

[48] Attin T, Hornecker E: Tooth brushing and oral health: How frequently and when should tooth brushing be performed? Oral Health Prev Dent 2005;3:135-140.

[49] Duckworth RM, Jones Y, Nicholson J, Jacobson AP, Chestnutt IG: Studies on plaque fluoride after use of F-containing dentifrices. Adv Dent Res 1994;8:202-207.

[50] Chesters RK, Huntington E, Burchell CK, Stephen KW: Effect of oral care habits on caries in adolescents. Caries Res 1992;26:299-304.

Permissions

All chapters in this book were first published in ICO, by InTech Open; hereby published with permission under the Creative Commons Attribution License or equivalent. Every chapter published in this book has been scrutinized by our experts. Their significance has been extensively debated. The topics covered herein carry significant findings which will fuel the growth of the discipline. They may even be implemented as practical applications or may be referred to as a beginning point for another development.

The contributors of this book come from diverse backgrounds, making this book a truly international effort. This book will bring forth new frontiers with its revolutionizing research information and detailed analysis of the nascent developments around the world.

We would like to thank all the contributing authors for lending their expertise to make the book truly unique. They have played a crucial role in the development of this book. Without their invaluable contributions this book wouldn't have been possible. They have made vital efforts to compile up to date information on the varied aspects of this subject to make this book a valuable addition to the collection of many professionals and students.

This book was conceptualized with the vision of imparting up-to-date information and advanced data in this field. To ensure the same, a matchless editorial board was set up. Every individual on the board went through rigorous rounds of assessment to prove their worth. After which they invested a large part of their time researching and compiling the most relevant data for our readers.

The editorial board has been involved in producing this book since its inception. They have spent rigorous hours researching and exploring the diverse topics which have resulted in the successful publishing of this book. They have passed on their knowledge of decades through this book. To expedite this challenging task, the publisher supported the team at every step. A small team of assistant editors was also appointed to further simplify the editing procedure and attain best results for the readers.

Apart from the editorial board, the designing team has also invested a significant amount of their time in understanding the subject and creating the most relevant covers. They scrutinized every image to scout for the most suitable representation of the subject and create an appropriate cover for the book.

The publishing team has been an ardent support to the editorial, designing and production team. Their endless efforts to recruit the best for this project, has resulted in the accomplishment of this book. They are a veteran in the field of academics and their pool of knowledge is as vast as their experience in printing. Their expertise and guidance has proved useful at every step. Their uncompromising quality standards have made this book an exceptional effort. Their encouragement from time to time has been an inspiration for everyone.

The publisher and the editorial board hope that this book will prove to be a valuable piece of knowledge for researchers, students, practitioners and scholars across the globe.

List of Contributors

Raquel Gonçalves Vieira-Andrade
Department of Pediatric Dentistry and Orthodontics, Federal University of Minas Gerais, Belo Horizonte, Minas Gerais, Brazil

Saul Martins de Paiva
Department of Pediatric Dentistry and Orthodontics, Federal University of Minas Gerais, Belo Horizonte, Minas Gerais, Brazil

Leandro Silva Marques
Department of Pediatric Dentistry and Orthodontics, Federal University of the Jequitinhonha and Mucuri Valleys, Diamantina, Minas Gerais, Brazil

Gaastra Carolin, Zamora Natalia, Paredes Vanessa, Tarazona Beatriz and Jose Luis Gandía
Department of Orthodontics, Faculty of Medicine and Dentistry, University of Valencia, Valencia, Spain

Andréa Cristina Barbosa da Silva, Diego Romário da Silva, Ana Marly Araújo Maia and Pierre Andrade Pereira de Oliveira
Center of Sciences, Technology and Health, State University of Paraiba, UEPB, Paraíba, Brazil

Daniela Correia Cavalcante Souza and Fábio Correia Sampaio
Center of Health Sciences, Federal University of Paraiba, Paraíba, Brazil

Hideki Ioi, Naohisa Murata and Ichiro Takahashi
Section of Orthodontics, Graduate School of Dental Science, Kyushu University, Fukuoka, Japan

Mizuho A. Kido
Department of Molecular Cell Biology and Oral Anatomy, Graduate School of Dental Science, Kyushu University, Fukuoka, Japan

Masato Nishioka
Nishioka Orthodontic Clinic, Fukuoka, Japan

Mikari Asakawa and Ryusuke Muroya
Faculty of Dentistry, Kyushu University, Fukuoka, Japan

Paulo Beltrão
French Board of Orthodontics, Portugal

Emilia Taneva, Budi Kusnoto and Carla A. Evans
Department of Orthodontics, College of Dentistry, University of Illinois at Chicago, IL, USA

Zouhair Abidine and Mourad Sebbar
Hospital Moulay Abdellah, Mohammedia, Morocco

Nassiba Fatene, Asmaa El Mabrak, Narjisse Laslami and Zakaria Bentahar
Department of orthodontics; Faculty of dentistry, Casablanca, Morocco

Farid Bourzgui and Hakima Aghoutan
Department of Dento-facial Orthopedic, Faculty of Dental Medicine, Casablanca Hassan II University, Morocco

Samir Diouny
Department of English, Faculty of Letters & Human Sciences, Chouaib Doukkali University, El Jadida, Morocco

Jong-Moon Chae
Department of Orthodontics, School of Dentistry, University of Wonkwang, Daejeon Dental Hospital, Wonkwang Dental Research Institute, Iksan, South Korea
The Korean Orthodontic Research Institute Inc, Daejeon and Seoul, South Korea
The Charles H. Tweed International Foundation, Tucson, Arizona, USA

Anas H. Al-Mulla
Department of Orthodontics, European University College, Dubai Health Care City, Dubai, United Arab Emirates

Index

www.ingramcontent.com/pod-product-compliance
Lightning Source LLC
Chambersburg PA
CBHW061950190326
41458CB00009B/2831

* 9 7 8 1 6 3 2 4 1 5 7 2 1 *